Clinical
Clerkship

▶in

Outpatient

Medicine

SECOND EDITION

D0831643

Clinical Clerkship

▸in
Outpatient
Medicine

SECOND EDITION

Stephen Bent, MD
Assistant Professor of Medicine in Residence
Department of Medicine
University of California, San Francisco
San Francisco, California

Lianne S. Gensler, MD
Rheumatology Clinical Fellow
Department of Medicine
University of California, San Francisco
San Francisco, California

Craig Frances, MD
Former Chief Resident
Department of Medicine
University of California, San Francisco
San Francisco, California

 Wolters Kluwer | Lippincott Williams & Wilkins
Health

Philadelphia • Baltimore • New York • London
Buenos Aires • Hong Kong • Sydney • Tokyo

Acquisitions Editor: Nancy Anastasi Duffy
Managing Editor: Cheryl W. Stringfellow
Marketing Manager: Jennifer Kuklinski
Production Editor: Kevin Johnson
Designer: Holly Reid McLaughlin
Compositor: Aptara, Inc.

Printed in the United States of America

First edition, 1999

Library of Congress Cataloging-in-Publication Data

Bent, Stephen.
  Saint-Frances guide : clinical clerkship in outpatient medicine / Stephen Bent, Lianne S. Gensler, Craig Frances.—2nd ed.
      p. ; cm.
  Rev ed. of: Saint-Frances guide to outpatient medicine / Craig Frances, Stephen Bent, Sanjay Saint. c1999.
  Includes bibliographical references and index.
  ISBN-13: 978-0-7817-6502-2
  ISBN-10: 0-7817-6502-1
  1. Ambulatory medical care—Outlines, syllabi, etc.   2. Internal medicine—Outlines, syllabi, etc.   I. Gensler, Lianne S.   II. Frances, Craig.   III. Frances, Craig. Saint-Frances guide to outpatient medicine.   IV. Title.   V. Title: Guide.
  [DNLM: 1. Ambulatory Care—Outlines.   2. Internal Medicine—Outlines. WB 18.2 B475s 2008]
  RC59.F73 2008
  616—dc22

                                                                    2007020781

Dedication

To my family: Christine, Blake, Chase, and Brooke, who
bring me eternal love and joy
Stephen Bent

To Scot, and our families, the Weners & Genslers
Lianne S. Gensler

To my mom, the most giving person I know
Craig Frances

Preface

· ·

Has this ever happened to you?

During a routine clinic visit, a patient reports the new onset of a headache that has persisted for approximately 3 weeks. Although you have taken care of many patients with headaches, you are never quite confident that you know all of the possible causes of headache, or how best to approach the work-up. You consider consulting the textbooks in your office for a quick review of the subject, but a glance at your watch reminds you that your next patient is due in 5 minutes. You decide to read about headache after clinic. By the end of the day, you've scribbled down four more disorders that you would like to learn more about. Later, while reading about headache, you realize that the patient may have a disorder that you don't usually consider. You wish that you had been aware of this possibility earlier so you could have ordered the necessary blood tests right away. Reading about headache took more time than you expected, and you decide to delay investigating the other four topics you had written down. What you wouldn't give to have a complete, concise approach to each of the common problems that you encounter daily!

If you take care of ambulatory patients, this scenario is probably familiar to you. Outpatient medicine can be as challenging as inpatient medicine, sometimes even more so! Consider the following:

- As a result of the rapid growth of managed care and its emphasis on cost containment, healthcare providers often treat patients in the outpatient setting for conditions that would have been grounds for admission to the hospital a few years ago.
- Physicians in the outpatient setting often have less information to use as a basis for making diagnostic and treatment decisions than physicians who are caring for hospitalized patients.
- It is generally much more difficult to provide follow-up care to patients who are being seen on an outpatient basis, so the consequences of making a mistake are often much greater.

These factors, combined with the fact that less time is being allotted for each office visit, have "raised the bar" for healthcare professionals wishing to provide high-quality ambulatory care.

If there is barely time to care for patients, how can a medical student, house officer, nurse practitioner, physician's assistant, or attending physician hope to know all that is critical to being a good healthcare provider? Invariably, questions arise during a patient visit that stimulate the provider to want to review a topic of interest, but the time it takes to read a textbook becomes a barrier to learning. At the other extreme, handbooks often miss the boat by providing a "laundry list" of information, instead of providing ways to remember the differential diagnosis and approach to the patient. One of our goals in writing the *Saint-Frances Guide to Outpatient Medicine* was to provide you with a concise resource containing useful mnemonics, algorithms, figures, and tables, so that when these brief learning opportunities arise, you will be able to take full advantage of them.

Like the *Saint-Frances Guide to Inpatient Medicine*, the *Saint-Frances Guide: Clinical Clerkship in Outpatient Medicine, 2nd edition*, was authored with the intent of providing a practical resource for house officers, medical students, nurse practitioners, and other healthcare professionals. Both books provide a useful framework for board review, and they may be used as a teaching tool by attending physicians. We have purposefully distinguished the care of inpatients from that of outpatients because the types of illnesses encountered and the approach to diagnosis, treatment, and follow-up often differ markedly.

We hope that this book will increase your confidence when you are faced with the vast array of medical disorders that are seen in the outpatient setting. Most importantly, we hope that this book helps you take better care of your patients and makes the practice of medicine much more fun.

ACKNOWLEDGMENTS

We would like to acknowledge the support and guidance of the incredibly talented clinicians at the San Francisco VA Medical Center and the University of California, San Francisco, including Andy Avins, Deborah Grady, Mike Shlipak, Lawrence Tierney, Jeff Kohlwes, Jody Garber, Ken Sack, and Ken Fye. We are grateful to the deserving patients at these two institutions, who have allowed us to practice evidence-based medicine and have provided us with experience. We are indebted to Sanjay Saint for his remarkable clinical skills and ability to succinctly summarize information, which formed a large part of the foundation for the original version of this book. We would also like to acknowledge Cheryl Stringfellow for her outstanding editorial work in this revised edition.

Stephen Bent
Lianne S. Gensler
Craig Frances

Contributors

Mateen Akhtar, MD
Cardiology Fellow
The Cleveland Clinic Foundation
Cleveland, Ohio
Part III: Cardiology

Jennifer Babik, MD, PhD
Chief Medical Resident
University of California, San Francisco
San Francisco, California
Part XII: Infectious Diseases

Bryan Cho, MD, PhD
Clinical Instructor in Dermatology
University of California, San Francisco
San Francisco, California
Part XIII: Dermatology

Allen Frances, MD
Emeritus Professor
Department of Psychiatry
Duke University
Durham, North Carolina
Part XIV: Psychiatry

Lianne S. Gensler, MD
Rheumatology Clinical Fellow
Department of Medicine
University of California, San Francisco
San Francisco, California
Part VIII: Orthopedics and Rheumatology

Samir Gupta, MD
Assistant Professor, Department of Medicine
Division of Digestive and Liver Diseases
University of Texas Southwestern
Dallas, Texas
Part V: Gastroenterology

S. Andrew Josephson, MD
Assistant Clinical Professor
Neurovascular and Behavioral Neurology
Department of Neurology
University of California, San Francisco
San Francisco, California
Part IX: Neurology

Christopher Keller, MD
Clinical Fellow, Division of Nephrology
University of California, San Francisco
San Francisco, California
Part VI: Nephrology and Urology

Grant Lee
UCLA School of Medicine
Los Angeles, California
Part II: Ophthalmology

Scott Lee
Chief Resident in Ophthalmology
UCSF School of Medicine
San Francisco, California
Part II: Ophthalmology

Kip Mihara, MD
Assistant Clinical Professor of Medicine
University of California, San Francisco
San Francisco, California
Part I: General Care of the Ambulatory Patient

Alison Oler, MD
Assistant Clinical Professor of Medicine
University of Pennsylvania
School of Medicine
Philadelphia, Pennsylvania
Part VII: Gynecology

Eric J. Seeley, MD
Fellow in Pulmonary and Critical Care
University of California, San Francisco
San Francisco, California
Part IV: Pulmonology

Eric Swagel, MD
Assistant Clinical Professor
Department of Medicine
San Francisco VA Medical Center
San Francisco, California
Part I: General Care of the Ambulatory Patient

Sunny Wang, MD
Fellow, Hematology/Oncology
University of California, San Francisco
San Francisco, California
Part X: Hematology

Melissa E. Weinberg, MD
Fellow in Endocrinology, Diabetes and Metabolism
University of California San Francisco
San Francisco, California
Part XI: Endocrinology

Contents

PART VI: NEPHROLOGY AND UROLOGY

PART VII: GYNECOLOGY

PART VIII: ORTHOPEDICS AND RHEUMATOLOGY

PART I

GENERAL CARE OF THE AMBULATORY PATIENT

1. Approach to the Patient and Medical Decision Making

 PATIENT—PROVIDER RELATIONSHIP. The relationship that exists between a patient and his healthcare provider is critical to the patient's well-being. The healthcare provider must be more than simply a master diagnostician. Trust between patient and provider is a great therapeutic tool and should be sought. The following principles have been shown to enhance the patient-provider relationship.

MNEMONIC

Enhancing the Patient-Provider Relationship ("WE CARE")

Warmly greet the patient (e.g., address her by the name she prefers)

Equalize the relationship by avoiding condescension

Care for the patient as a person, not just as a patient (e.g., express an interest in the patient's family, job, or hobbies)

Allow the patient to tell her story without frequent interruptions

Resist using jargon to explain things

Encourage questions by asking "What questions can I answer?" after every visit

---

HOT KEY Bad patient outcomes due to mistakes on the part of the healthcare provider sometimes occur. Affected patients are more likely to seek legal remedies if their relationship with the provider is poor.

II APPROACH TO DIAGNOSIS

A. Straightforward diagnoses. Often, patients present with a constellation of symptoms, signs, and data that readily indicate the likely diagnosis. In these cases, making a diagnosis is relatively straightforward because the patient's clinical presentation represents a **pattern of disease** with which the clinician is familiar. For example, when a patient presents with fever, cough productive of sputum, pleuritic chest pain, and a lobar infiltrate, the clinician quickly diagnoses the patient as having a pneumonia.

B. Diagnostic dilemmas. Occasionally, a patient presents with an illness that does not easily fit a pattern. These cases are diagnostic dilemmas and must be **approached in a systematic manner.**

    1. Generate a list of the patient's medical problems (e.g., low back pain, dyspnea, anemia). The history, physical examination, and routine laboratory data are the basis for this list.

    2. Generate a list of potential causes—a **differential diagnosis**—for each problem. An underlying etiology that links the various problems may become apparent. Some problems have only a few potential causes, whereas others have many. The mnemonic **"CHOPPED MINTS"** or the organ-based mnemonic **"ABCDEFGHIJK"** are useful ways to remember the potential causes of medical problems.

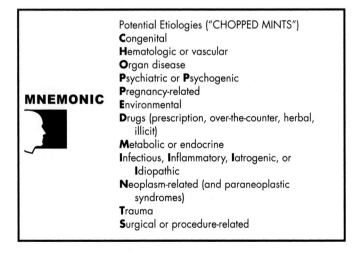

MNEMONIC	Potential Etiologies ("CHOPPED MINTS") **C**ongenital **H**ematologic or vascular **O**rgan disease **P**sychiatric or **P**sychogenic **P**regnancy-related **E**nvironmental **D**rugs (prescription, over-the-counter, herbal, illicit) **M**etabolic or endocrine **I**nfectious, **I**nflammatory, **I**atrogenic, or **I**diopathic **N**eoplasm-related (and paraneoplastic syndromes) **T**rauma **S**urgical or procedure-related

MNEMONIC 	Potential Etiologies ("ABCDEFGHIJK") **A**irway/Pulmonary **B**rain/CNS **C**ardiac **D**rugs **E**ndocrine/Metablolic **F**luids/Electrolytes **G**astrointestinal **H**ematologic/Oncologic **I**nfectious diseases **J**oint related/Rheumatologic **K**idney/Genitourinary

3. **Decide what tests you want to order** to evaluate a potential diagnosis. Section III discusses how to use diagnostic tests in an appropriate manner.
4. **Unifying diagnoses.** It is often difficult to recognize a single disease that accounts for all of the problems in a complex case. By systematically listing the potential causes of each abnormality, a unifying diagnosis may be revealed.
5. **Remember probabilities.** In complex cases it helps to take into account the probablilities of each disease for the patient population to which your patient belongs. The unifying diagnosis is more likely to be a common one.

HOT **KEY**	Often, in elderly patients or patients infected with HIV, no single diagnosis adequately explains all the of the patient's clinical manifestations.

HOT ▶ **KEY**	In a patient with multiple unexplained medical complaints, always consider depression and domestic violence.

III APPROACH TO MEDICAL DECISION MAKING

A. **Introduction.** Diagnoses tend to exist on the following continuum:

Probability of disease

0%   100%

Disease absent   **Disease present**

1. The probability of a given disease listed on an initial differential diagnosis will usually fall somewhere in the middle of this continuum.
2. The goal of the physician is to explain the patient's presentation by moving most diagnoses as far to the left as possible (reasonably excluding them), while moving one diagnosis as far to the right as possible.
3. The inappropriate use of diagnostic tests will leave many diagnoses frustratingly close to the midpoint of the continuum.

B. **Qualitative assessment.** The degree of certainty required to qualify a diagnosis as "reasonable" depends on:
   1. The severity of the condition under consideration
   2. The extent to which the condition is treatable
   3. The risks associated with diagnostic testing
   4. The risks associated with the treatment

C. **Quantitative assessment.** In order to really learn this approach, you must use it. Try it on your next patient and you'll be familiar with odds before you know it!
   1. The **pretest probability** is the probability of disease prior to testing.
      a. Consider the following three examples:
         (1) A 45-year-old man presents to your clinic with a history of paroxysmal, sharp, left-sided chest pain occurring both at rest and with exercise. He denies chest pressure occurring with exercise. The symptoms have been present for 2 months. A literature search reveals that 50% of 45-year-old men with atypical chest pain have coronary artery disease (CAD). Therefore, the pretest probability of CAD in this patient is 50%.
         (2) If the patient were a 30-year-old woman with atypical chest pain, the pretest probability of CAD would be 5%.
         (3) If the patient were a 60-year-old man with exertional chest tightness (typical angina), the pretest probability of CAD would be 95%.
      b. Suppose all three of these patients undergo an exercise treadmill test. Is CAD ruled in if the tests are positive? Is it ruled out if the tests are negative? In order to answer these questions, it is necessary to consider the likelihood ratio as well.
   2. The **likelihood ratio** is the strength of the diagnostic test result.

a. Sensitivity and specificity are the characteristics used most often to define diagnostic tests.

   (1) Sensitivity answers the question, "Among patients with the disease, how likely is a positive test?"

   (2) Specificity answers the question, "Among patients without the disease, how likely is a negative test?"

   (3) The **likelihood ratio** helps answer the clinically more important questions:

   (a) Given a positive test result, how likely is it that the disease is truly present?

   (b) Given a negative test result, how likely is it that the disease is truly absent?

b. Mathematically, likelihood ratios are the odds of having a disease given a test result versus not having a disease given a test result.

   (1) For example:

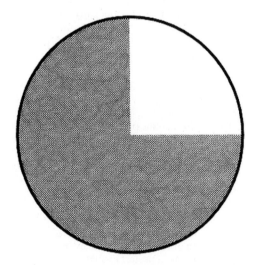

If the circle represents all patients with a positive test and the shaded portion represents the portion who actually have disease, then the likelihood ratio is 3.

$$\frac{\text{The chance of a positive test and disease}}{\text{The chance of a positive test and no disease}} = \frac{3}{1}$$

   (2) Consider another example. The likelihood ratio of a positive treadmill test is 3.5. In a large, heterogeneous population of patients, all of whom have had positive treadmill tests, 7 patients will actually have coronary artery disease for every 2 patients who do not. Therefore, if your patient has a positive treadmill test, the odds of him having coronary artery disease are 7 to 2, or 3.5 to 1. That is, given a positive treadmill test, it is **3.5 times more likely** that coronary artery disease is present.

c. Likelihood ratios can be found in epidemiology textbooks or calculated using the following formulas:

$$\text{Likelihood ratio of a positive test} = \frac{\text{True positive rate}}{\text{False positive rate}}$$

$$= \frac{(\text{Sensitivity})}{(1 - \text{Specificity})}$$

$$\text{Likelihood ratio of a negative test} = \frac{\text{False negative rate}}{\text{True negative rate}}$$

$$= \frac{(1 - \text{Sensitivity})}{(\text{Specificity})}$$

(1) Most diagnostic tests have likelihood ratios in the 2–5 range for positive results and in the 0.5–0.2 range for negative results. These types of tests are only very useful if the pretest probability of disease is in the middle of the scale (e.g., 30%–70%). At either end of the probability scale, diagnostic tests with small likelihood ratios do not change the pretest probability much.

(2) Good tests have positive likelihood ratios of 10 or more. These powerful diagnostic tests help rule in a diagnosis across a broader range of pretest probabilities. Unfortunately, these types of tests are often expensive or dangerous.

(3) In order for a test to truly rule in disease across the full range of pretest probabilities, it must have a likelihood ratio of 100 or more. Very few tests (e.g., some biopsies, exploratory laparotomy, cardiac catheterization) have likelihood ratios this high.

3. Calculating the posttest probability. Posttest probability is the probability that a specific disease is present after a diagnostic test. Once we have determined the **pretest probability** of disease (using clinical information and disease prevalence data) and the **likelihood ratio** of the diagnostic test result, we are ready to calculate the **posttest probability.**

First, however, the pretest probability must be converted to odds (the likelihood ratio is already expressed in odds).

a. Steps

(1) Pretest probability must be converted to pretest odds:

$$\text{Odds} = \frac{(\text{Probability})}{(1 - \text{Probability})}$$

(For example, a probability of 75% equals odds of 3:1.)

(2) Pretest odds are multiplied by the likelihood ratio to give posttest odds

(3) Posttest odds must then be converted back to posttest probability:

$$\text{Probability} = \frac{(\text{Odds})}{(\text{Odds} + 1)}$$

b. Examples

(1) In the 45-year-old man with the atypical chest pain and a positive treadmill test, the posttest probability of disease would be 78%:

(a) The 50% pretest probability is converted to pretest odds: $(0.5)/(1 - 0.5) = (0.5)/(0.5) = 1:1$

(b) The 1:1 pretest odds are multiplied by the likelihood ratio (3.5) to yield posttest odds of 3.5:1.

(c) The posttest odds are converted to a posttest probability: $(3.5)/(3.5 + 1) = (3.5)/(4.5) = 0.78$, or 78%. These steps can also be presented schematically:

Pretest probability	Likelihood ratio	Posttest probability
$50\% \longrightarrow$	$\frac{1}{1} \times \frac{3.5}{1} = \frac{3.5}{1}$	$\longrightarrow 78\%$

(2) In the 30-year-old woman with atypical chest pain and a positive treadmill test, the posttest probability would be 16%:

Pretest probability	Likelihood ratio	Posttest probability
$5\% \longrightarrow$	$\frac{1}{19} \times \frac{3.5}{1} = \frac{3.5}{19}$	$\longrightarrow 16\%$

(3) In the 60-year-old man with atypical chest pain and a positive treadmill test, the posttest probability would be 98.5%:

Pretest probability	Likelihood ratio	Posttest probability

$$95\% \longrightarrow \frac{19}{1} \times \frac{3.5}{1} = \frac{66.5}{1} \longrightarrow 98.5\%$$

HOT

▶

KEY

In order to gain diagnostic strength, several tests may be combined—as long as they are independent tests. The posttest probability after the first test then becomes the pretest probability for the next test.

References

Jaeschke R, Guyatt G, Sackett DL (for the Evidence-Based Medicine Working Group). Users' Guide to the Medical Literature: How to Use an Article about a Diagnostic Test, part A (Are the Results of the Study Valid?). *JAMA* 1994;271(5):389–391.

Jaeschke R, Guyatt G, Sackett DL (for the Evidence-Based Medicine Working Group). Users' Guide to the Medical Literature: How to Use an Article about a Diagnostic Test, part B (What are the Results and Will They Help Me in Caring for My Patients?). *JAMA* 1994;271(9):703–707.

2. Preoperative Evaluation

I INTRODUCTION

A. Each year, millions of patients in the United States undergo a major surgical procedure. Approximately 3%–10% of these patients experience significant morbidity, most of which results from cardiac, pulmonary, or infectious complications of surgery.

B. The role of the preoperative medical consultant includes evaluating the severity and stability of the patient's existing medical conditions, providing a surgical risk assessment, and recommending interventions to reduce risk.

II ROUTINE EVALUATION.

Patients younger than 50 years who do not have significant medical problems are at very low risk for perioperative complications. The preoperative evaluation of these patients should include:

A. A **complete history** and **physical examination,** with emphasis on assessment of functional status, exercise tolerance, and cardiopulmonary symptoms

B. A **12-lead electrocardiogram (EKG)** [for men older than 40 years and women older than 50 years] to look for evidence of silent myocardial ischemia

III PRE-EXISTING CARDIAC DISEASE.

Patients with advanced age, coronary artery disease (CAD), or congestive heart failure (CHF) are at highest risk for developing post-operative cardiac complications (e.g., myocardial infarction, CHF, cardiac death). Cardiovascular conditions that can place a patient at risk for developing complications following surgery include the following.

A. Coronary artery disease (CAD)

    1. Risk evaluation. Clinical predictors should be used to define a patient's risk of developing CAD-related post-operative complications. Figure 2-1 is an algorithm using both patient- and surgery-specific risks to guide this assessment and subsequent management.

    2. Perioperative management. Beta-blocker therapy has been shown to reduce CAD-related complications in at-risk surgical patients. Table 2-1 outlines recommendations for their perioperative use.

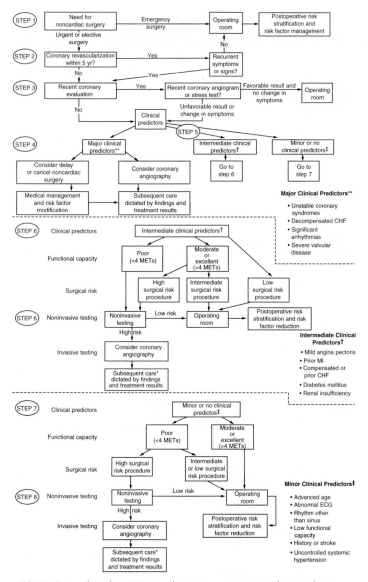

FIGURE 2-1. Algorithmic approach to pre-operative cardiac evaluation.
*Subsequent care may include cancellation or delay of surgery, coronary revascularization followed by noncardiac surgery, or intensified care. From Eagle et al. Used with permission.

TABLE 2-1. Recommendations for Perioperative Beta-Blocker Medical Therapy		
Strength of Recommendation	Recommendation	Indication*
Class I	Beta-blocker therapy should be continued in patients taking them for:	Angina Symptomatic arrhythmia HTN
	Beta-blocker therapy should be given to:	Vascular surgery patients with ischemia on pre-operative testing.
Class IIa	Beta-blocker therapy probably recommended for:	Vascular surgery patients with CAD. Vascular surgery patients with multiple clinical predictors (see Fig. 2-1) Patients with CAD or multiple clinical predictors undergoing high- or intermediate-risk surgery (see Fig. 2-1)
Class IIb	Beta-blocker may be considered	Patients with a single clinical predictor undergoing high- or intermediate-risk surgery Vascular surgery patients with low cardiac risk.

*Clinical predictors are shown in Figure 2-1.
   Adapted from ACC/AHA 2006 Guideline Update on Perioperative Cardiovascular Evaluation for Noncardiac Surgery: Focused Update on Perioperative Beta-Blocker Therapy. JACC Vol 47 No.11 2006.

B. Congestive heart failure (CHF)
   1. Risk evaluation. Decompensated CHF increases the patient's risk of perioperative pulmonary edema and cardiac death.
   2. Perioperative management. Preoperative control of CHF, including the use of diuretics and afterload-reducing agents, is likely to reduce the perioperative risk.

C. Valvular heart disease
   1. **Risk evaluation.** Patients with severe symptomatic aortic stenosis are clearly at increased risk for cardiac complications.
   2. **Perioperative management.** Candidates for valve replacement surgery or balloon valvuloplasty should have the corrective procedure performed prior to the noncardiac surgery.
D. Rhythm disturbances
   1. **Risk evaluation.** Rhythm disturbances are frequently associated with underlying structural heart disease, especially CAD and left ventricular dysfunction. Patients found to have a rhythm disturbance without evidence of underlying heart disease are at very low risk for perioperative cardiac complications.
   2. **Perioperative management.** Management of patients with arrhythmias in the preoperative period is similar to that for nonsurgical patients. Patients who have indications for a permanent pacemaker should have it placed prior to noncardiac surgery.
E. Hypertension
   1. **Risk evaluation**
      a. **Severe hypertension** (i.e., a systolic pressure greater than 200 mm Hg or a diastolic pressure greater than 110 mm Hg) appears to increase the risk of perioperative cardiac complications.
      b. **Mild** to **moderate hypertension** in the preoperative period does not appear to increase cardiac complication rates.
   2. **Perioperative management**
      a. Severe hypertension should be controlled prior to surgery
      b. Medication changes in patients with mild to moderate hypertension are generally not recommended immediately prior to surgery. However, chronic medications for hypertension should be continued up to and including the day of surgery.

IV PRE-EXISTING PULMONARY DISEASE

A. Risk evaluation. The most significant risk factors for postoperative pulmonary complications can be divided into two categories:
   1. **Patient factors:** Age >60, COPD, American Sociey of Anesthesiologists (ASA) class II or greater, functional dependence, serum albumin <35 g/L, and CHF.
   2. **Surgical Factors:** surgery > 3 hours; AAA repair, abdominal, thoracic, neuro-, vascular, or head and neck surgery; emergency surgery; and general anesthesia.

B. Perioperative management
1. Patients with risk factors should receive:
   a. post operative deep breathing exercises or incentive spirometry
   b. use of an NG tube for nausea or vomiting, abdominal distention, or intolerance of oral intake
2. Preoperative pulmonary function testing and chest x-ray should not be performed routinely to predict the risk of complications.
3. Right heart caterization and total parenteral nutrition should not be used solely to reduce the risk of post-operative pulmonary complications.

V PRE-EXISTING HEPATIC DISEASE

A. Cirrhosis. In patients with cirrhosis, the degree of hepatic dysfunction roughly correlates with surgical outcomes.
1. **Risk evaluation.** Class A cirrhosis (using Child's or Pugh's classification scheme) is associated with a mortality rate of less than 10%, while class C cirrhosis is associated with a mortality rate as high as 50%.
2. **Perioperative management.** A conservative approach would be to avoid elective surgery in patients with severe hepatic dysfunction.

B. Hepatitis
1. **Acute viral or alcoholic hepatitis.** Although data are limited, it appears that patients with acute viral or alcoholic hepatitis are at substantial risk for major complications (e.g., liver failure) during and after surgery. Elective surgery should be delayed at least until the acute episode has resolved.
2. **Symptomatic chronic hepatitis.** Patients may be at increased risk for perioperative complications and mortality. A prudent course would be to avoid elective surgery in these patients, although delaying urgent or emergent surgery is not supported by the available data.

VI PRE-EXISTING HEMATOLOGIC DISEASE

A. Anemia
1. **Risk evaluation.** When feasible, evaluation of the patient for anemia should be performed prior to surgery because certain types of anemia (particularly hemolytic anemias) may have implications for perioperative management. The morbidity and mortality rates associated with surgery increase as the preoperative hemoglobin level decreases, especially to levels below 9 g/dl.
2. **Perioperative management.** When considering preoperative transfusion, one must consider factors other than the absolute

hemoglobin level, including the presence of cardiopulmonary disease, the type of surgery, and the likelihood of surgical blood loss.

B. Bleeding disorders
   1. If there is no history of abnormal bleeding, no family history of bleeding disorders, and no indication of abnormal bleeding on physical examination, the patient's risk of having an occult bleeding disorder is very low. Laboratory tests of hemostatic parameters in these patients are generally not needed.
   2. When the bleeding history is unreliable or incomplete or abnormal bleeding is suggested, a formal evaluation of hemostasis should be performed prior to surgery. This evaluation should include the prothrombin time (PT), the partial thromboplastin time (PTT), the platelet count and possibly a platelet functional assay.

VII PRE-EXISTING VASCULAR DISEASE. Patients who undergo cardiac or peripheral vascular surgery and those with severe symptomatic carotid stenoses are at risk for perioperative stroke.

A. Patients who are already candidates for carotid endar- terectomy (e.g., those with severe symptomatic carotid stenosis) should undergo this surgery prior to having other, elective surgery.
B. Asymptomatic carotid bruits or stenoses are associated with little or no increased risk of postoperative stroke; therefore, prophylactic carotid endarterectomy in these patients is unlikely to be beneficial.

VIII PRE-EXISTING ENDOCRINE DISEASE

A. Diabetes mellitus. Perioperative glucose control is challenging in diabetic patients. Although the ideal blood glucose level during surgery is not known, maintaining a blood glucose level of 100–200 mg/dl is usually recommended.
   1. Management of patients with diabetes that is controlled by diet alone
      a. Avoid administration of glucose-containing solutions during surgery.
      b. Measure the blood glucose level every 4–6 hours throughout the procedure and administer regular insulin subcutaneously as needed to maintain a blood glucose level of less than 200 mg/dl.
   2. Management of patients with diabetes that is controlled by oral agents
      a. Discontinue the oral agent on the day of surgery.

TABLE 2-2. Recommendations for Supplemental Therapy in Surgical Patients at Risk for Adrenocortical Insufficiency

Degree of Stress	Dose on Day of Surgery
Mild (hernia repair)	25 mg hydrocortisone, then return to usual dose
Moderate (joint replacement, open cholecystectomy, lower extremity revascularization)	50–75 mg hydrocortisone, 1 day taper
Major (CT surgery, Whipple procedure, total colectomy)	100–150 mg hydrocortisone, 1 day taper
Critical Illness (i.e. sepsis, hypotension)	100 mg hydrocortisone q 8h, gradual taper

Adapted from: Krasner AS. Glucocorticoid-induced Adrenal Insufficiency. *JAMA* 1999;282:671–676. Used with permission.

    b. Measure the blood glucose level every 4-6 hours in the preoperative period and administer regular insulin subcutaneously as needed to maintain a blood glucose level of less than 200 mg/dl.

    c. Measure the blood glucose level every 4–6 hours (or more frequently as indicated) during surgery.

    d. While the patient is fasting, infuse 5% glucose-containing solution at a rate of approximately 100 ml/hour and continue until the patient resumes eating. Resume oral hypoglycemic therapy when the patient returns to his baseline diet.

   3. Management of patients with diabetes that is controlled by insulin is summarized in Table 2-3.

B. Adrenocortical insufficiency. Very rarely, patients with primary or secondary adrenocortical insufficiency develop perioperative complications (usually **hypotension).**

   1. Risk evaluation. There is no consensus regarding the identification of patients at risk for having adrenocortical insufficiency. The most conservative approach is to consider any patient who has received either the equivalent of 20 mg of prednisone daily for 1 week or the equivalent of 7.5 mg of prednisone daily for 1 month within the past year to be at risk for having adrenocortical insufficiency.

   2. Perioperative management. Table 2-2 outlines recommendations for supplemental glucocorticoid therapy for at-risk patients.

C. Hypothyroidism

   1. Severe hypothyroidism. Patients with severe hypothyroidism are at risk for **intraoperative hypotension.** Elective

TABLE 2-3. Perioperative Management of Patients with Diabetes That Is Controlled by Insulin

Method	Administration of Insulin and Intravenous Glucose	Blood Glucose Monitoring
Subcutaneous insulin	Administer one half to two thirds of the usual dose of insulin on the morning of surgery Infuse 5% glucose-containing solution at a rate of at least 100 ml/hour, beginning on the morning of surgery and continuing until the patient resumes eating.	Every 2–4 hours, beginning the morning of surgery
Continuous intravenous insulin infusion in glucose-containing solution	Infuse 5%–10% glucose-containing solution containing 5–15 U regular insulin per liter of solution at a rate of 100 ml/hour* on the morning of surgery; addition insulin may be added as needed to maintain a blood glucose level of less than 250 mg/dl	Every 2–4 hours during intravenous insulin infusion
Separate intravenous insulin and glucose infusions	Infuse intravenous regular insulin at a rate of 0.15–1.5 U/hour (dose may be adjusted as needed to maintain a blood glucose level of less than 250 mg/dl) Infuse 5%–10% glucose-containing solution at a rate of 100 ml/hour	Every 2–4 hours during intravenous insulin infusion

*This combination provides 0.5–1.5 U of insulin per hour.

surgery should be delayed in patients with severe hypothyroidism until adequate thyroid hormone replacement can be achieved. Adequate thyroid hormone replacement usually requires at least 1 month.

2. **Mild or asymptomatic hypothyroidism.** Patients with asymptomatic or mild hypothyroidism generally tolerate surgery well. In these patients, surgery need not be delayed.

IX PRE-EXISTING RENAL DISEASE

A. Risk evaluation. The **risk factors** for postoperative deterioration of renal function include:
   1. Aortic or cardiac surgery
   2. Preoperative jaundice
   3. Advanced age
   4. Preoperative renal insufficiency

B. Perioperative management
   1. In patients with risk factors for postoperative deterioration of renal function, it is important to maintain adequate intravascular volume during the perioperative period.
   2. Patients with end-stage renal disease should receive dialysis within 24 hours of undergoing surgery. Their serum electrolyte levels should be measured just prior to surgery and monitored closely during the postoperative period.

References

Eagle KA, et al. ACC/AHA Guideline Update on Perioperative Cardiovascular Evaluation for Noncardiac Surgery. *J Am Coll Cardiol* 2002;39:542–553.

Fleisher LA, et al. ACC/AHA 2006 Guideline Update on Perioperative Cardiovascular Evaluation for Noncardiac Surgery: Focused update on perioperative Beta-Blocker Therapy. *J Am Coll Cardiol* 2006;47(11) 1–13.

McFalls EO, et al. Coronary Artery Revascularization before Elective Major Vascular Surgery. *N Engl J Med* 2004;351:2795–2804.

Qaseem A, et al. Risk assessment for and strategies to reduce perioperative pulmonary complications for patients undergoing noncardiothoracic surgery: a guideline from the American College of Physicians. *Ann Int Med* 2006;144(8)575–581.

3. Pain Management

....

 APPROACH TO THE PATIENT

A. **Identify the cause.** Always strive to identify the source of pain and explain the cause to the patient.

B. **Assess the severity of the pain.** Have the patient rate the pain on a scale of 0–10 (0 no pain, 10 worst pain ever). Pain ratings of 1–4 are considered mild, 5–6 are considered moderate, and 7–10 are considered severe.

HOT

KEY

Remember that pain is entirely subjective and that different patients will experience different levels of pain in similar situations.

II **TREATMENT.** The goal of treatment is to reduce pain and maximize function while limiting side effects from medications.

A. **Pharmacologic therapy.** In 1986, the World Health Organization (WHO) released a set of guidelines for treating patients with chronic pain from cancer that remains the standard today. This **three-step system** is a useful guide for treating chronic pain from all causes. Tables 3-1 through 3-3 list the most commonly used agents; there are many other agents in these classes that are also effective and useful for certain patients.

1. **Step 1.** For patients with mild to moderate pain and no prior treatment, start with a step 1 agent (see Table 3-1). The choice of medications depends on the side effect profile and the patient's medical history.

2. **Step 2.** If the pain is not adequately controlled with a step 1 agent, move to a step 2 agent (see Table 3-2) and then reassess.

3. **Step 3.** If the pain cannot be controlled with a step 2 agent, move to a step 3 agent (see Table 3-3).

B. **General guidelines**

1. **Move quickly to eliminate pain.** For patients with severe pain, start with a step 2 or step 3 agent.

2. **Schedule the doses.** In patients with chronic pain, scheduled dosing of pain medications helps the patient erase the memory and expectation of pain.

3. **Monitor response to therapy** using the 0–10 numerical scale.

TABLE 3-1. Step 1 Agents: Nonopioid Analgesics

Agent	Equianalgesic Dose	Interval	Cautions
Acetaminophen	650 mg	Every 4–6 hours	Do not exceed 4 g in 24 hours. Avoid in patients with liver disease.
Aspirin	650 mg	Every 4–6 hours	Avoid in pregnant women, patients with gastrointestinal bleeding or bleeding disorders, postoperative patients, and patients younger than 18 years.
NSAIDs*			
Ibuprofen	400 mg	Every 6–8 hours	Monitor for gastropathy, renal dysfunction, and bleeding.
Naproxen	375 mg	Every 12 hours	

Modified with permission from World Health Organization: Cancer pain relief and palliative care: report of a WHO expert committee, technical report series 804. Geneva, Switzerland, World Health Organization, 1990.
NSAIDs = nonsteroidal anti-inflammatory drugs.
*NSAIDs other than the two examples given here are available.

4. **Allow the patient to decide the level of pain control.** Use the dose of medication that reduces pain to an acceptable level and minimizes side effects. There is no maximum dose for step 3 agents.
5. **Anticipate the need for stool softeners and laxatives in patients taking opiates.**
6. **Opt for the administration route that is easiest for the patient.**
   a. The **oral route** is simple and inexpensive, and permits rapid adjustment of doses.
   b. The **transdermal route** provides steady drug levels and obviates the need for frequent pill taking.
   c. The **rectal** or **sublingual routes** can be used in patients who are unable to tolerate oral or transdermal medicines.
   d. The **subcutaneous** and **intravenous routes** are used for patients with pain refractory to all other methods.

TABLE 3-2. Step 2 Agents: Opioid Analgesics for Mild to Moderate Pain

Agent	Equianalgesic Dose	Interval	Usual Dosage Form
Codeine	30–60 mg	Every 4–6 hours	Tylenol #3: Acetaminophen, 325 mg, plus codeine, 30 mg
Hydrocodone	5–10 mg	Every 4–6 hours	Vicodin: Acetaminophen, 500 mg, plus hydrocodone, 5 mg
Oxycodone	5–10 mg	Every 6 hours	Percodan: Acetylsalicylic acid, 325 mg, plus oxycodone, 5mg Percocet: Acetaminophen, 325 mg, plus oxycodone, 5 mg

Modified with permission from World Health Organization: Cancer pain relief and palliative care: report of a WHO expert committee, technical report series 804. Geneva, Switzerland, World Health Organization, 1990.

C. Nonpharmacologic therapy. Massage, biofeedback, relaxation and visualization, transcutaneous electrical nerve stimulation, acupuncture, and other treatments may help patients reduce or replace their dose of oral analgesics.

D. Special situations

   1. Neuropathic pain (see also Chapter 66) is caused by damage to central or peripheral nervous system structures and is associated with a variety of conditions, including diabetes, alcoholism, AIDS, cancer, and amputation.

   a. The pain is usually described as **"tingling," "burning," "electric,"** or **"needle-like."**

   b. Patients with neuropathic pain often respond to adjuvant agents (Table 3-4). Use of these agents can limit the use of step 2 and step 3 agents.

   (1) Tricyclic antidepressants are considered **first-line agents** for neuropathic pain.

   (2) Capsaicin cream is a substance P inhibitor that may improve pain when applied topically. Remind patients to wash their hands after applying this "hot pepper" derivative to their skin.

TABLE 3-3. Step 3 Agents: Opioid Analgesics for Moderate to Severe Pain

Agent	Equianalgesic Dose	Interval	Administration Route
Morphine*			
Short-acting	30 mg	Every 3–4 hours	Orally
Long-acting	90 mg	Every 12 hours	Orally
Hydromorphone**	7.5 mg	Every 3–4 hours	Orally
Fentanyl***	25–50 μg	Every 72 hours	Transdermal patch

Modified with permission from World Health Organization: Cancer pain relief and palliative care: report of a WHO expert committee, technical report series 804. Geneva, Switzerland, World Health Organization, 1990.

*Start with a rapid-acting preparation, then divide 24-hour total dose into two or three sustained-release doses. Continue administration of the rapid-acting preparation for breakthrough episodes.

**Hydromorphone has no specific advantage over morphine.

***Maximum effect is achieved only after 24 hours. Fentanyl has a long half-life (because the drug is absorbed by the skin and then slowly released into the blood stream) and is excellent choice for patients who cannot take oral medications.

TABLE 3-4. Agents for Neuropathic Pain

Agent	Starting Dose
Tricyclic antidepressants*	
Nortriptyline	10–25 mg at bedtime; increase as tolerated
Desipramine	10–25 mg at bedtime; increase as tolerated
Anticonvulsants	
Carbamazapine**	200 mg twice daily
Clonazepam	0.5 mg three times daily
Mexiletine	150 mg three times daily
Capsaicin 0.025% cream	Three times daily
Gabapentin	300 mg at bedtime on day #1; increase to 300–600 mg three times daily over a few days

*Both nortriptyline and desipramine have fewer side effects than amitriptyline

**Blood counts should be monitored in patients taking carbamazepine because of the risk of bone marrow suppression.

   2. Cancer pain. A number of specialized treatments are available for patients with cancer pain.
      a. Nerve compression and central nervous system (CNS) metastases. Pain may be relieved by **nonsteroidal anti-inflammatory drugs (NSAIDs)** and **steroids.**
      b. Bony metastases. Pain from bony metastases may be reduced by **pamidronate, strontium chloride,** and **calcitonin.**

III FOLLOW-UP AND REFERRAL. Patients should be seen as often as necessary to ensure rapid and optimum pain control.

A. Patients with unusual pain syndromes and those who do not respond to the standard treatment approach can be referred to a **specialized pain control center.**
B. Patients with pain from cancer should be referred to an **oncologist** for advice about chemotherapy, radiation therapy, and adjuvant agents.
C. Patients with known cancer and new back pain should be evaluated promptly to rule out metastatic disease to the spine.

Reference
Pain Management: Overview of Management Options. American Medical Association CME Library, found on-line at: http://www.ama-cmeonline.com/pain_mgmt/module02/index.htm

4. Preventive Medicine

....

I INTRODUCTION

A. Forms of preventive medicine. Prevention of illness takes three forms: primary prevention, secondary prevention, and tertiary prevention. This chapter focuses on primary and secondary prevention of disease. Tertiary prevention is covered in the chapters that discuss specific diseases.

   1. **Primary prevention** is the **prevention of disease.** Interventions used to achieve primary prevention include the following:

      a. **Immunization** reduces the patient's susceptibility to certain infectious diseases.

      b. **Counseling** involves patient education with the goal of changing a patient's high-risk behavior in order to prevent disease before it occurs.

      c. **Prophylactic drug therapy.** Certain medications can reduce the patient's risk of developing a disease [e.g., Aspirin can reduce the occurrence of non-fatal myocardial infarction in men].

   2. **Secondary prevention** is the **detection and treatment of disease in asymptomatic patients and in patients who have developed risk factors for a disease.** The goal is to cure or control the disease and risk factors in order to prevent complications from developing [e.g., treating hypertension before it leads to coronary artery disease (CAD)]. Secondary prevention is accomplished through **screening** for asymptomatic disease and risk factors (e.g., a Pap smear can detect cervical dysplasia at an early stage, thereby preventing the development of invasive cancer).

   3. **Tertiary prevention** is the prevention of complications caused by a disease already established in the patient (e.g., the prevention of retinopathy in a patient with diabetes).

B. Sources of recommendations

   1. **United States Preventive Services Task Force (USPSTF).** The preventive services recommended in this chapter are based on the recommendations in the updated USPSTF guidelines found online at the following address (www. preventiveservices.ahrq.gov). This group takes a systematic approach to evaluating the effectiveness of clinical preventive services, and their recommendations and review

of the evidence are based on a predetermined methodology. Using this evidence-based technique, they recommend only those interventions that have documented effectiveness.

2. Two other organizations, the **Canadian Task Force on Periodic Health Examination (CTFPHE)** and the **American College of Physicians (ACP),** take an approach similar to that of the USPSTF and make similar recommendations.

II IMMUNIZATIONS. The recommended adult immunizations are given in the prevention checklists that appear at the end of the chapter (Tables 4-1 and 4-2). Certain patients are at particularly high risk for contracting certain diseases or suffering from complications of the diseases; for these patients, immunization is critical.

A. **Influenza A virus.** Individuals at high risk include:
   1. Residents of chronic care facilities
   2. Healthcare providers seeing high-risk patients
   3. Patients with chronic cardiopulmonary disorders, metabolic disorders (including diabetes), hemoglobinopathies, immunosuppression, or renal dysfunction
   4. Patients aged $\geq$ 65 years

B. **Pneumococcal pneumonia.** Individuals at high risk include:
   1. Institutionalized patients who are > than 50 years
   2. Patients with chronic cardiopulmonary disease, diabetes mellitus, or anatomic asplenia [excluding sickle cell disease (SCD)]
   3. Patients with special high-risk living situations (e.g., Native American or Alaska Native populations)
   4. Immunocompromised patients
   5. Patients aged $\geq$ 65 years

C. **Hepatitis A.** Individuals at high risk include:
   1. Travelers to endemic areas
   2. Homosexual men
   3. Users of illegal drugs
   4. Military personnel
   5. Institutionalized patients and workers in these institutions.
   6. Certain hospital and laboratory workers

D. **Hepatitis B.** Individuals at high risk include:
   1. Young adults not previously immunized
   2. Homosexual men
   3. Injection drug users and their sex partners
   4. Patients with a history of multiple sex partners in the past 6 months and those who have recently acquired a sexually transmitted disease (STD)

TABLE 4-1. Preventive Medicine Checklist for Asymptomatic Women

IMMUNIZATIONS
- [ ] **Influenza A vaccine:** Age ≥ 65 years or at high risk*, **annually**
- [ ] **Pneumococcal vaccine:** Age ≥ 65 years or at high risk†, **once every 5–10 years**
- [ ] **Diphtheria tetanus (DT) vaccine:** Ensure completed series; **booster every 10 years**
- [ ] **Measles-mumps-rubeila (MMR) vaccine:** Women born after 1956 who lack evidence of immunity
- [ ] **Hepatitis A vaccine:** Women at high risk§
- [ ] **Hepatitis B vaccine:** Young women not previously immunized, and women at high risk‡
- [ ] **Varicella vaccine:** Healthy women with no history of previous varicella infection
- [ ] **Rubella vaccine:** Women of childbearing age (alternative is to screen, then vaccinate as needed)

COUNSELING
- [ ] Cessation of tobacco use
- [ ] Regular physical activity
- [ ] Diet
- [ ] Contraception and prevention of sexually transmitted disease
- [ ] Dental care
- [ ] Prevention of motor vehicle accidents
- [ ] Prevention of household and recreational injuries

PROPHYLACTIC MEDICATIONS TO CONSIDER
- [ ] Aspirin (women at high risk for myocardial infarction)
- [ ] Multivitamin or folic acid supplementation (women considering or capable of pregnancy)

SCREENING
- [ ] **Hypertension:** Evaluate blood pressure in all women 21 years or older, **at each visit** and **at least every 2 years**
- [ ] **Elevated cholesterol:** Evaluate cholesterol in all women age 45–69 years, **at least every 5 years**
- [ ] **Breast cancer:** Mammogram +/− clinical breast exam for all women age 50–69 years, **annually or binannually**
- [ ] **Colorectal cancer:** Annual fecal occult blood test +/− sigmoidoscopy for all women 50 years or older, at **3-** to **5-year intervals**

continued

TABLE 4-1. Preventive Medicine Checklist for Asymptomatic Women
(*Continued*)

☐ **Cervical cancer:** Pap smear **at onset of sexual activity**
   and **at least every 3 years**
☐ **Obesity:** Periodic height and weight determinations
☐ **Sexually transmitted diseases**
   Chlamydia trachomatis: Annual cervical culture or nonculture
   assay for all sexually active female adolescents
   Neisseria gonorrhoeae: Annual cervical culture for all high-risk
   women‖
☐ **Problem drinking:** History and questionnaire
☐ **Hearing and vision:** Elderly women
PATIENT-SPECIFIC PREVENTIVE SERVICES
☐ _____
☐ _____
☐ _____
☐ _____

*Residents of chronic care facilities; healthcare providers seeing high-risk
patients; patients with chronic cardiopulmonary disorders, metabolic disorders
(including diabetes), hemoglobinopathies, immunosuppression, or renal
dysfunction
†Institutionalized patients who are older lhan 50 years; those with chronic
cardiopulmonary disease, diabetes mellitus, or anatomic asplenia (excluding
sickle cell disease); those with special high-risk living situations;
immunocompromised patients
‡Injection drug users and their sex partners; patients with a history of multiple
sex partners in the past 6 months; patients who have recently acquired a
sexually transmitted disease (STD); travelers to endemic areas; recipients of
blood products; healthcare workers who are exposed to blood
§Travelers to endemic areas; injection drug users; military personnel;
institutionalized patients; certain hospital and laboratory workers
‖Commercial sex workers; women with a history of frequent *N. gonorrhoeae*
infection; women younger than 25 years with a history of two or more sex
partners in the lest year

5. Travelers to endemic areas
6. Recipients of blood products
7. Healthcare workers who are exposed to blood

III COUNSELING

A. Cessation of tobacco use. Convincing a patient to stop smoking is likely the most valuable method of disease prevention in

---

TABLE 4-2. Preventive Medicine Checklist for Asymptomatic Men

IMMUNIZATIONS

☐ **Influenza A vaccine:** Age ≥ 65 years or at high risk*, **annually**

☐ **Pneumococcal vaccine:** Age ≥ 65 years or at high risk[†], **once every 5 years**

☐ **Diphtheria tetanus (DT) vaccine:** Ensure completed series; **booster every 10 years**

☐ **Measles-mumphs-rubella (MMR) vaccine:** Men born after 1956 who lack evidence of immunity

☐ **Hepatitis A vaccine:** Men at high risk[§]

☐ **Hepatitis B vaccine:** Young men not previously immunized, and men at high risk[‡]

☐ **Varicella vaccine:** Healthy men with no history of previous varicella infection

COUNSELING

☐ Cessation of tobacco use

☐ Regular physical activity

☐ Diet

☐ Contraception and prevention of sexually transmitted disease

☐ Dental care

☐ Prevention of motor vehicle accidents

☐ Prevention of household and recreational injuries

PROPHYLACTIC MEDICATIONS TO CONSIDER

☐ Aspirin (men at high risk for myocardial infarction)

SCREENING

☐ **Hypertension:** Evaluate blood pressure in all men 21 years or older, at **each visit** and at **least every 2 years**

☐ **Elevated cholesterol:** Evaluate cholesterol in all men age 35–65 years, **at least every 5 years**

continued

---

adults. Counseling to stop or avoid starting should be given to all smokers and non-smokers respectively.

1. Specialized or group counseling may be useful and should be offered if it is available.

2. Nicotine gum, patches, inhaler, or nasal spray may be a useful adjunct.

3. Medications such as sustained-release bupropion, clonidine, or nortriptyline may be useful.

B. Diet. Certain patients should be advised to reduce their intake of dietary fat to less than 30% of their total daily caloric intake

---

TABLE 4-2. Preventive Medicine Checklist for Asymptomatic Men (*Continued*)

☐   **Colorectal cancer:** Annual fecal occult blood test $+/-$ sigmoidoscopy for all men 50 years or older, at **3-** to **5-year intervals**

☐   **Obesity:** Periodic height and weight determinations

☐   **Problem drinking:** Use history and questionnaire

☐   **Hearing and vision:** Elderly men

PATIENT-SPECIFIC PREVENTIVE SERVICES

☐   _____

☐   _____

☐   _____

☐   _____

---

*Residents of chronic care facilities; healthcare providers seeing high-risk palients; patients with chronic cardiopulmonary disorders, metabolic disorders (including diabetes], hemoglobinopathies, immunosuppression, or renal dysfunction

†Institutionalized patients who are older than 50 years; those wiih chronic cardiopulmonary disease, diabetes mellitus, or anatomic osplenia (excluding sickle cell disease); those with special high-risk living situations; immunocompromised patients

‡Homosexual men; injection drug users and their sex partners; patients with a history af multiple sex partners in the past 6 months; patients who have recently acquired c sexually transmitted disease; travelers to endemic areas; recipients af blood products; healthcare workers who are exposed to blood

§Travelers to endemic areas; homosexual men; injection drug users; military personnel, institutionalized patients: certain hospital ond laboratory workers

---

(saturated fat should be less than 10% of the total daily caloric intake).

1. Fruits, vegetables, grain products containing fiber, fish, poultry without skin, and low-fat dairy products should be emphasized.
2. Specialized counseling by dieticians and nutritionists may be useful, especially for patients who are having difficulty or who have other diet-related conditions (e.g., CAD, diabetes, obesity, hyperlipidemia).

C. Contraception and prevention of STDs. Counseling about risk factors for HIV and other STDs should be given to all patients.

1. All patients of reproductive age should be advised about effective methods of contraception (see Chapter 50).

2. Effective methods of preventing HIV and other STDs include abstinence, a mutually monogamous relationship between partners known to be free of HIV or other STDs, use of a latex condom, and avoidance of high-risk partners.

D. Prevention of motor vehicle accidents

1. All patients should be counseled about wearing seat belts (lap and shoulder, even if an air bag is present), properly using child safety seats, and not driving under the influence of alcohol or drugs.

2. Motorcyclists should be advised to wear approved helmets.

E. Prevention of household and recreational injuries

1. Prevention of household injuries

   a. All households. Smoke detectors should be installed and checked at regular intervals.

   b. Households with children. Parents should be encouraged to review safety recommendations with their child's pediatrician. Some safety measures include:

   (1) Setting hot water heaters at 120°–130°F

   (2) Putting children to bed in flame-resistant night clothing

   (3) Keeping medicines, cleaning supplies, and other toxic substances out of reach of children and in child-resistant containers

   (4) Keeping a fresh 1-ounce bottle of syrup of ipecac on hand

   (5) Displaying emergency telephone numbers

   (6) Installing fences around pools, windows, and stairs that pose a risk for injury

   c. Households with elderly family members

   (1) Elderly patients may benefit from counseling about reducing the risk of falling. Effective approaches include installing railings, ensuring that lighting is adequate, and completing balance training.

   (2) For frail patients, specialized programs or in-home "safety-checks" may be useful.

   (3) Prevention of recreational injuries. All patients who bicycle, in-line skate, or ride all-terrain vehicles should be encouraged to wear helmets.

F. Dental care. Patients should be encouraged to have regular check-ups with a dentist and to follow good dental hygiene habits.

IV Prophylactic Medications

A. Aspirin reduces the risk of a first myocardial infarction in men older than 50 years, but it increases the risk of bleeding. Although the USPSTF does not recommend for or against the use of aspirin for the primary prevention of myocardial infarction, asymptomatic patients with risk factors for myocardial infarction and without contraindications to aspirin use can be considered for prophylactic treatment. Treatment decisions should be based on individual risk and discussion of the risks and benefits with the patient.

B. Multivitamin or **folic acid supplementation** may be indicated for women considering or capable of pregnancy.

    1. In order to reduce the risk of neural tube defects in the fetus, the USPSTF recommends that women who are planning pregnancy take a multivitamin containing 0.4–0.8 mg of folic acid daily, beginning at least 1 month prior to conception and continuing through the first trimester.

    2. Women who are capable of pregnancy should take a multivitamin containing 0.4 mg of folic acid daily to prevent neural tube defects in the event of an unplanned pregnancy.

V SCREENING

A. Screening for cardiovascular disease

    1. Hypertension (see also Chapter 15). **Office sphygmomanometry** can accurately detect hypertension. Treatment of hypertension has been shown to reduce overall mortality as well as morbidity and mortality due to stroke and ischemic heart disease.

        a. Treatment is effective for both young and elderly patients.

        b. Patients at high risk for complications from hypertension (e.g., patients with diabetes or hypercholesterolemia) should be considered for early, aggressive therapy.

    2. Hypercholesterolemia. Providers may choose to use the **total cholesterol** and **High-density lipoprotein (HDL)** levels as an initial screen. In patients with elevated risk on the initial screening results, **low-density lipoprotein (LDL)** and triglyceride levels can then be obtained to further clarify the situation.

        a. It is reasonable to screen asymptomatic men between the ages of 35 and 65 years once every 5 years. Screening for asymptomatic women should begin at age 45 and take place every 5 years.

        b. Screening is also reasonable in younger patients with diabetes, a family history of premature cardiovascular disease, familial hyperlipidemia, or multiple coronary heart disease risk factors.

        c. Patients with multiple risk factors for CAD, or patients with borderline high test results can be considered for more frequent screening.

B. Screening for cancer
  1. **Cervical cancer.** Screening for cervical cancer is one of the great success stories of medical prevention. Since the implementation of widespread screening programs several decades ago, there has been a dramatic reduction in the number of women who have died from cervical cancer. All women should undergo a **Pap smear** within 3 years of the **onset of sexual activity** or **age 21** (whichever comes first), and then **once every 1–3 years thereafter.**
      a. Patients with multiple risk factors (early age at the onset of sexual intercourse, multiple sex partners, low socioeconomic status, history of cervical neoplasia, infection with HPV or other STD) should probably be screened annually, while patients without risk factors may be candidates for screening every 3 years.
      b. Patients who have had their cervix removed do not require screening (unless it was removed because of cervical cancer).
  2. **Breast cancer.** Screening techniques include **mammography** and **clinical breast examination.**
      a. **Women 40–69 years of age.** The efficacy of annual or biennial mammography is well documented and should be recommended to all patients. An annual or biannual clinical breast examination may also be performed at the discretion of the provider for women in this age group.
      b. **Women older than 69 years.** Providers may choose to screen women older than 69 years, especially those patients who do not have significant comorbid disease.
  3. **Colorectal cancer.** All patients older than 50 years should be screened. Proven methods of screening include **fecal occult blood testing (FOBT), periodic flexible sigmoidoscopy,** and colonoscopy.
      a. FOBT should be performed annually. Flexible sigmoidoscopy should be performed every 3–5 years. Colonoscopy may be performed at 10 year intervals or as a once-in-a-lifetime examination at age 55–65 years old.
      b. Earlier screening is reasonable in patients with a first-degree relative who is diagnosed with colorectal cancer before 60 years of age.
      c. The screening method or combination of methods used should be based on analysis and discussion of the risks and benefits with each patient.
      d. Patients with a history of familial syndromes of colon cancer, ulcerative colitis, previous colonic polyps, or colon cancer require more frequent screening and expert consultation.

4. Other types of cancer. Screening tests are available for a number of other kinds of cancer (e.g., prostate, lung, ovarian, testicular, bladder, pancreatic, oral, thyroid, and skin cancers). The current USPSTF guidelines do not include screening tests for these cancers, due to either insufficient evidence of efficacy of screening or evidence that the screening was ineffective. Providers may wish to review the information and develop their own interpretations.

C. Screening for other health problems

   1. Obesity. Periodic **height** and **weight determinations** are recommended as a screening test for obesity. Although weight loss alone has not been shown conclusively to decrease mortality, it has been demonstrated to reduce the risk of developing cardiovascular disease and other health problems.

   2. Problem drinking. Screening for problem drinking and brief counseling can reduce the amount of alcohol consumed by patients. Several questionnaires are available (see Chapter 89).

   3. Vision and hearing impairment. Screening for visual impairment and hearing difficulty in the elderly may improve the patient's quality of life and prevent injury.

   4. Osteoporosis. Screening for osteoporosis with bone mineral density measurements is recommended in all women over 65 years of age. The screening accurately predicts the risk for fractures in asymptomatic women and subsequently guides decisions on therapy.

   5. Depression. Screening for depression may decrease clinical morbidity in patients.

VI **PREVENTIVE MEDICINE CHECKLISTS.** The checklists in Tables 4-1 and 4-2 (for women and men, respectively) have been developed based on the USPSTF guidelines. Several points about these checklists are important to remember:

A. These checklists are not comprehensive and **should be modified to suit the individual needs of each patient.** Patients in certain high-risk groups require additional preventive services (e.g., intravenous drug users should be offered HIV screening). Primary care providers should review the information in the USPSTF *Guide to Clinical Preventive Services* to determine which preventive services they should offer to their patients.

B. The checklists deal only with primary and secondary prevention in adults. Patients with known disease often require additional preventive services (i.e., tertiary prevention), and the checklists can be updated to reflect those needs (e.g., annual screening for microalbuminuria to detect nephropathy in a patient with diabetes).

C. There are a number of preventive services that are available, but that have not been recommended by the USPSTF due to inconclusive evidence (e.g., screening for testicular cancer with a periodic physical examination). Providers may decide, after reviewing the evidence, that some of these services should be provided to their patients.

D. Checklists are only useful if they are actually used. These lists, or similar ones created by the primary care provider, should be posted in each patient's chart. Providers with access to computer charting may want to incorporate these checklists into a program that reminds providers when preventive services should be given.

Reference
United States Preventive Services Task Force. *Guide to Clinical Preventive Services,* 2nd ed. Baltimore: Williams & Wilkins, 1996 (updates at www.preventiveservices. ahrq.gov).

PART II

OPHTHALMOLOGY AND OTOLARYNGOLOGY

5. Urgent Eye Complaints

I **INTRODUCTION.** Because some ophthalmologic conditions can threaten vision, internists must be able to recognize and triage serious eye problems within an appropriate time frame.

A. Incidence. Acute ophthalmologic problems account for **3%–10% of presentations** in emergency rooms, urgent care centers, and primary care offices.

B. Major complaints. Most eye problems involve one of three major complaints: **impaired vision, red** or **painful eye,** or **ocular trauma.**

II **APPROACH TO THE PATIENT**

A. Obtain a patient history. Be sure to note the following:
1. **Symptoms.** What is the major complaint (change in vision, change in eye appearance, discomfort, or trauma)? Is there photophobia? (Iritis, corneal edema, glaucoma.) Are there flashing lights, a rush of floaters, a shadow over the vision? (Retinal detachment.) Does the patient see blood? (Vitreous hemorrhage.) What other symptoms does the patient have?
2. **Time course.** When did the symptoms begin?
3. **Past medical history.** What is the patient's vision status and past medical history? For example, does the patient have a history of hypertension, diabetes, or another systemic disease with possible ocular manifestations, or a history of eye surgery?

B. Perform a physical examination

HOT KEY

Pupillary dilatation should occur at the end of the examination because you cannot assess visual acuity or pupillary responses in a dilated eye.

1. **Visual acuity survey.** Visual acuity is evaluated by using the **Snellen chart**. If the vision is worse than 20/400 (big E) then the patient is asked to count fingers (CF), recognize hand motion (HM), or to perceive light (LP).
2. **Pupil examination.** The pupils' **size, shape,** and **reaction to direct and consensual light** should be noted.
3. **Adnexa and periorbital examination.** Evaluate the **lids, lashes,** and **orbital rim.**
4. **Neurologic examination. Facial** and **corneal nerve sensation** should be evaluated by lightly touching the face and cornea with a cotton swab before topical anethesia.
5. **Ocular mobility assessment.** Ask the patient to look up, down, and to each side.
6. **Visual field testing.** See if the patient can detect motion when you wiggle your fingers in the right and left upper and lower outer quadrants.
7. **Slit-lamp examination** is used to evaluate the cornea (using fluorescein stain) and the depth of the anterior chamber.
8. **Intraocular pressure evaluation.** Tonometry is contraindicated in patients with globe penetration, foreign bodies, trauma, or active infection. It is especially important in angle closure glaucoma.
9. **Direct ophthalmoscopy** allows the examiner to evaluate the red reflex, lens clarity, and the fundus. The red reflex is the reflection of the retinal vessels, which appear red in patients with a healthy eye during ophthalmoscopy.
C. **Treat or refer the patient to an ophthalmologist** as necessary. In general, consultation with an ophthalmologist is necessary if the patient's vision is acutely altered or threatened.

HOT KEY

When calling the ophthalmologist, never forget the visual acuity with correction (glasses), the pupil exam, and the intraocular pressure. These three are the vital signs for the eye.

 CAUSES OF IMPAIRED VISION. Table 5-1 summarizes causes of acute vision loss that may result in permanent

TABLE 5-1. Causes of Impaired Vision That Require Urgent Referral to an Ophthalmologist

Disorder	History	Physical Examination and Laboratory Findings	Treatment
Retinal artery occlusion	Rapid, profound, painless monocular vision loss Typical patient is an elderly man More common in early morning	Examination may be normal in early stages Late-stage findings include a "milky" retina around the optic disk, a pale fundus, and a cherry-red macula	Immediately refer (irreversible blindness can occur within 90 minutes of the onset of symptoms)
Retinal vein occlusion	Past medical history of diabetes, hypertension, hyperviscosity, glaucoma, or mild vision loss (from macular edema)	"Blood and thunder" retina (diffuse retinal hemorrhages and venous dilation; cotton-wool spots)	Refer within 24–48 hours Globe pressure-massage Have patient breathe into a paper bag to increase the $PaCO_2$
Temporal arteritis	Headaches, pain with chewing, myalgias	Tender temporal arteries High sedimentation rate	Oral prednisone (60 mg daily) until temporal artery biopsy can be performed
Vitreous hemorrhage	Painless vision loss Risk factors include trauma, diabetes mellitus, and retinal tear	Absent red reflex (i.e., vessels appear dull or black)	Immediately refer; increased intraocular pressure can threaten retinal circulation Laser therapy (patients with proliferative retinopathy associated with diabetes mellitus)

(Continued)

TABLE 5-1. Causes of Impaired Vision That Require Urgent Referral to an Ophthalmologist (*Continued*)

Disorder	History	Physical Examination and Laboratory Findings	Treatment
Retinal detachment	Acute "floaters," flashing lights, decreased or cloudy vision, "curtain" over the visual field Risk factors include advanced age, myopia, and a history of ocular surgery or retinal degeneration	Detached retina may look like bulging, floating folds within the vitreous humor, or appear grey with black vessels	Immediately refer for photocoagulation, cryotherapy, diathermy, scleral buckling, or air/silicon oil injections
Age-related macular degeneration	Sudden onset of central blurring or central distortion of straight lines Sudden decompensation can result from macular hemorrhage, proliferative retinopathy, or trauma	Vision impairment is noted only in line of focus (peripheral vision is normal)	Refer within 48 hours for evaluation and possible laser therapy

$PaCO_2$ = arterial carbon dioxide tension.

blindness if not adequately diagnosed and treated. Usually, the cause of a patient's vision loss can be traced back to one of six anatomic sites (think of the six sites from "outside-in").

A. Cornea. Corneal abrasion and ulcers are the most common causes of acute changes in vision.

B. Lens. Acute lens refractive error is most often caused by wide fluctuations in the blood glucose level in patients with diabetes. Rarely, medications (e.g., thiazide diuretics) cause lens edema.

C. Retina. Retinal artery or vein occlusion, retinal detachment, vitreous hemorrhage, and bleeding from age related macular degeneration are causes of acute vision loss that can result in permanent blindness if not quickly diagnosed and treated.

D. Optic nerve. Damage to the optic nerve can be idiopathic, or it may result from any number of disorders that impair circulation, cause inflammation, or damage the optic nerve directly (e.g., multiple sclerosis/optic neuritis, temporal arteritis, anterior ischemic optic neuropathy).

 HOT KEY Regardless of the cause, optic nerve damage results in a relative afferent pupillary nerve defects on examination (i.e., both pupils do not constrict equally when shining light in each eye and comparing each eye to the other).

E. Optic chiasm. Impingement of the optic chiasm by a pituitary mass or infarct can result in bitemporal hemianopia (Figure 5-1).

F. Area posterior to the optic chiasm. Loss of vision can also result from lesions of the lateral geniculate bodies, optic radiations, or the occipital cortex.

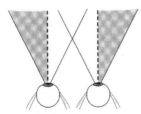 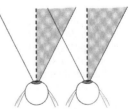

FIGURE 5-1. Hemianopia.

> **HOT**
> **▶**
> **KEY**
>
> Lesions posterior to the optic chiasm produce bilateral loss of vision on the same side of the vertical meridian (i.e., a homonymous hemianopia). Neurologic work-up [for cerebrovascular accident (CVA) or masses] is usually required.

IV **CAUSES OF RED EYE.** A red eye is an extremely common complaint with multiple causes.

A. **Inflammation of the lids, lashes, and glands (Blepharitis, hordeolum, chalazion,** and **dacryocystitis)** can usually be diagnosed by inspection alone.

1. **Blepharitis** is an inflammation of the eyelid margins, usually bilateral. The two most common causes are seborrhea, which causes greasy scales, and *Staphylococcus aureus* infection, which causes dry scales and more erythema.

2. A **hordeolum (stye)** is an acute inflammation of one of the glands lining the eyelid.

   a. An internal hordeolum results from inflammation of the meibomian glands and points toward the conjunctival surface.

   b. An external hordeolum results from inflammation of the Moll's glands or glands of Zeis and is located on the outer lid.

3. A **chalazion** is a chronic granulomatous inflammation of a meibomian gland. It is different from an internal hordeolum in terms of its time course (weeks versus days). Chalazia are usually painless and unaccompanied by signs of acute infection.

4. **Dacryocystitis** is an acute infection of the lacrimal sac, usually caused by *S. aureus* or β-hemolytic *Streptococcus*. Dacryocystitis presents with swelling below the medial canaliculus, pain, and tearing. It may be possible to express pus from the lacrimal duct.

B. **Conjunctivitis** is the most common cause of red eye seen in urgent care centers. Conjunctivitis has multiple causes (Table 5-2), but the **physical examination findings (normal vision, minimal photophobia, conjunctival injection, eyelid edema, tearing, intact pupillary light reflex)** are often similar regardless of the cause. Often, the cause is revealed by the patient history.

1. **Bacterial conjunctivitis** is most often caused by *Streptococcus pneumoniae, S. aureus, Haemophilus influenzae,* and *Neisseria gonorrhoeae.* Foreign bodies must be ruled out.

2. **Chlamydial conjunctivitis** is caused by *Chlamydia trachomatis.* Chronic chlamydial conjunctivitis, called **trachoma,**

TABLE 5-2. Conjunctivitis

Disorder	History	Physical Examination and Laboratory Findings	Treatment
Bacterial conjunctivitis	Thick crust on eyelid on awakening (unilateral or bilateral) No associated viral symptoms Patients with conjunctivitis caused by *Neisseria gonorrhoeae* are usually sexually active adults with a history of recent exposure to a patient with genital gonorrhea; may also be newborns who have been exposed during delivery	Gram stain of a conjunctival scraping may identify causative organism (indicated if patient's symptoms do not improve in 2–3 days)	Gentamicin or erythromycin eye drops every 2 hours Eye patches and topical steroid drops are contraindicated Patients with *N. gonorrhoeae* conjunctivitis require 1 g ceftriaxone IM or IV and ciprofloxacin eye drops Refer all patiens within 48 hours
Chlamydial conjunctivitis	Neonates infected during delivery present with red eye within 5–14 days 90% of women and 60% of men with chlamydial conjunctivitis also have genital chlamydia	Red eye, preauricular lymphadenopathy, and lid edema Giemsa stain of an epithelial scrape reveals intracellular inclusion bodies	Tetracycline (250 mg) or doxycycline (100 mg) four times daily for 14 days Azithromycin (1 g orally) for pregnant women Refer within 48 hours

(Continued)

TABLE 5-2. Conjunctivitis (Continued)

Disorder	History	Physical Examination and Laboratory Findings	Treatment
Viral conjunctivitis	Often bilateral and associated with red eye; a watery, nonpurulent discharge; and systemic symptoms (e.g., fever, preauricular adenopathy, pharyngitis)	Patients with adenoviral keratoconjunctivitis may have scattered, small corneal infiltrates and subconjunctival hemorrhage Slit-lamp examination with fluorescein staining may reveal dendritic keratitis in patients with conjunctivitis caused by HSV or herpes zoster virus	Symptoms are self-limited, although HSV conjunctivitis can be treated with Acyclovir, Valacyclovir, or Famciclovir No referral necessary, unless herpes zoster is suspected
Allergic conjunctivitis	Clear discharge bilaterally, itching, and lid edema often accompanied by rhinorrhea and a history of seasonal allergies or atopic dermatitis	Eosinophils on Giemsa stain are diagnostic	Removal of allergen Oral antihitamines or decongestants Naphcon A

HSV = herpes simplex virus; IM = intramuscularly; IV = intravenously.

is more prevalent in developing countries and can cause corneal scarring, cataracts, and blindness. Treatment is with a 6-week course of systemic and topical antibiotics.

3. **Viral conjunctivitis (pinkeye)** is most often caused by **adenoviruses, coxsackieviruses,** and **picornaviruses.** Viral conjunctivitis is **highly contagious** and patients often report contact with a patient with similar symptoms.

4. **Allergic conjunctivitis** is usually seen in patients with a history of seasonal allergies or atopic dermatitis.

C. **Causes of red eye requiring urgent referral** to an ophthalmologist are summarized in Table 5-3.

1. **Acute angle closure glaucoma** results from the acute blockage of aqueous humor flow in patients with shallow anterior chamber angles. Attacks can be precipitated by pupillary dilatation, which increases contact between the iris and lens. The increased contact blocks the flow of aqueous humor from the posterior to the anterior chamber (Figure 5-2), increasing the pressure behind the iris and causing the iris to bow forward. The bowed iris closes the anterior chamber angle, preventing drainage of the aqueous humor and increasing the intraocular pressure from its normal range of 10–20 mm Hg to 30–70 mm Hg. The increased intraocular pressure can damage the cornea, and optic nerve, posing a threat to vision.

2. **Uveitis** (i.e., intraocular inflammation) has multiple causes, including connective tissue disorders, infectious disorders, trauma, and malignancy. Recurrent uveitis can lead to synechiae or glaucoma.

   a. **Anterior uveitis** affects the iris **(iritis),** anterior chamber, or posterior chamber.

   b. **Intermediate uveitis** affects the vitreous body.

   c. **Posterior uveitis** affects the retina or choroid.

3. **Orbital cellulitis**

   a. Common causative organisms include ***H. influenzae,* S. *aureus, Streptococcus pyogenes,*** and ***S. pneumoniae.***

      (1) In immunocompromised patients (including those with diabetes), **mucormycosis** should be considered, especially if the patient has a history of sinusitis.

      (2) Consider computed tomography (CT) or magnetic resonance imaging to rule out an **abscess** that requires drainage.

   b. **Complications** of untreated orbital cellulitis include vision loss, cavernous sinus thrombosis, and intracranial infection.

4. **Corneal ulcer** can occur secondary to foreign body, entropion (and eyelid that turns inward), trichiasis (misdirection of eyelashes towards the globe), lagophthalmus (an inability to fully close the eyes), or conjunctivitis.

TABLE 5-3. Causes of Red Eye That Require Urgent Referral to an Ophthalmologist

Disorder	History	Physical Examination and Laboratory Findings	Treatment
Acute angle closure glaucoma	Red, painful eye Blurred vision Halos around lights (from corneal edema) Nausea or vomiting Initial symptoms may resemble those of a migraine headache	Shallow anterior chamber on slit-lamp examination Fixed, semi-dilated pupil Hazy cornea (from edema) High intraocular pressure on tonometry or palpation	Refer immediately for iridotomy Timolol (0.5% solution) to decrease intraocular pressure and aqueous humor formation Pilocarpine (1%–2% solution) to constrict pupil Acetazolamide (500 mg) or mannitol (1 mg/kg) IV to decrease intraocular pressure
Anterior uveitis (iritis)	Unilateral, painful red eye with limbic flush Photophobia Blurred vision (if clouded aqueous humor)	Small, poorly reactive pupil Consensual photophobia (i.e., pain with light in either eye, owing to consensual iris contraction in the affected eye) Cells and flare in anterior chamber on slit-lamp examination Preorbital swelling	Disorder is usually self-limited, but refer within 24–48 hours to avoid complications Ophthalmologist may prescribe a long-acting cycloplegic (e.g., atropine) or topical prednisolone acetate 1% to alleviate pain

Orbital cellulites	Dull, aching ocular pain; exophthalmos; fever; malaise	Limited extraocular motion Decreased vision	Refer immediately Initiate IV antibiotic therapy immediately, without waiting for a consult; use a first- or second-generation cephalosporin (with an antifungal agent if patient is immunocompromised)
Corneal ulcer	Pain, tearing, history of foreign body	Slit-lamp examination with fluroescein stain to rule out perforation Evert eyelids to rule out retained foreign body Culture to determine cause	Refer immediately Ophthalmologist may prescribe a short-acting cycloplegic (e.g., cyclopentolate) and gentamicin or tobramycin drops

IV = intravenous.

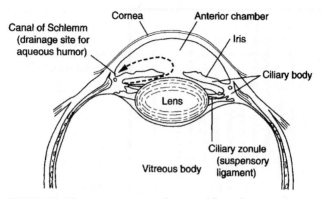

FIGURE 5-2. The *arrow* represents the normal flow of aqueous humor from the posterior chamber to the anterior chamber.

V **CAUSES OF EYE TRAUMA.** Primary physicians are often the first to evaluate patients with eye trauma.

A. Chemical exposures can threaten long-term vision. Exposures may be **acidic or alkali, the latter being worse for the eye.**

　1. Irrigation. The eye should be copiously irrigated with a minimum of 2L of normal saline, prior to performing a physical examination. After irrigating the eye, sweep the fornices with a moistened applicator to remove traces of any foreign body or chemical that may remain.

　　a. If the patient calls from home, he should be advised to irrigate the eye for 30 minutes prior to leaving for the emergency room.

　2. Physical examination

　　a. Examine the cornea for abrasions.

　　b. Evert the lids to rinse the conjunctiva and search for foreign bodies.

　3. Referral

　　a. If the examination is normal, a cycloplegic and topical antibiotic should be prescribed, and the eye should be patched using light pressure. The patient should see an ophthalmologist within 48 hours.

　　b. Patients with evidence of corneal or conjunctival scarring should be referred to an ophthalmologist.

B. Lid laceration

　1. Physical examination

　　a. Assess lid function by having the patient look up and down.

    b. If the lid is lacerated near the medial canthus, assess the eye for canalicular injury. These patients may require an urgent stent to prevent chronic tearing.

  2. Referral. Patients should be referred to an ophthalmologist immediately. Levator and canaliculus repair may require surgical exploration.

C. Blunt orbital trauma. A slit-lamp examination and visual acuity survey should be performed to evaluate for hyphema, vitreous hemorrhage, and retinal detachment. Patients should be referred to an ophthalmologist if history or physical examination findings suggest complications.

D. Blow-out fractures

  1. Physical examination may reveal soft-tissue swelling, diplopia, epistaxis, periorbital ecchymosis, crepitus, orbital emphysema, enophthalmos, exophthalmos, ptosis, or numbness over the maxillary region. Subcutaneous crepitus in the periorbital area may indicate communication with a sinus space, which can be caused by a blow-out fracture.

  2. Imaging studies

    a. Plain film radiographs may reveal the "teardrop" sign (caused by herniation of soft tissue into the sinus) or an air-fluid level in the ipsilateral sinus.

    b. CT scans may be indicated to search for bony fragments or herniation.

  3. Referral. Patients must be referred to an ophthalmologist immediately. In the meantime, ice compresses can be applied and systemic antibiotics can be initiated (to prevent orbital infection from the sinuses). Valsalva maneuvers should be avoided.

E. Ruptured globe can result from high impact trauma to the globe. Often if the orbit is intact, the globe may be ruptured and vice versa. Signs include vision loss, hyphema, vitreous hemorrhage, and an extremely deep or shallow anterior chamber.

  1. Once a diagnosis of ruptured globe is ascertained, the patient should not be further examined. **Place a metal eye shield over the eye and refer the patient to an ophthalmologist for immediate surgical repair.**

  2. Avoid topical eye ointments, because these agents can complicate surgical repair. **Systemic antibiotics may be prescribed** to prevent endophthalmitis.

Reference

Loewenstein J, Lee S. Ophthalmology, Just the Facts. New York, New York: McGraw Hill, 2004.

6. Hearing Loss

I **INTRODUCTION.** Hearing impairment is the most common chronic handicap in the United States.

A. An estimated 28 million Americans have some degree of hearing impairment.

B. Only 10% of people 65 years of age or older report having normal hearing.

II **CAUSES OF HEARING LOSS.** There are three types of hearing loss: conductive, sensorineural, and mixed.

A. **Conductive hearing loss** originates in the external or middle ear. Passage of sound to the cochlea is obstructed or reduced secondary to cerumen impaction, fluid, congenital deformities, tumors, trauma, or otosclerosis within the sound-conducting apparatus.

B. **Sensorineural hearing loss** occurs when the cochlea (inner ear) or the cochlear portion of cranial nerve VIII (i.e., the acoustic nerve) is affected, preventing the transmission of the auditory signal to the brain. The causes of sensorineural hearing loss are numerous and include ototoxicity, presbycusis, Meniere's disease, trauma, noise-induced hearing loss, multiple sclerosis, autoimmune disease, and tumors.

C. **Mixed hearing loss** includes components of both conductive and sensorineural hearing loss. The primary component should be identified. Causes of mixed hearing loss include trauma, otosclerosis, and chronic otitis media.

III **APPROACH TO THE PATIENT.** Identification of hearing loss requires diligence on the part of the physician because many patients deny or have trouble describing their hearing loss. First, determine that there is hearing loss, then classify it as conductive, sensorineural, or mixed (Figure 6-1).

A. **Patient history.** A thorough history is crucial to the proper diagnosis of hearing loss.

    1. **Signs and symptoms.** The presentation of a patient's hearing loss varies depending on the site of disease along the auditory pathway.

        a. Elderly patients may exhibit **isolation** and **dementia-like symptoms** as a result of deafness, which in many cases is reversible.

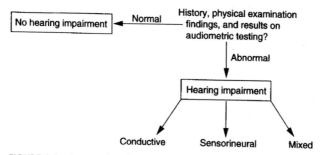

FIGURE 6-1. Approach to the patient with hearing loss.

    b. Vertigo, tinnitus, and **ear pressure** may accompany hearing loss.
  2. Questions to ask include the following:
    a. Was the onset of hearing loss sudden, progressive, or fluctuant?
    b. How long has the patient been aware of a change?
    c. Is the hearing loss unilateral or bilateral?
    d. What is the patient's family history?
    e. What is the patient's exposure to noise?
    f. What is the patient's medication history?
    g. Were there any precipitating events, such as an upper respiratory tract infection or trauma?

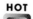

HOT KEY

Sudden hearing loss is a medical emergency.

B. Physical examination should focus on the ear, nose, and throat, with special attention to the ears and adjacent structures.
  1. Neurologic examination. Any abnormal findings on cranial nerve examination are suggestive of serious central nervous system (CNS) pathology.
  2. Otoscopic examination. In order to allow complete visualization of the external auditory canal and the tympanic membrane, the canal must be clear of cerumen.
    a. The **external auditory canal** should be examined for cerumen, exostosis, signs of infection (e.g., erythema), and dry skin.
    b. The **tympanic membrane** should be inspected for evidence of scars, perforation, color changes, or tympanosclerosis.

> **HOT**
> ▶
> **KEY**
>
> In an adult without a recent history of upper respiratory tract infection, the presence of fluid in the middle ear (evidenced by opacification or bulging of the tympanic membrane) necessitates referral to an otolaryngologist for a complete head and neck examination to rule out carcinoma.

3. **Tuning fork examination.** Although underutilized, tuning fork tests are a quick and useful way of differentiating between normal and abnormal hearing, and between conductive and sensorineural hearing loss.

   a. **Weber test.** The examiner strikes the tines of a 512-Hz tuning fork and then places the fork in the center of the patient's forehead or on the bridge of her nose. He then asks the patient if she hears the noise in the right ear, left ear, or both ears.

      (1) **Symmetric results** (i.e., the patient hears the noise in both ears) suggest that the patient has either normal hearing or bilaterally symmetric hearing loss.

      (2) **Lateralized results** (i.e., the patient hears the noise better on one side)

         (a) **Conductive loss.** The tone is louder in the poorer ear.

         (b) **Sensorineural loss.** The tone is louder in the better ear.

   b. **Rinne test.** This test can be used to detect conductive hearing loss and estimate its severity. A 512-Hz tuning fork is placed firmly against the mastoid bone. The examiner strikes the tines of the fork and asks the patient to compare the loudness of the bone conduction to the loudness of the sound when the tuning fork is held 2 centimeters away from the meatus of the external auditory canal.

      (1) **Bone conduction less than air conduction** - suggests normal hearing or sensorineural hearing loss in the tested ear.

      (2) **Bone conduction greater than air conduction**, suggests a conductive hearing loss of at least 20 dB in the tested ear.

> **HOT**
> ▶
> **KEY**
>
> Asymmetric hearing loss on tuning fork examination requires a referral to an otolaryngologist for additional evaluation.

TABLE 6-1. Differential Diagnosis of Hearing Loss

	Type of Hearing Loss	
Onset	Conductive	Sensorineural
Acute (<24 hours)	Foreign Body Trauma Burn Laceration Fracture Barotrauma Tympanic membrane perforation	Acoustic neuroma Vascular occlusion Meniere's disease Labyrinthitis (viral, bacterial)
Progressive (>24 hours)	Otitis externa Acute otitis media Tumor Otosclerosis Cerumen impaction	Presbycusis (age-related) Noise-induced hearing loss Acoustic neuroma Ototoxicity Inner ear autoimmune disease

   c. Table 6-1 narrows the possible diagnoses according to the type and onset of the hearing loss.

C. Audiometric testing is usually necessary for definitive diagnosis.

IV **TREATMENT.** The treatment of otitis media, otitis externa, and cerumen impaction are discussed in Chapters 7, 8, and 9, respectively.

V **FOLLOW-UP AND REFERRAL.** All patients with significant hearing loss should be referred to an otolaryngologist.

References

Cook JA, Hawkins DB. Hearing loss and hearing aid treatment options. Mayo Clinic Proceedings. 2006;81:234–237.

Palmer CV, Ortman A. Hearing loss and hearing aids. *Neurology Clinics* 2005;23: 901–918.

7. Otitis Media

I INTRODUCTION

A. There are **four general types** of otitis media, which represent different points along a continuum. Within each type, there are a number of phases. The four types are:
1. **Acute suppurative otitis media**
2. **Chronic suppurative otitis media**
3. **Acute serous otitis media**
4. **Chronic serous otitis media**

B. Otitis media is the most common diagnosis made by clinicians who care for children. The **peak prevalence** of otitis media is in **patients between the ages of 6 months and 3 years.**

II SUPPURATIVE OTITIS MEDIA

A. Acute suppurative otitis media
1. **Causes** include *Streptococcus pneumoniae, Haemophilus influenzae, Moraxella catarrhalis,* and **group A streptococci.**
2. **Clinical manifestations** – a diagnosis is established by the presence of three factors (all three must be present): 1) acute onset of ear pain, 2) evidence of inner ear effusion (noted by bulging or limited mobility of the tympanic membrane (TM), a visible air fluid level behind the TM, or evidence of otorrhea), and 3) evidence of inflammation by either visible erythema or acute pain.
3. **Differential diagnoses** include **otitis externa** and **acute mastoiditis** (i.e., inflammation of the mastoid air cells).

HOT KEY Consider acute mastoiditis when a patient with otitis media experiences worsening of symptoms along with mastoid tenderness, postauricular swelling and erythema, and prolapse or swelling of the posterior wall of the external canal.

4. **Treatment**
   a. **Antibiotic therapy** – recent studies suggest that many children with acute otitis media have resolution of symptoms without antibiotic therapy. Therefore, current guidelines recommend observation for 72 hours without antibiotics for children older than 6 months except for

those with severe illness, with treatment only if symptoms do not resolve. Children less than 6 months and those with severe illness should be treated upon presentation.

    (1) Amoxicillin (80 mg/kg/day, divided in 3 doses) is considered first-line therapy.

    (2) Second-line therapy – is reserved for children at higher risk for infection with resistant organisms, including antibiotic treatment within the past 30 days or concurrent conjunctivitis (which is often caused by penicillin-resistant strains of *Haemophilus influenzae*).

  b. Myringotomy (performed by an otolaryngologist) may be necessary for patients with persistent pain and high fever, facial nerve palsy, acute meningitis, labyrinthitis, or mastoiditis.

  5. Follow-up and referral. Consider referring adults with unilateral otitis media to an otolaryngologist for evaluation of the nasopharynx (to rule out an obstructing tumor).

B. Chronic suppurative otitis media

  1. Causes

    a. Cholesteatoma (i.e., a cyst-like mass or benign tumor with a lining of squamous epithelium trapped behind the tympanic membrane in the middle ear) can lead to infection and erosion of the ossicles and chronic suppurative otitis media.

    b. Conditions that cause irreversible changes to the middle ear mucosa and lead to adhesions and congestion around the eustachian tube (e.g., allergic rhinitis, sinusitis, immunodeficiency, adenoid infection in children) can lead to chronic ear drainage and chronic suppurative otitis media. Infection is usually caused by *Staphylococcus aureus, anaerobic bacteria,* or *Pseudomonas.*

  2. Clinical manifestations

    a. Chronic suppurative otitis media is characterized by the **chronic discharge of a mucoid, purulent, odorless exudate** (i.e., **chronic tympanic membrane perforation).** Periods of no drainage alternating with exacerbations are common.

    b. Conductive hearing loss is usually present.

    c. Pain is absent and the **patient's general condition is good.**

  3. Differential diagnoses also include **tuberculosis** and **carcinoma.**

  4. Treatment depends on whether the chronic suppurative otitis media is associated with a cholesteatoma (Figure 7-1).

    a. With cholesteatoma. These patients require referral to an otolaryngologist for **surgical treatment.**

    b. Without cholesteatoma. The goal of treatment is to resolve the infection. If the infection can be reversed with

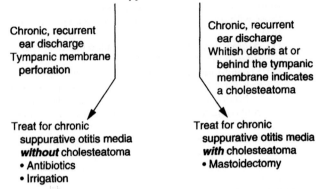

Chronic suppurative otitis media

Chronic, recurrent
  ear discharge
Tympanic membrane
  perforation

Chronic, recurrent
  ear discharge
Whitish debris at or
  behind the tympanic
  membrane indicates
  a cholesteatoma

Treat for chronic
  suppurative otitis media
  without cholesteatoma
  • Antibiotics
  • Irrigation

Treat for chronic
  suppurative otitis media
  with cholesteatoma
  • Mastoidectomy

FIGURE 7-1. Algorithm for determining treatment of chronic suppurative otitis media.

antibiotics and **irrigation,** then mastoidectomy can be avoided.

III SEROUS OTITIS MEDIA

A. Acute serous otitis media

1. **Causes.** Acute serous otitis media often precedes or follows an episode of acute suppurative otitis media. It may also be associated with conditions that cause eustachian tube dysfunction (e.g., upper respiratory tract infection, allergic rhinitis, sinusitis, nasopharyngeal masses).

2. **Clinical features** include a **feeling of pressure or fullness** in the ears, often accompanied by **hearing loss** and **crackling** or **popping** while swallowing. On otoscopic examination, the **tympanic membrane** may be **hyperemic** and an **amber color** can be appreciated behind it, with or without air bubbles.

3. **Differential diagnoses** include **acute suppurative otitis media** and **leakage of cerebrospinal fluid (CSF)** into the middle ear or mastoid air cells.

4. **Treatment** generally involves watchful waiting, as 80 percent of children will clear effusions in 2 months without treatment. Antihistamines, decongestants, and corticosteroids are not recommended and have not been shown to improve outcomes. There is limited data to support the use of antibiotics, though some experts recommend one 10–14 day course of antibiotics in children with significant hearing, language, or speech abnormalities or other forms of developmental delay.

   5. Follow-up and referral. Children with acute serous otitis media that has not resolved in 2 months should be referred to an otolaryngologist. Children with significant hearing, language, or speech abnormalities or other forms of developmental delay may warrant earlier surgical intervention. An adult patient with acute serous otitis media, particularly when it is unilateral and outside of the setting of an upper respiratory tract infection, may require referral to an otolaryngologist to rule out obstruction of the eustachian tube by a nasopharyngeal mass.

B. Chronic serous otitis media. By definition, the effusion is present for at least 3 months.

   1. Causes. Chronic serous otitis media results from eustachian tube dysfunction. Allergies or abnormalities of the adenoids, sinuses, or nasopharynx may be responsible.

   2. Clinical manifestations include a feeling of **fullness in the ear** and **hearing loss without pain.** Findings on physical examination are similar to those for acute serous otitis media.

   3. Differential diagnoses include **hemotympanum** and **CSF leak.**

   4. Treatment entails addressing the underlying cause of eustachian tube dysfunction, generally with a trial of decongestants and/or nasal steroids. Antibiotics have not been shown to be effective.

   5. Follow-up and referral. When effusions do not respond to therapy, referral to an otolaryngologist is indicated.

References

American Academy of Pediatrics Subcommittee on Management of Acute Otitis Media. Diagnosis and management of acute otitis media. *Pediatrics* 2004;113:1451–1465.

Pichichero ME, Casey JR. Acute otitis media: making sense of recent guidelines on antimicrobial treatment. *J Fam Prac* 2005;54:313–322.

8. Otitis Externa

I INTRODUCTION

A. Definition. Otitis externa **("swimmer's ear")** is an infection of the external auditory canal.

B. Pathogenesis. Particularly common during the summer months, otitis externa is caused by a breakdown in the protective barrier normally formed by the skin and cerumen.

1. Factors such as elevated heat and humidity, water maceration, allergy, and trauma (e.g., mechanical damage) cause atrophy of the sebaceous and ceruminous glands located in the outer third of the external auditory canal.

2. With the loss of the protective layer provided by these glands, the external auditory canal becomes dry and loses the chemical balance needed to prevent infection.

3. The most common pathogens are ***Pseudomonas aeruginosa*** and ***Staphylococcus aureus.***

II CLINICAL MANIFESTATIONS OF OTITIS EXTERNA

A. Four major symptoms
1. **Pain** (often severe)
2. **Pruritus**
3. **Hearing loss**
4. **Fullness** (e.g., a "plugged" sensation)

HOT KEY Pain when pressure is placed on the tragus (i.e., the semicircular piece of cartilage in front of the ear canal) is strongly suggestive of otitis externa. Inflammation and swelling of the pinna itself is indicative of a more severe infection (e.g., cellulitis, perichondritis, erysipelas) and an otolaryngology consultation is indicated.

B. Two stages
1. **Acute inflammatory stage.** During this stage, bacterial infection occurs and the patient experiences pain in the affected ear. As the infection becomes more severe, pain and swelling in the external auditory canal increase.

2. Chronic inflammatory stage. This stage is characterized by a marked thickening of the skin of the external auditory canal due to long-standing infection. Examination reveals flakes of dry, scaly skin in the canal. Often, the lumen of the canal is significantly narrowed.

III **APPROACH TO THE PATIENT.** The list of conditions similar to otitis externa is long. The following is a selected list of conditions that should always be ruled out:

A. Necrotizing external otitis (malignant otitis externa) is a **potentially lethal** infection usually found in elderly or immuno-compromised patients (e.g., those with diabetes, HIV infection, or chronic illness). The characteristic history is one of a long-standing case of otitis externa that continues to progress in severity despite seemingly adequate treatment.

1. Clinical manifestations. The patient often describes an ear discharge and severe "deep" or "boring" pain. The onset of new cranial nerve deficits may be detected on physical examination.

2. Treatment. Patients must be referred to an otolaryngologist.

B. Perichondritis and chondritis. Infections of the perichondrium or cartilage of the ear are serious, and require prompt attention.

1. Clinical manifestations. Patients often present with a diffusely swollen and exquisitely tender pinna.

2. Treatment. Intravenous antibiotics covering both aerobic and anaerobic organisms should be administered. Surgical debridement of necrotic cartilage may be necessary.

C. Furunculosis. These circumscribed swellings, which may be single or multiple, are noted in the cartilaginous portion of the external auditory canal.

1. Clinical manifestations. The swellings may be fluctuant, and tenderness is often noted when the tragus is pulled and when the ear speculum is inserted.

2. Treatment consists of draining fluctuant areas and applying topical antibiotics. Systemic antibiotics are only necessary if cellulitis or systemic symptoms are noted.

D. Dermatitis or **contact allergy of the ear** can be acute, chronic, or both.

1. Clinical manifestations
  a. In the **acute stage,** inflammatory findings are noted with associated pruritus, desquamation, and weeping.
  b. In the **chronic stage,** the skin of the external auditory canal is atrophic, dry, and scaly.

2. Treatment is with steroid creams or solutions.

      a. For patients with severe cases, betamethasone valerate or fluocinonide can be applied for a short time. If used too long, these agents can cause atrophy of the epithelium.

      b. For patients with chronic cases, a 1% hydrocortisone cream or solution can be used.

E. Herpes zoster oticus (Ramsay Hunt syndrome) is caused by infection of the cranial nerve ganglia by the virus that causes chicken pox.

    1. Clinical manifestations. Painful herpetic lesions are noted on the auricle and in the external auditory canal. In severe cases, facial nerve paralysis (Bell's palsy), hearing loss, and balance disorders may occur.

    2. Treatment. Bell's palsy can progress to a severe, complete facial nerve paralysis; therefore, cortico-steroid therapy and referral to an otolaryngologist is warranted for these patients.

F. Otomycosis (external mycotica) is a fungal infection of the external auditory canal.

    1. Clinical manifestations. Symptoms are similar to those of otitis externa, except that pruritus is more common than pain. A whitish exudate and black spots suggest *Aspergillus niger* infection.

    2. Treatment consists of acidifying the ear canal.

IV TREATMENT

HOT KEY Regardless of the stage of otitis externa, frequent and thorough cleaning of the external auditory canal is essential for effective treatment. If associated pain or swelling prevents thorough visualization and cleaning of the external auditory canal, the patient should be referred to an otolaryngologist.

HOT KEY In order for treatment to be successful, the external auditory canal must be kept dry. Insertion of silicon earplugs or petroleum jelly-coated cotton balls into the external auditory canal prior to bathing will keep the canal dry.

A. Acute inflammatory stage. Proper treatment depends on the extent of the infection.

    1. Mild infection

      a. If an exudate is present, the external auditory canal must be thoroughly cleaned (by **suctioning,** to avoid introducing water into the canal).

    b. An **antibiotic eardrop combined with a steroid** (e.g., poly-mixin, neomycin, and hydrocortisone as in Cortisporin) is recommended to cover both *Pseudomonas and S. aureus* infection. Typical treatment is one dropperful three times daily for 3–5 days, **until the symptoms resolve.** Oral antibiotics are not required.

  2. Moderate to severe infection. Because patients with moderate to severe infection require thorough de-bridement of the external auditory canal and edema may interfere with the installation of drops, referral to an otolaryngologist is recommended.

B. Chronic inflammatory stage. Treatment consists of the following measures:

  1. Repeated cleaning of the external auditory canal

  2. Administration of combination antibiotic and steroid eardrops

  3. Culture of the external auditory canal to ensure that the causative organisms are being effectively treated

---

HOT

▶

KEY

Injection of betamethasone valerate cream into the external auditory canal may be necessary to suppress pruritus.

V FOLLOW-UP AND REFERRAL

A. Acute inflammatory stage

Patients with drainage should be referred to an otolaryngologist. More severe infections should be seen every 1–3 days until the condition improves substantially.

B. Chronic inflammatory stage. If the condition improves with treatment, referral is not required. The patient should be followed every 1–2 weeks until the condition resolves.

References

Block SL. Otitis externa: providing relief while avoiding complications. *J Fam Prac* 2005;54:669–676.

Rosenfeld RM, Singer M, Wasserman JM, Stinett SS. Systematic review of topical antimicrobial therapy for acute otitis externa. *Otolaryn Head Neck Surg* 2006;134 (4 Suppl):S24–S48.

9. Cerumen (Earwax) Impaction

I INTRODUCTION

A. Cerumen is a waxy yellowish-brown substance consisting of secretions from the sebaceous and ceruminous glands, desquamated epithelium, hair, and dirt particles. Cerumen has an acidic pH and is bacteriostatic and fungistatic.

B. Collections of cerumen and debris are unusual if the self-cleaning mechanism of the external auditory canal is not disturbed. The habit of cleaning the external auditory canal is counterproductive and eventually leads to the development of chronic otitis externa. Additionally, cotton swabs tend to drive wax deeper into the canal, leading to impaction.

II CLINICAL MANIFESTATIONS OF CERUMEN IMPACTION

A. **Conductive hearing loss** in the affected ear is the most common symptom. Deafness gradually develops as the external auditory canal becomes progressively occluded by cerumen.

B. **Other symptoms** may include a **sense of "fullness," tinnitus, dizziness,** and **ear discomfort.**

III APPROACH TO THE PATIENT

A. **Rule out** a **foreign body, suppurative otitis externa** or **otitis media** (evidenced by a purulent exudate), and a **skin plug.**

B. **Determine whether the tympanic membrane is perforated.** Is there a history of blood, odor, or discharge? How does the tympanic membrane appear on otoscopic examination?

IV TREATMENT (Figure 9-1)

A. **Perforated tympanic membrane.** Do not attempt to perform cerumenectomy if perforation of the tympanic membrane is suspected. Instead, refer the patient to an otolaryngologist.

B. **Intact tympanic membrane**
  1. **Cerumenectomy**
     a. To soften hard or impacted wax, have the patient instill Cortisporin eardrops or mineral oil two to three times daily for 1 week prior to returning for treatment.

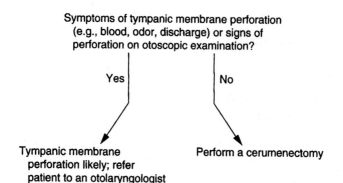

FIGURE 9-1. Treatment of a patient with cerumen impaction depends on whether typanic membrane perforation is likely.

    b. When the wax is softened, the canal is irrigated with warm water [i.e., water at body temperature (37°C)], using a large-bore irrigator tip to minimize the water pressure. The tip of the syring should not be inserted past the lateral third of the ear canal, and the stream should be directed upwards, towards the roof of the canal.

    c. After irrigating, the moist external auditory canal should be gently dried with a cotton applicator to avoid otitis externa.

2. Over-the-counter eardrops. Patients may attempt to manage wax themselves with eardrops that emulsify and disperse earwax (e.g., triethanolamine). The drops are instilled in the external auditory canal for 15–30 minutes at a time, causing the wax to dissolve. The dose may be repeated if necessary.

V **FOLLOW-UP AND REFERRAL.** The patient should be re-evaluated in 6–12 months.

References

Dimmitt P. Cerumen removal products. *J Pediatr Health Care* 2005;19:332–336.

Guest JF, Greener MJ, Robinson AC, Smith AF. Impacted cerumen: composition, production, epidemiology and management. *QJM* 2004;97:477–488.

10. Sinusitis

I INTRODUCTION

A. **Acute sinusitis** is inflammation of the mucosal lining of the sinus cavities from any cause.

   1. **Bacterial sinusitis** is most often caused by *Streptococcus pneumoniae, Haemophilus influenzae, Moraxella catarrhalis,* and group A streptococci.

   2. **Viral sinusitis** is a self-limited condition that occurs in approximately 80% of patients with the common cold and only rarely progresses to bacterial sinusitis (roughly 1 in 200 patients).

   3. **Fungal sinusitis.** Fungal infection of the sinuses may occur in immunocompromised patients, including those with diabetes, leukemia, and HIV infection. Commonly implicated organisms include *Mucor* and *Aspergillus* species. These infections are often invasive and difficult to cure and require emergent surgical–debridement.

B. **Chronic sinusitis** is defined as sinusitis that persists for longer than 3 months.

   1. The infection may be caused by the same organisms responsible for acute bacterial sinusitis, but anaerobic bacteria (e.g., *Bacteroides* species, peptostreptococci) also commonly cause chronic sinusitis.

   2. Chronic sinusitis may result from mechanical obstruction by a polyp, tumor, or deviated nasal septum.

II CLINICAL MANIFESTATIONS OF SINUSITIS

A. **Acute sinusitis**

   1. A **frontal headache** and **sinus pain that worsens when the patient leans forward** is the classic presentation. The location of the pain depends on the sinuses involved (Table 10-1).

   2. In addition, patients often report a **purulent nasal discharge, fever,** and **malaise.**

B. **Chronic sinusitis**

   1. Patients report a long history of **nasal congestion,** often associated with **postnasal drip, cough,** or the **sensation of being unable to clear the throat.**

   2. **Fever** and **sinus pain** are less common components.

TABLE 10-1. Pain Location in Sinusitis	
Affected Sinus	**Pain Location**
Maxillary	Cheeks, hard palate, teeth
Frontal	Low on the forehead
Ethmoid	Retro-orbital, upper or lateral nose
Sphenoid	Retro-orbital

III **COMPLICATIONS OF SINUSITIS.** Because of the proximity of the sinuses to the eyes and intracranial structures, complications can be extremely dangerous.

A. **Osteomyelitis** of the facial bones can occur and results in **Pott's puffy tumor** (i.e., a circumscribed area of edema surrounding areas of osteomyelitis of the skull). The involved bone has a "doughy" consistency.

B. **Periorbital infections** can result from the local spread of infection. The eyelids are often swollen and red. Pain with eye motion, ptosis, or proptosis suggests **periorbital cellulitis.**

C. **Cavernous sinus thrombophlebitis** occurs if the infection spreads via venous drainage of the ethmoid or sphenoid sinuses. Patients are usually severely ill and may have impaired ocular movement or a dilated pupil due to palsies of cranial nerves III, IV, and VI.

D. **Brain abscess** or **meningitis** can result from the intracranial spread of infection.

IV **DIFFERENTIAL DIAGNOSIS**

A. **Acute sinusitis**
   1. The main differential diagnoses are **viral sinusitis** (i.e., the **common cold,** see Chapter 12) and **allergic rhinitis.**
   2. **Migraine** or **cluster headache, dental abscess,** and **temporal arteritis** are occasionally confused with acute sinusitis.

B. **Chronic sinusitis**
   1. Chronic sinusitis may be confused with **allergic rhinitis,** which can be differentiated from chronic sinusitis on the basis of a history of seasonal symptoms and the presence of itching of the eyes, nose, and throat.
   2. When patients do not respond to therapy and have no evidence of mechanical obstruction, **rare systemic disorders** should be considered [e.g., **cystic fibrosis, Kartagener's syndrome, Wegener's granulomatosis, temporomandibular joint (TMJ) syndrome**].

V APPROACH TO THE PATIENT

A. History and physical examination
1. Perform a complete examination of the head and neck.
   a. Examine the nasal cavity for discharge and the presence of polyps, tumors, or septal deviation.
   b. Examine the cranial nerves and the eyes thoroughly; abnormalities suggest the spread of infection to periorbital structures or to the cavernous sinus.
2. The presence of at least five of the following six features—three detected as part of the history and three detected on physical examination—strongly suggests the presence of sinusitis. Always "TAP TAP" over the sinuses when examining a patient for sinusitis.

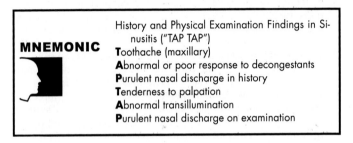

| **MNEMONIC** | History and Physical Examination Findings in Sinusitis ("TAP TAP")
Toothache (maxillary)
Abnormal or poor response to decongestants
Purulent nasal discharge in history
Tenderness to palpation
Abnormal transillumination
Purulent nasal discharge on examination |

B. Laboratory studies. Patients with a high fever, severe symptoms, or any sign of complicating infection should have a complete blood count (CBC) and serum chemistries.

C. Imaging studies
1. **Acute sinusitis.** Patients with clinical signs that suggest that the infection has spread beyond the sinus cavities should be evaluated using computed tomography (CT) or magnetic resonance imaging (MRI) of the sinuses. Routine imaging in patients with acute sinusitis and no signs of complications is generally not necessary.
2. **Chronic sinusitis.** Patients with chronic sinusitis who do not respond to therapy should have a CT scan to rule out mechanical obstruction and plan possible surgical intervention.

VI TREATMENT

A. Acute bacterial sinusitis
1. **Antibiotics.** The optimal duration of antibiotic therapy is controversial, but patients should be treated for 3–14 days with an antibiotic that covers the main bacterial pathogens (e.g.,

trimethoprim-sulfamethoxazole, 1 double-strength tablet twice daily).
   2. **Decongestants**
      a. **Topical decongestant sprays** (e.g., phenylephrine, 2 sprays per nostril every 3–4 hours or oxymetazoline, 2–3 sprays per nostril twice daily) can be used for a **maximum of 3 days.** Longer treatment may result in rebound nasal congestion.
      b. **Oral decongestants** (e.g., pseudoephedrine, 60 mg every 6 hours) can be used for up to 1 week.
B. **Chronic sinusitis**
   1. **Antibiotics.** The utility of antibiotics for the treatment of chronic sinusitis is not clear because the condition often results from a mechanical obstruction. If antibiotics are used, they should cover anaerobic organisms. For example, amoxicillin-clavulanate, 500 mg orally three times daily, could be used. Patients are often treated for 3 weeks or more.
   2. **Nasal steroids** (e.g., fluticasone (50 mcg/spray) 1 puff in each nostril twice a day) may reduce swelling and edema and improve sinus drainage.

VII FOLLOW-UP AND REFERRAL

A. Patients who respond appropriately to therapy do not require a follow-up visit.
B. Patients who do not respond to therapy and those with chronic sinusitis thought to be caused by a mechanical obstruction should be referred to an otolaryngologist.
C. Patients with clinical findings suggestive of complications or fungal sinusitis should be admitted to the hospital for the intravenous administration of antibiotics and urgent consultation with an otolaryngologist. Patients with periorbital cellulitis require urgent ophthalmologic consultation.

References
Klossek JM, Federspil P. Update on treatment guidelines for acute bacterial sinusitis. *Int J Clin Prac* 2005;59:230–238.
Sande MA, Gwaltney JM. Acute community-acquired bacterial sinusitis: continuing challenges and current management. *Clin Infect Dis* 2004;39:S151–S158.

11. The Common Cold

I INTRODUCTION

A. The common cold (i.e., **viral infection of the upper respiratory tract)** is one of the most common illnesses seen in outpatient medicine, and it is the **leading cause of absenteeism from work in the United States.**

B. Common causes include **rhinovirus, coronavirus, adenovirus, influenza virus,** and **parainfluenza virus.**

"The flu" generally refers to influenza virus infection, which often causes **severe systemic symptoms** (e.g., a high fever, myalgia, malaise) in addition to upper respiratory symptoms. However, clinical signs and symptoms are not very effective for distinguishing between influenza and other viral infections, and most cases of influenza are diagnosed during known outbreaks.

II CLINICAL MANIFESTATIONS OF THE COMMON COLD

A. Symptoms. Patients may present with any or all of the following symptoms:
1. **Nose:** congestion, rhinorrhea (i.e., clear nasal discharge), sneezing
2. **Throat:** scratchy or sore throat, hoarse voice
3. **Ears and sinuses:** congestion and pressure
4. **General:** headache, fever, myalgias, malaise

B. Signs include **erythema** and **edema of the mucosa** in the oropharynx and nasopharynx. A **transient middle ear effusion** is often present due to impaired drainage through the eustachian tube.

Patients with marked erythema or impaired mobility of the tympanic membrane should be treated for otitis media (see Chapter 7).

66

III **APPROACH TO THE PATIENT.** The goal in evaluating patients with symptoms of the common cold is to **rule out other disease processes with similar symptoms.** The main considerations are **bacterial sinusitis, bacterial pharyngitis,** and **allergic rhinitis** (Table 11-1).

HOT KEY

Allergic rhinitis can present similarly to the common cold, but it may be distinguished by a history of itching (of the eyes, nose, or throat) and seasonal or allergen-induced symptoms.

HOT KEY

Some viruses that infect the upper respiratory tract can also cause pneumonia (e.g., influenza virus). The lungs should be auscultated in all patients; abnormalities may warrant a chest radiograph.

TABLE 11-1. Features of Infections Often Confused with the Common Cold

	Bacterial Sinusitis	Bacterial Pharyngitis	Allergic Rhinitis
History	Maxillary toothache Poor response to decongestants Purulent nasal discharge	Recent exposure to group A streptococci Positive throat culture for group A streptococci in past year No rhinorrhea or cough	Itchy eyes, nose, throat Tearing Seasonal or allergic pattern
Physical examination	Purulent discharge Tender sinuses Abnormal transillumination	Temperature >101°F Anterior cervical lymphadenopathy Tonsilar exudates	Pale, edematous nasal mucosa (in contrast to erythematous mucosa associated with viral infections)

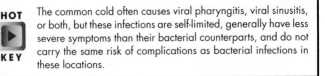

HOT KEY The common cold often causes viral pharyngitis, viral sinusitis, or both, but these infections are self-limited, generally have less severe symptoms than their bacterial counterparts, and do not carry the same risk of complications as bacterial infections in these locations.

IV **TREATMENT** for the common cold, as well as for the entities most often confused with the common cold, is described below.

A. Common cold. Antibiotics are not effective in patients with a common cold. Therapy centers on minimizing the patient's symptoms.

   1. Zinc lozenges or vitamin C. Taking zinc lozenges or vitamin C when cold symptoms are present may reduce the duration of illness.

      a. Zinc lozenges. Regular use of zinc lozenges (e.g. one lozenge containing 13.3 mg of zinc every 2 hours while awake) may reduce the duration of the common cold by several days.

      b. Vitamin C. The efficacy is controversial, but some experts suggest that Vitamin C (1 g per day) may reduce the duration of the illness by approximately 1 day.

   2. Fluids help prevent dehydration and may loosen secretions.

   3. Drugs that can alleviate the symptoms of the common cold are shown in Table 11-2.

      a. Expectorants have not been proven to have any benefit.

      b. Antihistamines are generally not used because they dry the nasal mucosa and prevent adequate drainage, although they may be useful as a sleeping aid.

HOT KEY α-Agonist nasal sprays, such as phenylephrine, should not be used for more than 3 days because extended treatment may cause rebound congestion (rhinitis medicamentosa) when the medication is stopped.

B. Allergic rhinitis. Patients with history and physical examination findings consistent with allergic rhinitis may be treated as follows (listed in the recommended order of therapy):

   1. Topical corticosteroids (e.g., beclomethasone, 1 spray in each nostril twice daily) are very effective at reducing nasal symptoms. Symptoms generally improve only after 1–2 weeks of treatment.

TABLE 11-2. Selected Symptomatic Treatments for the Common Cold			
Class of Drug	Examples	Dose	For Relief Of	Warnings
Oral decongestants	Pseudoephedrine	60 mg orally every 6 hours	Nasal congestion	Causes vasoconstriction and may elevate blood pressure; use with caution in patients with coronary artery disease
Decongestant nasal sprays	Phenylephrine	2 sprays per nostril every 3–4 hours	Nasal congestion	Long-term therapy (i.e., greater than 3 days) associated with rebound congestion
Analgesics	Acetaminophen	650 mg orally every 4–6 hours	Fever and pain	Be aware of specific contraindications for each agent (e.g., avoid aspirin in patients younger than 18 years)
	Ibuprofen	400 mg orally every 4–6 hours		
	Aspirin	650 mg orally every 4–6 hours		
Cough suppressants	Dextromethorphan	10 ml orally every 4 hours	Sleeplessness due to night-time cough	Can cause constipation
	Codeine	10 ml orally every 4 hours		

2. **Antihistamines.** Nonsedating, long-acting agents (e.g., loratadine, 10 mg orally once daily) may be useful when the patient's symptoms are not controlled with nasal steroids.

HOT KEY Astemizole and terfenadine should not be given with drugs that impair their metabolism (e.g., erythromycin, ketoconazole) because doing so may precipitate QT prolongation and torsade de pointes.

---

3. **Cromolyn sodium nasal spray** (1 puff in each nostril 3–4 times daily) may be useful, especially before contact with a known allergen.
4. **Ipratropium nasal spray** (0.03%, 2 puffs in each–nostril 2–3 times daily) is effective for reducing nasal congestion.
5. **Immunotherapy.** Antigen testing and immunotherapy may be used in patients who do not respond to other treatments.
C. **Bacterial sinusitis.** The treatment for bacterial sinusitis is discussed in Chapter 10 VI A.
D. **Bacterial pharyngitis.** The treatment for bacterial pharyngitis is discussed in Chapter 12 IV.

V FOLLOW-UP AND REFERRAL

A. Patients with a common cold do not need scheduled follow-up, although they should be advised to return if symptoms worsen or do not improve within approximately 1 week.
B. Patients with allergic rhinitis that does not respond to medical therapy may be referred to an allergist for antigen testing.

References
Eccles R. Understanding the symptoms of the common cold and influenza. *Lancet Infect Dis* 2005;5:718–725.
Pratter MR. Cough and the common cold: ACCP evidence-based clinical practice guidelines. *Chest* 2006;129(1suppl):72S–74S.

12. Pharyngitis

I INTRODUCTION

A. "Sore throat" resulting from pharyngitis is a common complaint in ambulatory medicine, accounting for **2%–3% of office visits.**

B. Viruses are the most common cause, but **group A streptococci** account for as many as 10% of cases of pharyngitis in adult patients. Because untreated group A streptococcal infection has a number of dangerous complications (e.g., acute rheumatic fever, peritonsillar abscess, acute glomerulonephritis), it is important to identify and treat this subset of patients.

II CAUSES OF PHARYNGITIS

A. **Rhinovirus, coronavirus, adenovirus, influenza virus,** and **parainfluenza virus infection.** The same viruses responsible for the upper respiratory viral infections that produce the common cold are the most common cause of pharyngitis. Rhinorrhea, cough, headache, and malaise commonly accompany the sore throat.

B. **Group A** *Streptococcus* **infection** is often characterized by a severe sore throat accompanied by fever and odynophagia. Cough, rhinorrhea, and hoarseness are not usually present.

C. **Groups C, G,** and **F** *Streptococcus, Mycoplasma,* and *Chlamydia* **infection** are uncommon, self-limited, bacterial causes of sore throat with similar presenting features (i.e., severe sore throat, fever, odynophagia).

D. *Neisseria gonorrhoeae* **pharyngitis** may develop after orogenital contact with an infected person.

E. *Corynebacterium diphtheriae* **infection** is characterized by a sore throat and a grey-white exudate (a "pseudomembrane") that coats the pharynx. Patients who have not been immunized are most at risk.

F. **Epstein-Barr virus infection.** Acute infection causes infectious mononucleosis and is most common in children and adolescents. Patients present with a sore throat, pharyngeal edema and exudate, and cervical lymphadenopathy. Prodromal symptoms of headache, fatigue, and fever are common. Splenomegaly occurs in approximately 50% of patients.

III APPROACH TO THE PATIENT. The goal of the evaluation is to identify patients with group A streptococcal

TABLE 12-1. Clinical Findings Suggestive of Group A Streptococcal Infection

History
    Recent exposure to known group A *Streptococcus* infection
    History of group A streptococcal infection in the past year
    Absence of cough, hoarseness, or rhinorrhea
Physical examination
    Temperature >101°F
    Tonsillar exudates
    Anterior cervical adenopathy

infection so that proper treatment can be initiated to prevent the development of complications.

A. History and physical examination
   1. The oropharynx should be examined for exudate, erythema, tonsillar swelling, and mucosal lesions.
      a. Group A streptococcal infection is more likely if the features shown in Table 12-1 are present; however, diagnosis of group A streptococcal infection cannot usually be made on the basis of clinical findings alone.
      b. Asymmetry of the soft palate, a fluctuant mass, or deviation of the uvula suggests peritonsillar abscess.
      c. A history of dyspnea, stridor, or odynophagia out of proportion to the physical examination findings suggests epiglottitis.

HOT

▶

KEY

Immediate consultation with an otolaryngologist is required when peritonsillar abscess or epiglottitis is suspected.

   2. Adolescents or children with prodromal features of mononucleosis should be examined for splenomegaly.
B. Laboratory studies. Patients with none of the features shown in Table 12-1 and symptoms consistent with the common cold have a very low probability of group A streptococcal infection and can be treated for the common cold without testing. Laboratory studies are indicated for patients with suspected group A streptococcal infection or mononucleosis.
   1. Group A streptococcal infection
      a. Group A *Streptococcus* antigen testing is indicated for patients with one or more of the features listed in Table 12-1.

Most "rapid strep tests" have a sensitivity and specificity
of approximately 80% and 95%, respectively.

   (1) Patients with a positive test should be treated with
   antibiotics and do not require a throat culture.

   (2) Patients with a negative test should be considered
   for throat culture, especially if the patient has several signs and symptoms suggestive of streptococcal
   infection.

   b. Throat culture is considered the gold standard test, although results are not available for 1–3 days.

2. Mononucleosis. Patients with historical and examination features suggestive of mononucleosis should have a **monospot
test.** False-negative results are possible within 3 weeks of infection, so patients with suggestive features and a negative
test should return for repeat testing.

IV TREATMENT

A. Antibiotic therapy

1. *Corynebacterium* **infection.** Therapy with **antitoxin** [which
can be obtained from the Centers for Disease Control
(CDC)] and **erythromycin** (500 mg orally 4 times daily) is
indicated.

2. *Neisseria* **infection** in adults can be treated with a single injection of **ceftriaxone** (125 mg intramuscularly).

3. Group A streptococcal infection. Although group A streptococcal pharyngitis is self-limited, antibiotic treatment reduces
the duration of symptoms and prevents the development of
some complications.

HOT KEY

Antibiotic treatment does not appear to prevent the development of acute glomerulonephritis in association with group A
streptococcal infection.

---

   a. Duration of therapy. Ten days of treatment are required
   for optimal prevention of complications.

   b. Selection of agents. Empiric treatment may be considered
   when 5 or 6 of the clinical features of group A streptococcal
   infection are present, although antigen testing is generally
   preferred to guide treatment and has been shown to reduce antibiotic overuse. The following antibiotic choices
   are all highly effective for patients with a positive test.

(1) Benzathine penicillin G (1.2 million units administered intramuscularly once) has a higher incidence of severe allergic reaction, but eliminates adherence problems.

(2) Penicillin V (250 mg orally 3 times daily for 10 days) can be used.

(3) Erythromycin (333 mg orally 3 times daily for 10 days) is indicated for patients who are allergic to penicillin or who live in an area with known high resistance patterns to penicillin. Alternatively, a **cephalosporin** (e.g., cefuroxime axetil, 250 mg orally twice daily for 10 days) may be used.

HOT KEY

It is not known whether antibiotic treatment is of any benefit when pharyngitis is caused by group C, G, or F streptococci, *Mycoplasma*, or *Chlamydia*.

B. Symptomatic therapy
   1. **Mild analgesics** (e.g., ibuprofen, 400 mg every 6 hours or acetaminophen, 650 mg every 6 hours) are useful for pain relief and reduction of fever.
   2. **Throat lozenges** or **sprays** may provide some relief.

V FOLLOW-UP AND REFERRAL

A. Patients who have complete relief of symptoms do not require scheduled follow-up.

B. Patients with more than 6 documented group A streptococcal infections per year can be considered for tonsillectomy.

References
Humair JP, Revaz SA, Bovier P, Stalder H. Management of acute pharyngitis in adults: reliability of rapid streptococcal tests and clinical findings. *Arch Intern Med* 2006;166:640–644.
Vincent MT, Celesin N, Hussain AN. Pharyngitis. *Am Fam Phys* 2004;69:1465–1470.

PART III
....

CARDIOLOGY

• •

13. Chest Pain
....

INTRODUCTION. Because chest pain (including "discomfort") is common and its causes range from a life-threatening myocardial infarction (MI) to benign musculoskeletal pain, a simple and reliable approach to the patient is necessary.

HOT ▶ **KEY** Patients who present with chest pain must be seen immediately. If there are any signs or symptoms suggestive of acute coronary ischemia, urgent transfer to an emergency department for monitoring and treatment is required while the initial evaluation is being completed.

II CAUSES OF CHEST PAIN. One way to remember the causes of chest pain is to take an "outside-in" approach.

A. Skin. Varicella-zoster virus infection (shingles) often causes pain before vesicular lesions are noted. The pain usually occurs in a dermatomal distribution.

B. Chestwall. Musculoskeletal pain may result from shoulder arthritis or bursitis, intercostal injury, metastatic disease to the bones or chest wall, or costochondritis. Breast pathology (e.g., tumors, fibrocystic disease) and nerve root compression (from cervical disk herniation) may also cause chest pain.

C. Lungs. Spontaneous pneumothorax, pulmonary embolus (PE), infection, malignancy, or a connective tissue disorder can cause pleural inflammation, which is usually associated with pleuritic chest pain (i.e., the pain worsens with inspiration or coughing).

D. Heart and great vessels. Pericarditis, myocardial ischemia and infarction, and aortic dissection can all cause chest pain.

E. Gastrointestinal tract. Esophageal disorders (including esophagitis, spasm, and rupture) are common causes of chest pain. Other gastrointestinal causes of chest pain include gastric and duodenal ulcers, pancreatitis, and biliary disease.

> **HOT** **KEY**
>
> 5 "Killer" Chest Pains
> Myocardial infarction or ischemia
> Pulmonary embolism
> Aortic dissection
> Spontaneous pneumothorax
> Esophageal rupture

III APPROACH TO THE PATIENT. First, quickly screen for the "killer" chest pains, then perform a more in-depth evaluation if the cause of the chest pain is still unclear.

A. Screen for the "killer" chest pains.

1. **"Eyeball" the patient.** A patient who is clutching his chest, diaphoretic, and ashen can be presumptively diagnosed from across the room as suffering from myocardial ischemia or infarction. Even if the presentation is not so classic, you can often decide on who looks "sick," and may need a rapid evaluation in a more monitored setting.

2. **Establish intravenous access and cardiac rhythm monitoring** immediately in patients who appear ill or who have cardiac risk factors.

3. **Evaluate the patient's vital signs.**

> **HOT** **KEY**
>
> Any abnormality of the vital signs should alert you to the possibility that the chest pain has a potentially serious cause.

    a. **Check the blood pressure in both arms.** Although a difference in pressure of 10 mm Hg or more may be seen in patients with aortic dissection, local atherosclerosis can also produce pressure differences. Therefore, the blood pressure reading is neither sensitive nor specific for aortic dissection.

    b. **Check the respiratory rate and oxygen saturation.** A low oxygen saturation may accompany spontaneous pneumothorax, PE, and MI (with pulmonary edema).

      (1) A **low oxygen saturation** (e.g., <92%) is often an indication that an arterial blood gas (ABG) should be ordered immediately.

      (2) A **normal oxygen saturation** may still be accompanied by a significant alveolar-to-arterial (A-a) oxygen gradient during hyperventilation. Therefore, ABG

testing to evaluate the possibility of PE may still be necessary if the rest of the evaluation is unrevealing.

4. **Interpret the electrocardiogram (EKG).** Obtaining and interpreting an EKG should not be delayed.

   a. **EKG abnormalities** that suggest **MI** or **ischemia** are always grounds for admission. Make sure the patient has intravenous access, a cardiac rhythm monitor, supplemental oxygen, and has been administered aspirin (usually 325 mg chewed) orally.

   b. **Normal EKG.** Because a normal EKG does not rule out a MI or ischemia, **nitroglycerin** (0.3–0.6 mg sublingually or via aerosol) may be administered and the dose repeated every 3–5 minutes as both a diagnostic challenge and as potential therapy.

5. **Take a preliminary history.**

   a. **Cardiac history and risk factors.** First, ask about any prior cardiovascular problems.

      (1) If there is a history of coronary artery disease (CAD), the patient has ischemia until proven otherwise.

HOT **KEY** In patients with a history of CAD or cardiac risk factors and no alternative explanation for the chest pain after careful evaluation, an admission to rule out myocardial infarction (ROMI) is usually appropriate.

---

      (2) If the patient's cardiac history is negative, you can quickly establish the pretest probability of MI by assessing cardiac risk factors:

         (a) Age > 45 years (in men) or 55 years (in women)
         (b) Male gender
         (c) History of smoking
         (d) Diabetes mellitus
         (e) Hypertension
         (f) High cholesterol
         (g) Obesity
         (h) Family history of an MI in a first-degree male relative younger than 55 years or female relative younger than 65 years

   b. **Other risk factors.** The preliminary history can also help elucidate any factors that may predispose the patient to the other "killer" chest pains. For example, a history of cancer or inactivity may suggest PE, and uncontrolled hypertension may increase the likelihood of aortic dissection or MI.

6. **Perform a preliminary physical examination.** Inspect the neck veins, listen to the heart and lungs, palpate the upper abdomen for tenderness, and evaluate the pulses in the arms and legs.

7. **Evaluate the chest radiographs.** Always compare the new films to old films, if they are available.

   a. **Spontaneous pneumothorax** can be subtle and you need to look carefully, especially in the apices.

   b. **Esophageal rupture** may lead to air in the mediastinum (pneumomediastinum).

   c. **MI** or **aortic dissection** may be accompanied by enlargement of the heart or mediastinum, respectively; however, these structures are often exaggerated on anteroposterior films. The presence of pulmonary edema may also be suggestive of MI.

B. **Further define the cause of the chest pain.**

   1. **Take a more detailed patient history.**

      a. **Type of chest pain.** PE frequently presents with pleuritic chest pain, MI may present with "crushing" chest pain or only a mild "discomfort," and aortic dissection often is characterized by a ripping pain that radiates to the back.

      b. **Radiation of chest pain.** Pain that radiates to the neck, left arm, or both arms should be considered cardiac in origin until proven otherwise.

         (1) Atypical patterns may also indicate ischemia and include pain, tingling, or numbness in the left fingertips unaccompanied by arm pain and pain in the outer left shoulder.

         (2) It is wise to consider any neck, upper abdominal, or upper back pain as cardiac in origin until proven otherwise.

      c. **Onset of chest pain.** Spontaneous pneumothorax, aortic dissection, and PE usually present with abrupt pain, whereas pain from MI or ischemia may build more gradually. Spontaneous pneumothorax and PE often occur while the patient is at rest, whereas aortic dissection and MI may occur with rest or exertion.

      d. **Duration of chest pain.** Pain that only lasts seconds or that has been constant for more than 24 hours, without positive biomarkers, is usually not caused by one of the four "killer" chest pains. An MI is almost always associated with more than 20 minutes of chest pain.

      e. **Associated symptoms.** Dyspnea, diaphoresis, lightheadedness, or syncope should alert you to a probable serious cause of chest pain.

   f. Aggravating and mitigating factors

     (1) Deep inspiration often aggravates pain from the pleura or pericardium (e.g., pleurisy from a PE or pericarditis).

     (2) Exertion may worsen the pain from MI or aortic dissection. **Rest** may ease the pain from cardiac ischemia, usually gradually.

     (3) Position. Patients with pericarditis often feel worse when supine, and better sitting up. Patients with musculoskeletal pain may feel worse in certain positions. The pain of an MI is usually unaffected by changes in position.

     (4) Food intake. Odynophagia localizes the problem to the gastrointestinal tract. Chest pain after a meal may indicate gastrointestinal pathology, but it also may occur with an MI.

     (5) Nitroglycerin. Improvement of chest pain after administration of sublingual nitroglycerin is not specific for cardiac ischemia since esophageal spasm may also respond to this therapy.

2. Perform a complete physical examination. Pay extra attention to the following parts of the exam:

   a. Jugular venous pressure. An elevated jugular venous pressure should alert you to the possibility of a serious disorder (e.g., MI, PE, or tension pneumothorax), but a normal jugular venous pressure does not exclude these disorders.

   b. Cardiac examination

     (1) Heart sounds. Listen carefully for a third heart sound (S_3) or fourth heart sound (S_4) gallop, which may indicate impaired ventricular contractility or ventricular relaxation, respectively. Both impaired ventricular contractility and impaired relaxation can accompany cardiac ischemia.

     (2) Murmurs may also increase the likelihood of a cardiac etiology of chest pain. A mitral regurgitant murmur may accompany an MI with papillary muscle ischemia, whereas an ejection murmur may indicate aortic stenosis or hypertrophic cardiomyopathy (both of these conditions may predispose the patient to ischemia).

     (3) Rubs. A pericardial friction rub may be heard in acute pericarditis, acute cardiac ischemia, or aortic dissection.

   c. Lung examination. Listen carefully for rales (e.g., from MI with pulmonary edema) and pleural friction rubs (e.g., from PE, infection, or other pleural processes).

    d. Chest wall examination. Minimal tenderness to palpation is nonspecific, but if the chest pain is exactly and reliably reproduced (especially in a well-localized area), a musculoskeletal cause is likely. Briefly inspect the skin for lesions.

    e. Abdominal examination. Palpate for any upper abdominal tenderness that may indicate a gastrointestinal cause of the chest pain.

    f. Pulses. Check pulses in the arms and legs bilaterally.

C. Diagnostic pearls

  1. Myocardial infarction

    a. Because CAD is such a common disease, it is always better to rule out MI if there is any doubt as to the diagnosis, even in young patients.

    b. More than 20 minutes of unexplained chest pain may represent an MI. Chest pain that lasts less than 20 minutes but increases in frequency or duration or occurs with minimal exertion often represents unstable angina. Both patterns are indications for admission.

    c. Frequently, patients with chest pain are given an antacid and lidocaine swish-and-swallow ("GI cocktail") to assess for reflux esophagitis. Many patients who "benefit" from this "diagnostic test" may actually have ischemic pain that is improving spontaneously or as a result of bed rest and oxygen therapy.

  2. Pulmonary embolus. Clinical suspicion is critical. There is often no evidence of deep venous thrombosis (DVT), and subtle symptoms and signs may be inappropriately rationalized away. If you have a high clinical index of suspicion, administer heparin to the patient before sending him for diagnostic tests.

  3. Aortic dissection

    a. The greater curvature of the aorta is the site for most dissections. With proximal spread, aortic dissection can involve the right coronary artery. If the patient has pain that radiates to the back, unequal blood pressures, or a widened mediastinum accompanied by evidence of right coronary ischemia (i.e., inferior or right ventricular ischemia), aortic dissection should be considered.

    b. Computed tomography (CT), transesophageal echocardiography, and magnetic resonance imaging (MRI) are used in the evaluation of aortic dissection. The choice of diagnostic modality depends on the patient (e.g., poor renal function may weigh against a CT scan) and institutional preferences. If clinical suspicion is high, a surgeon should be consulted immediately for input regarding subsequent evaluation. Transthoracic echo is not sensitive enough to rule out aortic dissection.

IV TREATMENT IS DIRECTED TOWARD THE UNDERLYING DISORDER.

A. **"Killer" chest pains.** Patients require **admission to the hospital** for intensive monitoring and treatment.

B. **Shingles.** Early treatment reduces the incidence of post-herpetic neuralgia and may reduce the duration of the painful rash.

1. **Acyclovir** (800 mg orally 5 times daily) is commonly used (the dosage should be adjusted for patients with renal insufficiency).

2. **Steroids** reduce pain and may help the patient resume normal activities, but they do not have an effect on post-herpetic neuralgia. A 3-week taper of prednisone (starting at 60 mg orally once daily) should be considered for immunocompetent patients.

C. **Musculoskeletal pain** usually responds to limitation of strenuous activity and a 5- to 10-day course of non-steroidal anti-inflammatory drugs (NSAIDs). An ice pack applied to the painful area for 20 minutes, 2–4 times daily, may also be helpful.

D. **Gastrointestinal disorders**

1. **Esophagitis.** Therapy is discussed in Chapter 34 IV C 1.

2. **Peptic ulcer disease.** Therapy is discussed in Chapter 35 IV A.

3. **Esophageal spasm** that is recurrent may respond to sublingual nitroglycerine (0.4 mg sublingually once for an episode of pain, not to exceed 3 tablets daily), oral nitrates (e.g., isosorbide dinitrate, 10–30 mg 3 times daily), or calcium channel blockers (e.g., long-acting nifedipine, 30–90 mg daily).

V FOLLOW-UP AND REFERRAL

A. **"Killer" chest pains.** These patients should be seen within a few days of being discharged from the hospital so that their progress can be monitored and long-term treatment plans can be discussed. Specialty consultation is usually indicated.

B. **Shingles.** Patients should be re-examined in 1 week to ensure that the rash is improving and not infected.

C. **Musculoskeletal disorders.** Patients should be seen in 1–2 weeks to ensure that the problem has been resolved. Patients with persistent symptoms may require further evaluation.

D. **Gastrointestinal disorders.** Follow-up depends on the specific disorder.

References

Chun AA, McGee SR. Bedside diagnosis of coronary artery disease: a systemic review. *Am J Med* 2004;117(5):334–343.

Swap CJ, Nagurney JT. Value and limitations of chest pain history in the evaluation of patients with suspected acute coronary syndromes. *JAMA* 2005;294(20):2623–2639.

14. Syncope

I. INTRODUCTION

A. Syncope is a transient loss of consciousness and postural tone that is caused by inadequate cerebral blood flow.

B. Syncope is extremely common, accounting for approximately 5% of medical admissions and 3% of emergency room visits. The lifetime incidence approaches 50% in some groups.

II. CAUSES OF SYNCOPE.
There are many causes of syncope, but the most important can be remembered using the mnemonic, "SYNCOPE."

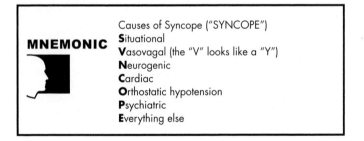

MNEMONIC

Causes of Syncope ("SYNCOPE")
Situational
Vasovagal (the "V" looks like a "Y")
Neurogenic
Cardiac
Orthostatic hypotension
Psychiatric
Everything else

A. Situational causes include micturition, defecation, swallowing, coughing, subclavian steal, and carotid sinus hypersensitivity.

B. Vasovagal syncope, also known as the "common faint," is the most common cause of syncope in young patients and is often preceded by a painful or emotional stimulus.

C. Neurogenic causes include autonomic insufficiency and transient ischemic attacks (TIAs).

    1. Autonomic insufficiency is common in elderly patients and patients with diabetes.

    2. TIAs are extremely rare causes of syncope. For syncope to occur, the vertebrobasilar circulation must be involved.

D. Cardiac causes

    1. Obstructive disorders. Aortic, mitral, or pulmonic stenosis, hypertrophic obstructive cardiomyopathy (HOCM), atrial myxoma, and pulmonary embolism may interfere with cardiac output and precipitate a syncopal attack.

    2. Arrhythmias. Disorders that cause bradycardia [e.g. sick si-
nus syndrome, second- and third-degree atrio-ventricular
(AV) block] or tachycardia (e.g. ventricular fibrillation, ventricular tachycardia, torsade de pointes, supraventricular
tachycardia) can also interfere with cardiac output.

    3. Ischemic disorders can precipitate an episode of syncope.

E. Orthostatic hypotension can cause syncope.

F. Psychogenic syncope is a diagnosis of exclusion.

G. Everything else

    1. Medications (e.g., vasodilators, hypnotics, sedatives, nitrates,
diuretics, α-blockers)

    2. Drugs (e.g. cocaine, alcohol)

III   **APPROACH TO THE PATIENT.** The evaluation of a patient
with syncope must be approached in a rigorous, stepwise fashion to avoid missing life-threatening disease.

A. History and physical examination. A thorough history and physical examination is a very important aspect of the evaluation and
may establish the diagnosis in many patients.

    1. Situational. Was the episode preceded by urination, defeca-
tion, swallowing, coughing, exertion of arm muscles (subclavian steal), or manipulation of the neck (carotid sinus hypersensitivity)?

    2. Vasovagal. Did a painful or emotional stimulus precede the
event?

    3. Neurogenic. Was there a transient loss of neurologic func-
tion, such as numbness, weakness, visual changes, dysarthria,
or poor coordination? Any abnormality in the neurologic
examination must be fully evaluated.

HOT KEY

Convulsions, bowel or bladder incontinence, or signs suggestive of a postictal state (e.g., confusion after the episode) are
suggestive of a seizure, not syncope.

---

    4. Cardiac

        a. A cardiac cause is more likely if the patient has any history
suggestive of cardiac disease:

            (1) Has the patient complained of feeling lightheaded dur-
ing exercise (suggestive of an obstructive cause)?

            (2) Has the patient complained of "palpitations" (sugges-
tive of an arrhythmic cause)?

       (3) Has the patient complained of symptoms suggestive of cardiac ischemia (e.g., substernal chest pain or pressure, chest pain radiating to the arms or neck, or left arm pain)?

       (4) Does the patient have a family history of cardiac disorders (e.g., long QT syndrome, Brugada sydrome, or hypertrophic cardiomyopathy)?

   b. Abnormalities found during the cardiac examination may suggest specific diagnoses and lead to more extensive testing (e.g., systolic murmur or delayed carotid pulse may suggest aortic stenosis).

5. Orthostatic. Does the patient report that he "got up too quickly"? Always check orthostatic vital signs in patients admitted with syncope.

6. Psychogenic. A psychogenic cause for the syncope (e.g., panic disorder) should be considered after all other causes have been excluded.

7. Everything else. What prescription, over-the-counter, or illicit drugs might the patient have used prior to the syncopal episode?

B. Imaging studies. All patients should have an electrocardiogram (EKG), although fewer than 10% of causes of syncope are identified in this manner. Look for evidence of acute or remote myocardial infarction, pre-excitation syndromes, arrhythmias, and conduction system disease.

C. Risk assessment. Patients should be classified as belonging to one of two groups: those without evidence of heart disease, and those who have known heart disease or some evidence of heart disease.

   1. No evidence of heart disease. Patients who meet **all of the following criteria** after a thorough history, physical examination, and EKG are at low risk for having a cardiac disorder as the cause of their syncope, and additional cardiac testing may not be indicated. However, some patients may require additional evaluation and treatment. The criteria are:

      a. Age younger than 50 years

      b. No history of coronary artery disease (CAD), congestive heart failure (CHF), or arrhythmias

      c. Normal EKG

   2. Evidence of heart disease or CAD. Anyone who does not meet the criteria described in III C (1) is included in this group, and the likelihood that an underlying cardiac defect is responsible for the syncope is greater. If there is suspicion of an ischemic or arrhythmic cause, admission and EKG monitoring are indicated. Additional diagnostic tests that may be appropriate include the following:

a. **Ambulatory EKG monitoring** is widely used, but it establishes a diagnosis in only a small percentage of patients. Event or loop recorders may improve the diagnostic yield.

b. **Exercise treadmill testing** can rule out exercise- or ischemia-induced syncope.

c. **Echocardiography** allows assessment of structural heart disease, as well as left ventricular size and function.

d. **Electrophysiologic testing** is especially useful in patients at high risk for a ventricular arrhythmia (i.e., those with poor left ventricular function) when a diagnosis cannot be established using noninvasive methods.

e. **Tilt table test.** This test can be useful for documenting vasovagal syncope, but a positive test does not mean that a more serious disorder (e.g., ventricular arrhythmia) is not present.

f. **Carotid sinus massage** is useful in the diagnosis of carotid sinus hypersensitivity. It requires cardiac monitoring and is contraindicated in the presence of cerebrovascular disease or carotid bruits.

g. **Signal-averaged EKG (SAEKG)** is a non-invasive method of detecting patients at risk for reentrant arrhythmias. Its utility is limited by low sensitivity.

HOT
▶
KEY

Syncope in a patient with a history of myocardial infarction or systolic dysfunction is ventricular tachycardia until proven otherwise.

IV TREATMENT

A. **Cardiac syncope.** The treatment of any correctable cardiac abnormality should be the first consideration. If indicated, placement of a permanent pacemaker or implantable cardioverter-defibrillator (ICD) should be considered in consultation with a cardiologist.

B. **Vasovagal syncope**
1. Avoidance of any precipitating stimulus (e.g., veni-puncture, prolonged standing) may be useful.
2. Patients with recurrences or a positive tilt-table test may be treated with a trial of β blockers (e.g., atenolol, 50–100 mg orally, once daily). Consultation with a cardiologist is recommended.

C. **Orthostatic hypotension**
1. Patients should be instructed to stay well-hydrated (by drinking eight 8-ounce glasses of water daily, in addition to normal

fluids), increase salt intake, and avoid abrupt changes from a supine to an upright position.

2. Compression stockings may be useful.

3. A trial of fludrocortisone (0.1–1 mg/day) may increase intravascular volume and relieve symptoms. Close monitoring of electrolytes and renal function is required when starting this agent.

D. Medication-induced syncope. Therapy with drugs that may cause syncope should be stopped or changed in affected patients, if possible.

V FOLLOW-UP AND REFERRAL

A. Patients with suspected or known heart disease should be followed in consultation with a cardiologist.

B. Patients with a suspected neurogenic cause for their syncope (e.g., TIA) require prompt referral to a neurologist.

C. A scheduled visit and re-examination is suggested for all other patients within 2 weeks of the syncopal episode.

HOT KEY All patients who have had a syncopal episode should be instructed not to drive and a report should be filed with the Department of Motor Vehicles (DMV). The patient's license can be reactivated if a full evaluation reveals that the patient is not at risk for a recurrence while driving.

Reference
Benditt DG, van Dijk JG, Sutton R, et al. Syncope. *Curr Probl Cardiol* 2004;29(4):152–229.

15. Hypertension

I INTRODUCTION

A. Hypertension is an extremely **common disorder,** affecting almost 50 million Americans (1 out of every 4 adults).

B. Patients who consistently have a **systolic blood pressure > 140 mm Hg** or a **diastolic blood pressure >90 mm Hg** are considered to be hypertensive.

C. Patients with systolic blood pressure between 120 to 139 or diastolic blood pressure between 80 to 89 are considered to be "**prehypertensive.**"

D. Hypertension is an important cause of **cerebrovascular, renal,** and **cardiac disease.**

II TYPES OF HYPERTENSION

A. Primary (essential) hypertension has no identifiable cause. Primary hypertension accounts for **95% of cases of hypertension.**

B. Secondary hypertension has an identifiable cause and must be considered in patients with **characteristic signs** or **symptoms,** the onset of hypertension at a **very young** or **old age,** or an elevated blood pressure that is **refractory to medical therapy.** The causes of secondary hypertension can be remembered using the following memory aid:

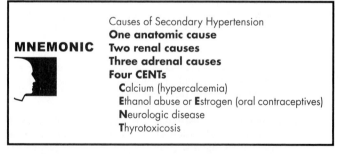

MNEMONIC

Causes of Secondary Hypertension
One anatomic cause
Two renal causes
Three adrenal causes
Four CENTs
   Calcium (hypercalcemia)
   Ethanol abuse or **E**strogen (oral contraceptives)
   Neurologic disease
   Thyrotoxicosis

1. One anatomic cause. Aortic coarctation, a congenital disorder characterized by aortic constriction at the origin of the left subclavian artery, usually presents in children or young adults and can lead to hypertension.

2. Two renal causes
   a. Intrinsic renal disease. Almost any parenchymal kidney disorder can lead to hypertension, usually as a result of

increased intravascular volume and increased activity of the renal-angiotensin-aldosterone system.

  b. Renal artery stenosis, a relatively common cause of secondary hypertension, is usually caused by fibromuscular dysplasia in young adults and atherosclerosis in older patients. The stenosis leads to decreased renal blood flow, which leads to increased renin release and hypertension.

HOT KEY Always consider renal artery stenosis as the cause of hypertension when a patient shows a dramatic increase in serum creatinine after starting angiotensin-converting enzyme (ACE) inhibitor therapy.

---

  3. Three adrenal causes

    a. Primary hyperaldosteronism, an uncommon cause of secondary hypertension, is caused by an aldosterone-secreting adenoma or bilateral adrenal hyperplasia.

HOT KEY Suspect primary hyperaldosteronism if a hypertensive patient is hypokalemic and not taking diuretics.

---

    b. Cushing's syndrome. Excess glucocorticosteroids (from any source) often lead to hypertension. Usually, other clinical manifestations of glucocorticoid excess are present.

    c. Pheochromocytoma is a norepinephrine- and -epinephrine-secreting tumor that may be malignant. Other manifestations include headache, glucose intolerance, and flushing.

  4. Four CENTs

    a. Calcium. Hypercalcemia is an uncommon cause of hypertension but should be considered in those who have underlying diseases that may lead to hypercalcemia (see Chapter 79).

    b. Ethanol abuse or **estrogen.** The most common causes of secondary hypertension are the use of **alcohol** and **oral contraceptive agents.** Hypertension from **pregnancy** requires careful evaluation.

    c. Neurologic disease. Any process that leads to **increased intracranial pressure (ICP)** can lead to the triad of hypertension, bradycardia, and irregular respiration (known as Cushing's triad).

    d. Thyrotoxicosis. Hyperthyroidism can also cause hypertension.

C. Hypertensive crises
1. **Hypertensive urgencies** are situations in which the patient has a systolic blood pressure > 220 mm Hg or a diastolic blood pressure > 120 mm Hg and no evidence of end-organ damage.
2. **Hypertensive emergencies** are those situations in which the elevated blood pressure leads to end-organ damage. A hypertensive emergency is hypertension accompanied by one of the following:
   a. **Hypertensive encephalopathy** (altered mental status)
   b. **Intracranial hemorrhage**
   c. **Aortic dissection**
   d. **Myocardial infarction**
   e. **Unstable angina**
   f. **Hypertensive nephropathy** (progressive acute renal failure with proteinuria and hematuria)

III APPROACH TO THE PATIENT

A. Goals of evaluation include the:
1. Assessment of the presence and extent of end-organ disease (i.e., renal, cardiovascular, or cerebrovascular disease)
2. Identification of factors that could lead to secondary hypertension (primary hypertension is a diagnosis of exclusion)
3. Identification of comorbid conditions, which can affect management of the hypertension
B. Patient history. The history should focus on the following areas:
1. The duration and severity of the hypertension
2. Symptoms or a history of comorbid conditions (e.g., cardiac disease, stroke, peripheral vascular disease, diabetes mellitus, kidney disease)
3. Medication history (over-the-counter and prescription drugs)
4. Use of alcohol, tobacco, or illicit drugs (e.g., cocaine)
5. Lifestyle and dietary habits (e.g., regularity of exercise, stress levels, salt intake)
C. Physical examination. The initial physical examination should focus on confirming the presence of elevated blood pressure in both arms. A complete examination also includes the following elements:
1. Assessment of heart rate and weight
2. Funduscopic examination
3. Thyroid examination
4. Evaluation of the heart and lungs
5. Evaluation of bruits over the renal arteries
6. Evaluation of the extremities
7. Neurologic assessment

D. Laboratory and imaging studies
  1. The following studies should be ordered for most patients with hypertension, at least initially:
     a. A complete blood count (CBC)
     b. Urinalysis
     c. Chemistry panel (i.e., sodium, potassium, creatinine, fasting glucose, and total cholesterol levels)
     d. Electrocardiogram (EKG)
  2. More specific studies (e.g., thyroid function tests, echocardiogram) may be necessary to rule out secondary causes of hypertension or complications caused by hypertension.

IV TREATMENT

A. Primary (essential) hypertension. The goal of treatment is to decrease the patient's risk of stroke, cardiovascular disease, and renal disease by lowering the systolic and diastolic blood pressures to at least 140 mm Hg and 90 mm Hg, respectively (Figure 15-1). A blood pressure less than 130/80 mm Hg is desirable in patients with diabetes or chronic kidney disease.
  1. **Lifestyle modifications.** All patients with prehypertension or hypertension should be advised to:
     a. Increase physical activity to at least 30 minutes daily
     b. Stop smoking (if applicable)
     c. Lose weight (if applicable)
     d. Limit alcohol intake to less than 1 or 2 drinks per day
     e. Reduce sodium intake to less than 2400 mg per day
     f. Increase fruit and vegetable consumption and reduce intake of saturated and total fat
  2. **Pharmacologic therapy** should be started if the blood pressure is greater than 140/90 mm Hg after 3 months of lifestyle modification, or if the initial blood pressure is greater than 160/100 mm Hg. Five major categories of drugs are available to control blood pressure (Table 15-1). These categories are as easy to remember as "ABCDE."

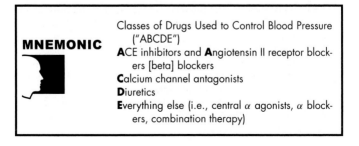

MNEMONIC

Classes of Drugs Used to Control Blood Pressure ("ABCDE")
ACE inhibitors and **A**ngiotensin II receptor blockers [beta] blockers
Calcium channel antagonists
Diuretics
Everything else (i.e., central α agonists, α blockers, combination therapy)

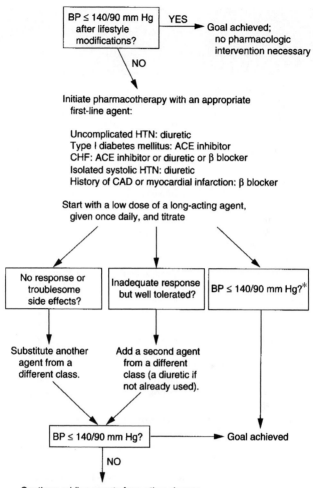

FIGURE 15-1. Algorithm for the management of hypertension. *ACE* = angiotensin-converting enzyme; *BP* = blood pressure; *CAD* = coronary artery disease; *CHF* = congestive heart failure; *HTN* = hypertension. (Modified with permission from Joint National Commission on Prevention, Detection, Evaluation, and Treatment of High Blood Pressure: The seventh report of the joint national commission on prevention, detection, evaluation, and treatment of high blood pressure. JAMA 2003;289(19):2560–2572.)

TABLE 15-1. Selected Agents Used for Management of Hypertension		
Generic Name	Trade Name	Usual Dose Range Total Dose (mg/day)/ # of Doses per Day
Angiotensin-converting enzyme (ACE) inhibitors		
Captopril	Capoten	25–150/2–3
Enalapril maleate	Vasotec	5–40/1–2
Lisinopril	Zestril	5–40/1
Angiotensin II receptor blockers		
Losartan potassium	Cozaar	25–100/1–2
Valsartan	Diovan	80–320/1
β blockers		
Metoprolol	Lopressor	50–200/2
Atenolol	Tenormin	50–100/1
Calcium channel antagonists		
Diltiazem	Cardizem SR	120–360/2
	Cardizem CD	120–360/1
Verapamil	Isoptin SR	90–480/2
	Calan SR	120–480/1
Amlodipine	Norvasc	2.5–10/1
Nifedipine	Procardia XL	30–120/1
	Adalat CC	30–120/1
Diuretics		
Hydrochlorothiazide	Hydrodiuril	12.5–50/1
	Esidrix	12.5–50/1
Other		
Clonidine	Catapres	0.2–1.2/2–3
Prazosin	Minipress	2–30/2–3

    a. In patients with **uncomplicated hypertension,** a thiazide-type **diuretic** is often used as a **first-line agent** because of its long-term efficacy, low cost, and utility in combination drug treatment programs.

    b. In patients with a **comorbid condition,** another type of drug may be considered for a first-line therapy (Table 15-2).

    c. If the initial blood pressure is greater than 160/100 mm Hg, treatment may be initiated with two drugs (one of these is usually a diuretic).

B. **Secondary hypertension.** Treatment is aimed at the underlying cause.

TABLE 15-2. Antihypertensive Agents That May Be Considered for First-Line Therapy in Patients with Comorbid Conditions

Comorbid Condition	First-Line Agents
Angina	β Blocker and/or calcium channel blocker
Benign prostatic hyperplasia	Prazosin
Bradycardia or heart block	Diuretic, ACE inhibitor, or angiotensin II receptor antagonist
Congestive heart failure (diastolic)	Diuretic and/or β blocker or calcium channel blocker
Congestive heart failure (systolic)	ACE inhibitor and/or diuretic or β blocker
Diabetes mellitus (type I)	ACE inhibitor
Edematous conditions	Diuretic
Gout (recurrent)	Any agent except a thiazide diuretic
Headaches (vascular)	β Blocker or calcium channel blocker
Impotence	ACE inhibitor, angiotensin II receptor antagonist, or calcium channel blocker
Myocardial infarction (history)	β Blocker
Pregnancy	Methyldopa
Reactive airway disease (severe)	Any agent except a β blocker
Renal insufficiency (chronic)	ACE inhibitor, diuretic, or angiotensin II receptor antagonist

ACE = angiotensin-converting enzyme

C. Hypertensive crises

  1. **Hypertensive urgency.** Patients are usually treated with **oral antihypertensive agents** (e.g., nifedipine, clonidine, captopril) in the emergency room. Once the blood pressure is decreased to an acceptable level, these patients can usually be discharged, although they require very close follow-up.

HOT KEY

Sublingual nifedipine should be avoided in almost all patients with hypertensive urgency because this drug may precipitate an abrupt decrease in blood pressure.

2. Hypertensive emergency. Patients usually require admission to the intensive care unit (ICU) and the administration of **parenteral antihypertensives** (e.g., nitroprusside, nitroglycerin, labetalol, esmolol, or hydralazine).

V FOLLOW-UP AND REFERRAL

A. A home blood pressure monitoring device can be used to monitor the blood pressure and evaluate the effectiveness of therapy.
   1. The patient should check his blood pressure daily until it is under control, and weekly thereafter.
   2. Once the blood pressure is adequately controlled, an office visit every 3–6 months is appropriate.
B. Referral to a hypertension specialist should be considered in the following situations:
   1. The blood pressure cannot be controlled adequately
   2. The patient is noncompliant
   3. The primary physician is having difficulty identifying a secondary cause of hypertension when one is strongly suspected.

Reference

Joint National Commission on Prevention, Detection, Evaluation, and Treatment of High Blood Pressure: The seventh report of the joint national commission on prevention, detection, evaluation, and treatment of high blood pressure. *JAMA* 2003;289(19):2560–2572.

16. Coronary Artery Disease

I INTRODUCTION. Coronary artery disease (CAD) is the **leading cause of death in the United States;** therefore, prevention and treatment of CAD is a major part of every primary care practice.

II CLINICAL MANIFESTATIONS OF CORONARY ARTERY DISEASE (CAD)

A. **Angina** is chest pain that results when oxygen supply to the myocardium is inadequate, usually reflecting reduced blood flow in the coronary arteries due to atherosclerotic plaques.

   1. **Stable angina** is a pattern of chest pain that has not changed. Patients generally report chest pain that occurs after certain amounts of exertion (e.g., walking up several flights of stairs, heavy housework) and resolves after resting or taking sublingual nitroglycerin (0.4 mg dissolved under the tongue).

   2. **Unstable angina** is an increase in the frequency or duration of angina, or chest pain that occurs with rest. Unstable angina is always an indication for urgent hospital admission and further work-up.

B. **"Anginal equivalents"** are symptoms other than chest pain (e.g., dyspnea, arm or jaw pain) that may occur with exertion and are likely caused by myocardial ischemia. This presentation is more common in diabetic patients. In patients with known CAD, anginal equivalents should be considered ischemic in origin until proven otherwise.

III RISK FACTORS FOR CORONARY ARTERY DISEASE (CAD)

	Risk Factors for CAD ("Must Start Helping CAD Fast")
MNEMONIC	**M**ale Gender
	Smoking
	Hypertension
	Cholesterol (hyperlipidemia)
	Age
	Diabetes mellitus
	Family history of CAD

A. Male gender is an unmodifiable risk factor for CAD. Following age 70, men and women have a nearly equal risk of developing CAD.

B. Smoking. People who smoke >1 pack per day are three times more likely to develop CAD than nonsmokers. The risk increases with the number of cigarettes smoked per day.

C. Hypertension increases the likelihood of developing CAD. Every 20/10 mm Hg elevation above goal blood pressure doubles the risk of CAD.

D. Hyperlipidemia. A 1% reduction in low-density lipoprotein (LDL) cholesterol levels reduces the risk of developing CAD by 2%.

E. Age 45 years or older in men and **55 years or older in women** is an unmodifiable risk factor for the development of CAD.

F. Diabetes mellitus is associated with a two-fold increase in the incidence of CAD in men, and a three-fold increase in risk in women.

G. Family history of CAD in a first-degree male relative younger than 55 years or a first-degree female relative younger than 65 years is another unmodifiable risk factor.

H. Biomarkers of Inflammation including C-reactive protein, lipoprotein (a), and homocysteine are increasingly being recognized as markers of cardiovascular risk.

Ⅳ APPROACH TO THE PATIENT

A. Prevention

1. Primary prevention.

a. All patients should receive counseling regarding lifestyle modifications (e.g., quitting smoking, increasing exercise, and eating a healthy diet) (see Chapter 4 III A–C).

b. Screening for hyperlipidemia should be done every 5 years in adults beginning at age 20.

2. Secondary prevention. Modifiable risk factors for CAD should be treated aggressively **to prevent the development of clinical cardiovascular disease**.

a. Smoking. Complete cessation is the goal. Provide **counseling, nicotine replacement therapy,** and referrals to **formal cessation programs** as necessary.

b. Hypertension. The goal is a blood pressure of less than 140/90 mm Hg. In patients with known CAD, diabetes, or chronic renal failure, the goal of therapy is a blood pressure of less than 130/80. **Lifestyle modifications** and **pharmacologic therapy** are discussed in Chapter 15 IV A 1–2.

TABLE 16-1. Treatment Goals in Patients with Hyperlipidemia

Number of CAD Risk Factors	Treatment Goal LDL Level (mg/dl)	Begin Diet Therapy* LDL Level (mg/dl)	Begin Drug Therapy LDL Level (mg/dl)
0–1	<160	≥160	≥160–190†
≥2	<130	≥130	≥130–160†
Documented CAD	≤70–100	>100	≥100†

CAD = coronary artery disease; LDL = low-density lipoprotein.
*American Heart Association (AHA) step II diet: ≤30% fa, ≤7% fat, <200 mg cholesterol per day.
†Lower range of LDL level advised in patients at higher risk for CAD.

    c. Hyperlipidemia may be primary or secondary. Secondary causes of hyperlipidemia are less common and include metabolic causes, drugs, and alcohol.

        (1) Management goals. The number of risk factors a patient has for CAD determines the cholesterol management goal. Smoking, hypertension, an HDL level < 40 mg/dl, age ≥ 45 years (or ≥ 55 years in women), diabetes mellitus, and a family history of CAD are each assigned 1 point. If the HDL is ≥ 60 mg/dl, subtract 1 point from the total.

        (2) Management strategies include **diet modification** and **pharmacologic therapy.** The choice of diet or pharmacologic therapy depends on both the number of risk factors and the patient's LDL level (Table 16-1). Patients with ≥ 2 risk factors are started on drug therapy at lower LDL levels than patients with < 2 risk factors. Pharmacologic therapy should be started if diet modification does not achieve the treatment goal within 3–6 months.

            (a) Diet modification. Patients should be placed on the American Heart Association (AHA) step II diet (i.e., **≤ 30% fat, ≤ 7% saturated fat, ≤ 200 mg/day cholesterol).**

            (b) Pharmacologic therapy is usually initiated with one agent (Table 16-2). Combination drug therapy may be needed if the LDL goal is not reached.

    d. Diabetes mellitus. It is not certain whether excellent **glycemic control** reduces diabetic patients' risk of developing CAD. However, **aggressive modification of**

TABLE 16-2. Selected Cholesterol-Lowering Medications

Drug	Starting Dose	Maximum Dose	Therapeutic Effects	Indications	Side Effects
HMG-CoA reductase inhibitors			$\downarrow$ LDL $\uparrow$ HDL $\downarrow$ TG	First-line drugs for most patients	Elevated liver transamines, myopathy, rhabdomyolysis*
Simvastatin	5–10 mg daily	80 mg daily			
Pravastatin	10–20 mg daily	80 mg daily			
Lovastatin	20 mg daily	80 mg daily			
Fluvastatin	20 mg daily	40 mg daily			
Atorvastatin	10 mg daily	80 mg daily			
Rosuvastatin	10 mg daily	40 mg daily			
Niacin	100 mg twice daily	1–2 g three times daily	$\downarrow$ LDL $\uparrow$ HDL	Best drug for increasing HDL levels	Flushing†, worsening of glycemic control (in patients with diabetes), hyperuricemia
Niaspan	500 mg daily	2000 mg daily			
Fibric acids‡			$\downarrow$ TG $\uparrow$ HDL	May be useful for patients with very high TG levels	Myalgias, elevated liver transaminases, nausea, abdominal discomfort
Gemfibrozil	300–600 mg twice daily	600 mg twice daily			
Clofibrate	500 mg four times daily	500 mg four times daily			

Bile acid-binding resins§			↓ LDL		Bloating, constipation, vitamin K deficiency
Cholestyramine	4 g daily	4 g four times daily			
Colestipol	2 g daily	4 g four times daily			
Cholesterol Absorption Inhibitor					
Ezetimibe	10 mg daily	10 mg daily	↓ LDL ↑ HDL ↓ TG	Usually as adjunct to – statins	

HDL = high-density lipoproteins; HMG-CoA = 3-hydroxy-3-methylglutaryl coenzyme A; LDL = low-density lipoproteins; TG = triglycerides.

*Monitor with liver function tests and creatine kinase levels every 4–6 months

†Flushing can be prevented by giving the patient aspirin (≥81 mg) 30 minutes prior to each dose.

‡Drugs in this class should not be used with HMG-CoA inhibitors due to an increased risk of myopathy.

§Drugs in this class impair the absorption of many other medications and should be used with caution

other cardiac risk factors (e.g., smoking, hypertension, hyperlipidemia) in diabetic patients is associated with greater CAD risk reduction than in non-diabetic patients.

HOT KEY Aspirin (325 mg once daily) is recommended for patients with moderate to high risk for CAD, and has been shown to decrease the risk of first myocardial infarction in men older than 50 years by more than 40%.

3. **Tertiary prevention.** The goal of tertiary prevention is to **prevent the development of further morbidity** and **mortality** in patients who have **already experienced a myocardial infarction**.

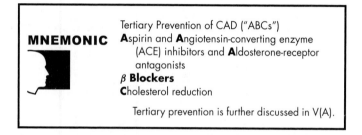

MNEMONIC

Tertiary Prevention of CAD ("ABCs")
Aspirin and **A**ngiotensin-converting enzyme (ACE) inhibitors and **A**ldosterone-receptor antagonists
β **Blockers**
Cholesterol reduction

Tertiary prevention is further discussed in V(A).

B. **Risk stratification** is the **process of using diagnostic tests to evaluate the extent of CAD in a patient**. This **allows determination of appropriate therapy** (i.e., revascularization versus specific medical therapy).
1. **Assess the extent of the CAD.** The patient is first categorized as "high-risk," "intermediate-risk," or "low-risk" based upon the pre-test probability of CAD, as formulated from history, physical examination, electrocardiogram (EKG), and laboratory biomarkers.
   a. **High-risk patients** are those who have a history of CAD, present with EKG changes suggestive of cardiac ischemia (e.g., ST-segment elevation or depression), positive cardiac biomarkers or enzymes (e.g., troponin, CK-MB, or CK), or present with congestive heart failure, recurrent episodes of ischemia, or high-risk arrhythmias (e.g., ventricular fibrillation, ventricular tachycardia). All of these patients must undergo **urgent or emergent cardiac catheterization** to determine if they are candidates for revascularization.

b. **Intermediate-risk patients** may have a history of CAD or several cardiac risk factors but may lack high-risk features described above. These patients should undergo **either noninvasive testing or cardiac catheterization** to evaluate the extent of CAD.

c. **Low-risk patients** typically have few cardiac risk factors, atypical chest pain, and no EKG changes suggestive of ischemia. These patients should undergo **noninvasive testing** to evaluate the possibility of CAD.

HOT KEY

For certain intermediate-risk patients, it may be appropriate to proceed straight to cardiac catheterization. Consultation with a cardiologist may be useful for these patients.

---

(1) **Noninvasive testing methods**

(a) **Exercise electrocardiography.** The patient exercises on a treadmill while his 12-lead EKG is continuously monitored. The test may be non-diagnostic if the patient is unable to achieve 85% of age-predicted maximum heart rate. The baseline EKG must be interpretable for ischemic changes (i.e., patients with left bundle branch block or ST segment devations are excluded). Horizontal or downsloping ST segment depression greater than 1 mm, or ST segment elevation greater than 1 mm indicates significant ischemia. Exercise testing is contraindicated in the setting of uncontrolled hypertension (>200/110 mm Hg), active cardiac ischemia, decompensated heart failure, or severe aortic stenosis.

(b) **Myocardial perfusion scintigraphy** is often performed in conjunction with exercise electrocardiography. A radioactive tracer [e.g., thallium-201 (^{201}Tl)] is injected into a peripheral vein while the patient exercises, and then again while the patient rests. **Well-perfused myocardial cells** take up the tracers and will **"light up"** when imaged.

(i) **Reversible defects** are areas of the heart that "light up" at rest, but show less tracer uptake with exercise (indicating ischemia with exertion).

(ii) **Fixed defects** are areas of the heart that do not take up tracer, even at rest (indicating infarcted tissue).

    (c) Pharmacologic stress tests can be used for patients who are unable to exercise on a treadmill. Agents such as **dipyridamole** dilate the coronary arteries. Those arteries with more atherosclerotic plaque are unable to dilate as much in response to these agents, leading to lower uptake of tracer in regions supplied by diseased coronaries.

    (d) Stress echocardiography. The patient exercises (or is given a drug that increases the heart rate and contractility, such as dobutamine) while undergoing echocardiography. Inducible regional wall motion abnormalities suggest significant CAD.

    (e) Computed tomography coronary angiography is a new non-invasive method of visualizing major coronary arteries. It has a high specificity and high negative predictive value for CAD, making it useful for "ruling out" CAD in low-risk patients and certain intermediate-risk patients. It has variable sensitivity and is not suitable for high-risk patients who are likely to require coronary intervention.

(2) Interpretation of noninvasive testing

    (a) Patients who have markedly positive results on noninvasive testing should be referred for cardiac catheterization and possible revascularization.

    (b) Patients with negative studies or only mild abnormalities may be managed with medical therapy alone.

    (c) Always keep the test characteristics (e.g., negative predictive value) in mind when deciding whether your risk stratification is adequate.

HOT

KEY

A negative study in a patient with a high pre-test probability for CAD does not necessarily rule out CAD.

---

2. Assess left ventricular function. Echocardiography or **multiple-gated acquisition scanning (MUGA)** is indicated for all patients after myocardial infarction to assess the left ventricular ejection fraction.

    a. Patients with an ejection fraction < 40% are candidates for ACE inhibitor therapy and aldosterone-receptor antagonists. Electrolytes and renal function should be monitored closely.

    b. Patients with a mural thrombus, ventricular aneurysm, or very low ejection fraction may be candidates for anticoagulation therapy to prevent the development of thrombus and embolic stroke.

c. Patients with ischemic cardiomyopathy and an ejection fraction of < 30% following myocardial infarction may be candidates for implantable cardioverter-defibrillator (ICD) placement.

V TREATMENT

A. Medical treatment can improve the quality of life for all patients with CAD and is generally aimed at increasing the myocardial oxygen supply (by dilating the coronary arteries) and decreasing the myocardial oxygen demand (by decreasing the heart rate, contractility, preload, or afterload).

1. **Aspirin** inhibits platelet aggregation and coronary thrombosis, thereby decreasing the patient's risk of a second myocardial infarction. Aspirin (325 mg once daily) is recommended for all patients with documented CAD.

2. **Clopidogrel** also inhibits platelet aggregation. It is required for a period of time following percutaneous coronary intervention and may be used as an adjunctive anti-platelet agent in patients with refractory ischemia.

3. **ACE inhibitors.** Following infarction, ACE inhibitors reduce mortality and recurrent myocardial infarction in patients with reduced left ventricular systolic function (i.e., an ejection fraction < 40%). They also attenuate post-infarction ventricular dilatation and remodeling.

4. **β Blockers** prevent recurrent myocardial infarction by reducing the heart rate and contractility. β Blockers reduce mortality following myocardial infarction and are a cornerstone of therapy for CAD.

   a. **Commonly used β blockers** include **metoprolol** (25–100 mg orally, twice daily) and **atenolol** (25–100 mg orally once daily). The initial dose should be at the low end of the range, with the goal of reducing the resting heart rate to approximately 60 beats/min. The dose may be increased until symptoms are controlled, side effects develop, or the maximum dose is reached.

   b. **Indications.** β Blockers are indicated for all patients who have had an infarction and can tolerate the medication.

   c. **Contraindications** include bradyarrhythmias and uncontrolled CHF. β blockers may be beneficial in patients with controlled CHF. These agents must be used with caution in patients with chronic obstructive pulmonary disease (COPD) or asthma.

    d. Side effects include postural hypotension, depression, and sexual dysfunction.

5. HMG-CoA reductase inhibitors and **niacin** have been shown to decrease the recurrence of myocardial infarction. In patients with known CAD, more aggressive lipid control is necessary; the goal is an LDL level of 70 mg/dl or less.

6. Aldosterone-receptor antagonists have been shown to reduce mortality following myocardial infarction in patients with New York Heart Association class III or IV heart failure and depressed left ventricular ejection fraction ≤40%.

7. Nitrates increase oxygen supply by vasodilating the coronary arteries and decrease oxygen demand by decreasing the preload and afterload. Nitrates provide symptomatic relief from angina but have no mortality benefit.

    a. Short-acting nitrates (e.g., **nitroglycerin,** 0.4 mg sublingually or by aerosol) can be used for immediate therapy of angina prophylaxis.

        (1) Immediate therapy. Patients should be instructed to take nitroglycerin every 3–5 minutes until the pain is relieved; if the pain is not relieved in 15 minutes, they should call for an ambulance.

        (2) Angina prophylaxis. The dose is taken 5 minutes before beginning an activity known to result in angina.

    b. Long-acting nitrates (e.g., **isosorbide dinitrate,** 10–40 mg orally three times daily) can provide prolonged relief.

        (1) A nitrate-free interval of approximately 8–10 hours daily is needed to prevent tachyphylaxis.

        (2) Headaches frequently occur with the initiation of nitrate therapy, but they can be managed conservatively and frequently resolve within 1–2 weeks.

8. Calcium channel blockers lower oxygen demand (by decreasing the heart rate, contractility, and afterload) and may increase oxygen supply (by inducing coronary artery vasodilation). These drugs have not been shown to decrease mortality from myocardial infarction so β blockers should always be considered before calcium channel blockers for patients with CAD.

    a. In order of decreasing effect on lowering systemic vascular resistance and increasing effect on myocardial inotropy and chronotropy, agents include:

        (1) Nifedipine (30–120 mg once daily)

        (2) Diltiazem (120–540 mg once daily)

        (3) Verapamil (120–480 mg once daily)

9. Enhanced external counterpulsation (EECP) is a noninvasive mechanical outpatient procedure that has been shown to improve symptoms of chronic angina by improving coronary blood flow.

   10. Unproven therapies
      a. Antioxidant vitamins. Beta carotene, vitamin E, and vita-
         min C have not definitively been found to reduce the risk
         of cardiovascular disease.
      b. Folate supplementation may reduce the risk of CAD in
         patients with high homocysteine levels. Its value in patients
         with normal homocysteine level is equivocal.
B. Revascularization. The indications for **percutaneous translumi-
nal coronary angioplasty (PTCA)** or **coronary artery bypass
graft (CABG) surgery** depend upon the location of lesions and
number of vessels involved.
   1. CABG is generally the treatment of choice for patients with
      left main CAD (>50% occlusion), three-vessel CAD (>70%
      occlusion), multi-vessel CAD in diabetic patients, or when
      large areas of myocardium are at risk.
   2. PTCA with drug-eluting stents is ideal for single-vessel or
      two-vessel CAD, or elderly patients with a high operative
      mortality from CABG.

VI FOLLOW-UP AND REFERRAL

A. Primary prevention. Patients can be seen annually or semi-
annually for counseling.
B. Secondary prevention. Patients should be seen regularly for risk
factor modification.
   1. Patients with 2 or more risk factors should be seen at least
      every 1–3 months until risk factors are adequately controlled.
   2. Consultation with an endocrinologist is appropriate for pa-
      tients with severe or refractory dyslipidemia.
C. Tertiary prevention and symptomatic control. Patients must be
treated aggressively because they are at high risk for recurrent
myocardial infarction and death.
   1. Weekly visits are appropriate until symptoms are controlled
      and all preventive measures have been employed, and then
      regular visits every 2–4 months are indicated.
   2. Consultation with a cardiologist is advised for patients with
      persistent symptoms despite medical therapy, or when non-
      invasive testing or revascularization is being considered.

References

National Cholesterol Education Program (NCEP) Expert Panel on Detection, Evaluation, and Treatment of High Blood Cholesterol in Adults (Adult Treatment Panel
   III). *Circulation* 2002;106:3143–3421.
Sleight P. Current options in the management of coronary artery disease. *Am J Cardiol*
   2003;92:4N–8N.
Snow V, Barry P, Fihn SD, et al. Primary care management of chronic stable angina
   and asymptomatic suspected or known coronary artery disease: a clinical practice guideline from the American College of Physicians. *Ann Intern Med* 2004;
   141(7):562–567.

17. Congestive Heart Failure

....

I INTRODUCTION

A. Definition. Congestive heart failure (CHF) occurs when the heart is unable to pump sufficient amounts of blood at normal filling pressures to keep pace with the metabolic demands of the body.

B. Clinical manifestations classically include fatigue, lethargy, dyspnea on exertion or rest, paroxysmal nocturnal dyspnea (PND), orthopnea, weight gain, and leg swelling.

C. Incidence. CHF is a common disorder, primarily affecting older individuals (10% of the population of the United States older than 65 years have CHF). Over 500,000 new cases are diagnosed each year.

II CLASSIFICATION. There are many different classification schemes. The most useful include the following:

A. New York Heart Association (NYHA) functional classification
  1. **Class I:** Symptomatic only with greater than normal physical activity
  2. **Class II:** Symptomatic during normal activity
  3. **Class III:** Symptomatic with minimal activity
  4. **Class IV:** Symptomatic at rest

B. Left-sided versus right-sided failure. The distinction between left-sided and right-sided failure is based primarily on signs found during physical examination.
  1. **Left-sided failure.** Signs of left-sided failure may include **hypoxia**, **tachypnea**, **rales**, **pleural effusions**, **wheezes** ("cardiac asthma," a manifestation of interstitial edema), and a **left-sided third heart sound (S_3).**
  2. **Right-sided failure.** Signs of right-sided failure may include a **right-sided S_3**, an **elevated jugular venous pressure, presence of hepatojugular reflux, ascites, hepatomegaly**, and **peripheral edema.**
     a. Often, evidence of biventricular failure is found on physical examination because **the most common cause of right-sided failure is left-sided failure.**
     b. Other causes of right-sided failure include:
        (1) **Pulmonary hypertension** [most commonly caused by chronic obstructive pulmonary disease (COPD)]

    (2) Right ventricular infarction (usually occurring in the setting of inferior wall infarction)

    (3) Tricuspid or Pulmonic Valve Disorders

C. Systolic versus diastolic dysfunction. Left ventricular failure can be either systolic or diastolic. This is the most important distinction to make because it affects treatment.

  1. Systolic dysfunction means that the heart's ability to pump is compromised and the left ventricular **ejection fraction is below normal** (usually < **40%**). Causes of systolic dysfunction include:

    a. Myocardial infarction and **ischemic heart disease**

    b. Dilated cardiomyopathies [i.e., disorders of the myocardial cell that are not caused by coronary artery disease (CAD), hypertension, or valvular disease] (see mnemonic below)

    c. Valvular heart disease that chronically increases left ventricular volume (e.g., mitral regurgitation or aortic insufficiency)

    d. "Burned out" hypertensive or valvular heart disease that chronically increases left ventricular pressure (e.g., aortic stenosis). Initially, these disorders lead to diastolic dysfunction, but with time, the heart dilates and the ejection fraction decreases.

    e. Myocarditis

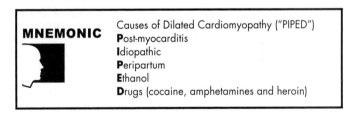

MNEMONIC

Causes of Dilated Cardiomyopathy ("PIPED")
Post-myocarditis
Idiopathic
Peripartum
Ethanol
Drugs (cocaine, amphetamines and heroin)

  2. Diastolic dysfunction means that the heart is able to pump adequately, but its ability to relax and allow adequate filling during diastole is compromised. These patients have a **normal or supranormal ejection fraction.** Causes of diastolic dysfunction include:

    a. Ischemia

    b. Disorders that lead to left ventricular hypertrophy, such as:

      (1) Hypertension

      (2) Aortic stenosis

      (3) Hypertrophic cardiomyopathy

   c. **Restrictive cardiomyopathy.** This disorder is usually caused by infiltrative diseases (e.g., hemochromatosis, amyloidosis, sarcoidosis, scleroderma).

3. In most patients, evidence of both diastolic and systolic dysfunction coexist; however, 20% of patients have predominantly diastolic dysfunction. Both types of dysfunction have similar clinical manifestations.

HOT
KEY
CHF with a low ejection fraction = systolic dysfunction. CHF with a normal or high left ventricular ejection fraction = diastolic dysfunction.

III APPROACH TO THE PATIENT

A. Assess how symptomatic the patient is.
B. On the basis of the patient's history, physical examination findings, and chest radiographs, categorize the failure as predominantly left-sided, right-sided, or biventricular.
C. If the patient has left-sided CHF, determine whether the dysfunction is predominantly systolic or diastolic, using the ejection fraction as a basis for the determination. This can be assessed using echocardiography, multiple gated acquisition (MUGA) scans, or cardiac catheterization. **Remember, if a patient with a normal ejection fraction has cardiogenic pulmonary edema, then the dysfunction is diastolic.**
D. Determine the underlying cause of the CHF (e.g., CAD, valvular disease, hypertension, cardiomyopathy).
E. Any potentially reversible causes of CHF must be treated appropriately (e.g., revascularization, valve replacement/repair, drug cessation program).
F. If the patient's symptoms have worsened, you must decide what precipitated the CHF exacerbation:

MNEMONIC

Factors that Can Exacerbate CHF ("FAILURE")
Forgot meds
Arrhythmia or **A**nemia
Infections, **I**schemia, or **I**nfarction
Lifestyle (e.g., increased sodium intake, stress)
Upregulators (e.g., thyroid disease, pregnancy)
Rheumatic valve or worsening of other valvular diseases
Embolism (pulmonary)

IV TREATMENT

A. **Goals** of treatment for CHF (and most other diseases) are two-fold:
   1. **Reduce symptoms**
   2. **Reduce mortality**
B. **Chronic systolic dysfunction.** Medical management of chronic CHF includes:
   1. **Vasodilators.** Systemic hypertension should be treated aggressively in patients with CHF. Peripheral arterial vasodilators (Table 17-1) have been shown to reduce both symptoms and mortality. These agents reduce afterload by decreasing systemic vascular resistance. Usually, therapy is initiated with a low dose and is then titrated upward based upon the patient's blood pressure and symptoms.
   2. **Diuretics** are useful for treating symptoms of fluid overload (e.g., rales, peripheral edema).
      a. In patients with very mild fluid overload, a thiazide diuretic (e.g., hydrochlorothiazide) at a dose of 25–50 mg daily may be all that is needed.
      b. For most patients with CHF, a loop diuretic (e.g., furosemide, 20–120 mg once or twice-daily) is required. Dosing and frequency depends upon the degree of fluid overload.
   3. **Diet.** Counseling patients to maintain a low-sodium diet (less than 2 grams per day) is important in preventing fluid overload.
   4. **Beta Blockers** block neurohormonal activation and have been shown to improve symptoms and survival. Typical oral

TABLE 17-1. Vasodilators Used to Treat Patients With Systolic Dysfunction

Drug	Dose Range (mg/day)	Dose Frequency (times/day)	Typical Dose
ACE inhibitors			
Captopril	6.25–150	3	50 mg 3 times daily
Enalapril	2.5–20	2	10 mg 2 times daily
Lisinopril	2.5–40	1	20 mg 1 time daily
Hydralazine	10–300	3	75 mg 3 times daily
Isosorbide dinitrate	5–160	3	40 mg 3 times daily
Amlodipine	2.5–10	1	10 mg 1 time daily

ACE = angiotensin-converting enzyme.

agents include carvedilol (3.125 mg twice daily, titrated up to 25 mg twice daily) and long-acting agents dosed daily.

HOT KEY Every patient with systolic dysfunction should be taking an ACE inhibitor (or angiotensin receptor blocker) and a beta-blocker, unless there is a compelling reason for the patient to avoid these agents.

---

   5. **Digoxin.** This age-old treatment for CHF has been shown to reduce symptoms, but has no effect upon mortality.
      a. Digoxin may be used in patients who are symptomatic in spite of other therapy.
      b. Doses vary, depending on the patient's weight and degree of renal function. The usual range is 0.125–0.375 mg/day, taken orally.
   6. **Aldosterone receptor antagonists** have been shown to reduce morbidity and mortality in patients with NYHA Class III or IV heart failure with EF < 40%. These patients who are already taking a β-blocker and an ACE inhibitor should also be started on one of these agents, often in consultation with a cardiologist. Commonly used agents include spironolactone (25–50 mg daily) and eplerenone (25–50 mg daily). Side effects may include hyperkalemia and gynecomastia.
   7. **Devices.** Cardiology consultation is recommended.
      a. Certain patients with severe cardiomyopathy (EF < 30–35%) may benefit from an **implantable cardioverter-defibrillator (ICD)** for prevention of sudden cardiac death.
      b. Pacemaker implantation for **cardiac resynchronization therapy** is also beneficial in selected patients.
   C. **Chronic diastolic dysfunction.** Treatment involves "3 Ds"—diuretics, diet, and diltiazem. Digoxin and vasodilators do not play a role in the treatment of patients with primarily diastolic dysfunction.
      1. **Diuretics** are given in doses similar to those used for patients with systolic dysfunction.
      2. **Diet.** Like patients with systolic dysfunction, patients with diastolic dysfunction should limit sodium intake.
      3. **Diltiazem** (a calcium channel blocker) or a β-blocker can reduce the heart rate and thereby improve ventricular filling. Doses vary but are similar to those recommended for the treatment of hypertension (see Chapter 16, Table 16-1).

V **PROGNOSIS.** Despite therapeutic advances, the annual mortality rate is 20% for all patients with CHF and 50% for patients who are symptomatic at rest.

VI REFERRAL AND FOLLOW-UP

A. Patients taking ACE inhibitors, Angiotensin Receptor Blockers, loop diuretics, or aldosterone receptor antagonists should have a serum electrolyte panel every 6 months (or sooner if the dose has been changed).

B. Patients whose symptoms result in significant limitations despite maximal management with routine agents should be referred to a cardiologist.

References

ACC/AHA 2005 guideline update for the diagnosis and management of chronic heart failure in the adult: a report of the American College of Cardiology/American Heart Association Task Force on Practice Guidelines. *J Am Coll Cardiol* 2005; 46(6):e1-82.

Aurigemma GP, Gaasch WH. Diastolic heart failure. *N Engl J Med* 2004;351:1097–1104.

18. Atrial Fibrillation

I INTRODUCTION

A. Epidemiology. Atrial fibrillation is the most common chronic arrhythmia, occurring in 2% of the general population. The incidence varies with age:

1. Rare in people younger than 50 years
2. One out of 20 people older than 60 years
3. One out of 10 people older than 80 years

B. Terminology. A number of terms are used to describe the types of atrial fibrillation.

1. **"Valvular"** refers to atrial fibrillation that is **secondary to valve disease,** most commonly rheumatic mitral stenosis. In the past, **rheumatic heart disease** accounted for most cases of atrial fibrillation, but currently accounts for few cases.
2. **"Nonvalvular"** applies to atrial fibrillation that is not accompanied by rheumatic or other valvular disease.
3. **"Isolated"** refers to atrial fibrillation that is secondary to another illness (e.g., hyperthyroidism, pneumonia, pulmonary embolism) and resolves when the illness is treated.
4. **"Paroxysmal"** refers to intermittent episodes of atrial fibrillation unrelated to an acute illness.
5. **"Chronic"** or "Persistent" refers to atrial fibrillation when it is the predominant rhythm.
6. **"Lone"** refers to atrial fibrillation in the absence of structural heart disease [e.g., left ventricular hypertrophy, congestive heart failure (CHF), valve disease, cardiomyopathy] or hypertension.

II CLINICAL MANIFESTATIONS OF ATRIAL FIBRILLATION

A. Patient history. Atrial fibrillation causes an increased heart rate and loss of atrial contraction, which results in decreased ventricular filling, decreased cardiac output, and an increase in cardiac demand. The most common symptoms reflect these processes:

1. **Palpitations**
2. **Fatigue**
3. **Dyspnea**
4. **Dizziness or syncope**
5. **Chest pain**

B. Physical examination findings

1. An **irregularly irregular pulse** is the hallmark of atrial fibrillation.

2. **Pulse of varying intensity** and **pulse deficit.** Because diastolic filling varies in length and is often reduced, pulses are of varying intensity and not all audible ventricular beats are palpable peripherally.

3. **Absent a waves.** These jugular venous pulsations, which normally represent atrial contraction, are not seen in patients with atrial fibrillation.

4. **Variation in the intensity of the first heart sound (S_1).** Due to variations in the filling time and end-diastolic volume, the pressure that closes the mitral and tricuspid valve varies, resulting in variations in the intensity of S_1.

C. Electrocardiography

1. **f Waves** (fine fibrillation of the atria at a rate of 350–600 beats/min) may be noted and are best visualized in lead V_1.

2. **P waves** are absent.

3. The **ventricular response** will be **irregularly irregular,** although this may be difficult to appreciate at higher heart rates.

III **CAUSES OF ATRIAL FIBRILLATION INCLUDE THE FOLLOWING:**

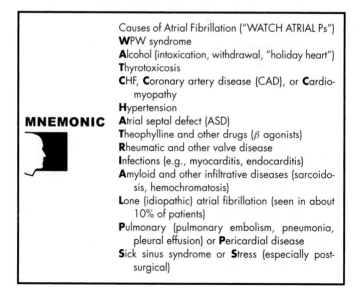

MNEMONIC	Causes of Atrial Fibrillation ("WATCH ATRIAL Ps")
	WPW syndrome
	Alcohol (intoxication, withdrawal, "holiday heart")
	Thyrotoxicosis
	CHF, **C**oronary artery disease (CAD), or **C**ardiomyopathy
	Hypertension
	Atrial septal defect (ASD)
	Theophylline and other drugs (β agonists)
	Rheumatic and other valve disease
	Infections (e.g., myocarditis, endocarditis)
	Amyloid and other infiltrative diseases (sarcoidosis, hemochromatosis)
	Lone (idiopathic) atrial fibrillation (seen in about 10% of patients)
	Pulmonary (pulmonary embolism, pneumonia, pleural effusion) or **P**ericardial disease
	Sick sinus syndrome or **S**tress (especially postsurgical)

> **HOT**
> ▶
> **KEY**
> Because many of the causes of atrial fibrillation are correctable, a thorough search for the underlying cause is required.

IV **COMPLICATIONS OF ATRIAL FIBRILLATION.** The overall risk of **stroke** in all patients with atrial fibrillation is approximately 5% per year, five times the risk in those without atrial fibrillation. The risk of stroke in a patient with atrial fibrillation depends on the presence of five clinical variables and two echocardiographic variables. It is important for patients to have their risk factors "CHASED" down, so that risk can be defined and treatment can be planned.

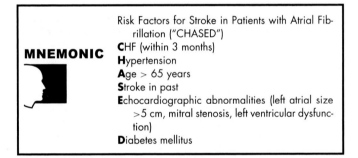

MNEMONIC

Risk Factors for Stroke in Patients with Atrial Fibrillation ("CHASED")
CHF (within 3 months)
Hypertension
Age > 65 years
Stroke in past
Echocardiographic abnormalities (left atrial size >5 cm, mitral stenosis, left ventricular dysfunction)
Diabetes mellitus

A. Patients with atrial fibrillation but no risk factors for stroke are at approximately the same risk for stroke as the general population.
B. Patients with one or two risk factors carry a risk of stroke of approximately 5% per year.
C. Patients with three or more risk factors carry a risk of stroke of roughly 20% per year.

V **TREATMENT**

A. Acute treatment. The goal of acute treatment is **rate control.** Patients with rapid atrial fibrillation and life-threatening problems (e.g., ischemia, severe hypotension, severe pulmonary edema) should undergo immediate **cardioversion.** Patients with rapid atrial fibrillation but no life-threatening problems should be treated with pharmacologic therapy.

1. **Cardioversion** can be **initiated with 100 J in the synchronized mode,** but **360 J may be necessary.** Unless there is an emergent indication, no patient with atrial fibrillation should be cardioverted until 3 weeks of anticoagulation therapy have been completed or until atrial thrombus has been excluded using transesophageal echocardiography (TEE).

   a. As a result of this stipulation, cardioversion is usually contraindicated in patients who are thought to have "new onset" atrial fibrillation because it is difficult to estimate the length of time the patient has been in atrial fibrillation from the patient history.

   b. Patients who are cardioverted without undergoing anticoagulation therapy have a 3%–5% risk of stroke within 30 days.

2. **Pharmacologic therapy**

   a. **Atrioventricular (AV) node blocking agents** include **calcium channel blockers** (e.g., verapamil, diltiazem), **β blockers** (e.g., esmolol), and **digoxin.**

      (1) Dosages are given in Table 18-1.

      (2) Intravenous administration of a calcium channel blocker or β blocker is thought to be more effective than digoxin for regaining rapid control of an accelerated heart rate in a patient with atrial fibrillation, although all of these agents may cause hypotension, bradycardia, conduction defects, and CHF. Short-acting agents are always preferred, and monitoring is required for all patients.

      (3) Digoxin may be the best choice for patients with heart failure.

B. **Chronic treatment.** The goals of chronic treatment of atrial fibrillation are **alleviation of symptoms** and **reduction of the risk for stroke.**

HOT

▶ It is useful to think of **three categories of treatment: rate control, rhythm control,** and **clot control.**

KEY

---

1. **Rate control.** The goal is a resting heart rate lower than 90 beats/min. **Pharmacologic treatment** should be selected after considering the patient's other medical problems. For example:

   a. In patients with hypertension or CAD, a β blocker (e.g., atenolol, 50–100 mg daily) is a good choice because it addresses these problems as well as the atrial fibrillation.

TABLE 18-1. Pharmacologic Therapy for Atrial Fibrillation

Drug	Initial Dose	Maintenance Dose
Diltiazem*	15–20 mg (0.25 mg/kg) intravenously over 2 minutes; repeat in 15 minutes at 20–25 mg if necessary	5–20 mg/hr intravenously
Verapamil*	2.5–5.0 mg administered as an intravenous bolus over 1–2 minutes, followed by 5–10 mg in 15–30 minutes if necessary; maximum dose is 30 mg	0.05–0.2 mg/min intravenously
Esmolol*	500 μg/kg intravenously over 1 minute	50-200 μg/kg/min intravenously
Digoxin	0.25–0.5 mg intravenously	0.25 mg intravenously every 6 hours to a total dose of 1 mg completes loading, followed by 0.125 mg-0.25 by PO or IV daily

*These agents may cause bradycardia, hypotension, conduction delay, or congestive heart failure (CHF) and should only be used in monitored settings.

However, in patients with asthma or chronic obstructive pulmonary disease (COPD), a β blocker may not be a good choice because it may induce bronchoconstriction.

   b. In patients with CHF, digoxin can control the heart rate as well as improve symptoms of CHF. However, in patients with chronic renal insufficiency, digoxin levels must be monitored closely.

2. Rhythm control. Theoretically, conversion to normal sinus rhythm returns the risk of stroke to baseline and relieves all rate-related symptoms.

HOT

KEY

Studies comparing rate control plus anticoagulation to rythm control in patients with atrial fibrillation have found a trend towards a reduced risk of stroke with the rate control plus anticoagulation strategy, suggesting that this is the preferred approach. Situations that might warrant an attempt at rythm control include persistent symptoms after rate control, an inability to maintain rate control, or patient preference.

a. **Cardioversion.** Elective cardioversion should be performed only after a 3-week course of therapeutic anticoagulation has been completed or after atrial thrombus has been excluded using TEE. Cardioversion should be followed by 4 more weeks of anticoagulation therapy.

b. **Pharmacologic therapy.** Rate must be controlled prior to the initiation of any antiarrhythmic medication because antiarrhythmic medications can increase conduction through the AV node (and accelerate the rate of atrial fibrillation).

    (1) **Amiodarone** is a Class III antiarrhythmic agent with beta-blocking properties. Unlike several other antiarrhythmic agents, it is not associated with proarrhythmic effects.

        (a) Although amiodarone is associated with significant side effects (e.g., optic neuropathy, hypo- and hyperthyroidism, pulmonary fibrosis), it is often the antiarrhythmic of choice in patients with left ventricular dysfunction.

        (b) Thyroid function tests and a liver panel should be obtained prior to initiating amiodarone and every 6 months while on therapy. Pulmonary function tests should be measured at baseline.

    (2) **Propafenone** (150-300 mg orally twice daily) and **flecainide** (50-150 mg orally twice daily) are Class IC antiarrhythmic agents that may be used in patients without coronary artery disease or left ventricular dysfunction.

        (a) Using a **"pill-in-the-pocket"** treatment approach, selected symptomatic patients with recurrent atrial fibrillation may convert to sinus rhythm by taking a single oral dose of propafenone (450-600 mg) or flecainide (200-300 mg) at the onset of symptoms.

HOT **KEY**

Consultation with a cardiologist is suggested before initiating treatment with antiarrhythmic agents.

---

c. **Radiofrequency catheter ablation** of pulmonary veins or **AV node ablation with pacemaker implantation** can be considered for symptomatic patients who do not respond to medical therapy.

3. **Clot control.** Stroke is a major cause of morbidity and mortality in patients with atrial fibrillation. As a rule of thumb,

all patients with **atrial fibrillation** should receive long-term **anticoagulant therapy** with warfarin unless they are young (less than 65 years old) and have none of the risk factors described above, or unless there is a major contraindication to the use of warfarin. The risks and benefits of anticoagulation therapy must be assessed on an individual basis.

  a. Aspirin (325 mg daily) alone is a consideration for patients without risk factors for stroke who are less than 65 years old.

  b. Warfarin. Although warfarin therapy places the patient at a slightly increased risk for major bleeding, the benefits from a reduced risk of stroke usually outweigh the risk of bleeding. Warfarin can reduce the risk of stroke by 40%–90%. The target international normalized ratio (INR) is 2.0–3.0.

VI FOLLOW-UP AND REFERRAL. Consultation with a cardiologist, who can assist with decisions regarding cardioversion, rate-controlling agents, and antiarrhythmic therapy, is recommended for most patients.

A. Patients with new-onset atrial fibrillation generally require hospitalization for rate control and determination of the cause of the arrhythmia.

B. Stable patients with chronic atrial fibrillation can be seen as needed (usually once a month) to monitor anticoagulation therapy and rate and symptom control. Anti-arrhythmic therapy should be re-evaluated every 1–3 months.

References

Falk RH. Atrial fibrillation. *N Engl J Med* 2001;344:1067–1078.

Hersi A, Wyse DG. Management of atrial fibrillation. *Curr Probl Cardiol* 2005;30(4): 175–233.

19. Heart Murmur

....

I **INTRODUCTION.** Auscultation of a heart murmur presents a challenging problem for the primary care provider. Some murmurs are benign, but others represent conditions that can lead to permanent damage and disability if left untreated.

A. Pathogenesis. A murmur is produced by turbulent blood flow that causes vibration of cardiac structures, usually heart valves.

B. Classification. Murmurs can be broadly classified as systolic, diastolic, or continuous.

1. Systolic murmurs occur between the first and second heart sounds (S_1 and S_2).

2. Diastolic murmurs occur between the second and first heart sounds (S_2 and S_1).

3. Continuous murmurs occur throughout systole and diastole.

C. Presentation

1. Most murmurs are detected during a routine clinical examination in asymptomatic patients.

2. Patients who present with symptoms suggestive of certain types of valve disease (e.g., exertional dyspnea, angina, syncope) and are found to have a murmur require prompt evaluation.

II **CAUSES OF HEART MURMURS.** Selected major causes of the three murmur types are shown in Table 19-1.

III **APPROACH TO THE PATIENT.** The goal is to differentiate benign conditions from those that require specific therapy to prevent complications and symptoms.

A. Patient history. Focus on the following:

1. Symptoms suggestive of cardiac disease (e.g., angina, shortness of breath, exercise intolerance, syncope)

2. Past medical history of **conditions that can affect the heart** (e.g., rheumatic fever, intravenous drug use) or **increase blood flow** (e.g., anemia, hyperthyroidism, renal failure, arteriovenous fistula)

B. Physical examination must include a complete cardiac examination.

TABLE 19-1. Selected Causes of Murmurs	
Murmur Type	**Causes**
Systolic	Increased flow
	Anemia
	Thyrotoxicosis
	Sepsis
	Renal failure
	Arteriovenous fistula
	Abnormal structure
	Stenosis (aortic or pulmonic)
	Regurgitation (mitral or tricuspid)
	Mitral valve prolapse
	Hypertrophic cardiomyopathy
	VSD, ASD
Diastolic	Stenosis (mitral or tricuspid)
	Regurgitation (aortic or pulmonic)
Continuous	Patent ductus arteriosus
	Coarctation of the aorta
	Arteriovenous fistula

ASD = atrial septal defect, VSD = ventricular septal defect.

1. Classify the murmur as systolic, diastolic, or continuous to narrow the differential diagnosis (see Table 19-1).
2. Use the following characteristic physical examination findings to arrive at a specific diagnosis:
   a. **Aortic stenosis**
      (1) The carotid upstroke is diminished and delayed ("**pulsus parvus et tardus**").
      (2) A harsh, crescendo-decrescendo systolic ejection murmur is best heard at the right upper sternal border and radiates to the carotids.
      (3) The intensity of the S_2 is decreased.
   b. **Aortic regurgitation**
      (1) A diastolic decrescendo murmur is heard immediately following S_2.
      (2) The murmur is best heard with the patient sitting up, leaning forward, and holding his breath after a full expiration.
   c. **Mitral stenosis**
      (1) An opening snap is often followed by a subtle mid-diastolic rumble.
      (2) The murmur is best heard at the apex using the bell of the stethoscope.

    d. Mitral regurgitation
        (1) A blowing, holosytolic murmur is auscultated at the apex, often with radiation to the axilla.
        (2) The murmur may increase when the patient firmly clenches his fists.
    e. Tricuspid stenosis. The murmur is best heard at the left lower sternal border and increases with inspiration.
    f. Tricuspid regurgitation. This harsh, holosystolic murmur increases when the patient inhales or when gentle pressure is applied continuously to the right upper quadrant of the abdomen.
    g. Pulmonic stenosis is rare in adults. The murmur is best heard at the left sternal border in the second intercostal space.
    h. Pulmonic regurgitation occurs in the setting of pulmonary hypertension. The murmur may be difficult to distinguish from that of aortic regurgitation and is best heard at the left sternal border in the second intercostal space.
    i. Hypertrophic cardiomyopathy.
        (1) This harsh, crescendo-decrescendo murmur is best heard at the left lower sternal border.
        (2) The murmur intensity increases with Valsalva maneuver or standing and decreases with passive leg elevation or when the patient moves from a standing to a squatting position.
    j. Mitral valve prolapse is usually diagnosed by detecting a systolic click, which may or may not be accompanied by a mitral regurgitation murmur.
    k. Ventricular septal defect (VSD). This holosystolic murmur is best heard at the left lower sternal border and often radiates to the right sternal border. The intensity does not change with inspiration.
    l. Atrial septal defect (ASD) results in fixed splitting of the S_2. The murmur is best heard at the left sternal border in the second intercostal space.
C. Imaging studies. An **echocardiogram** is indicated:
    1. For all patients with suspected **systolic murmur** when the diagnosis cannot be established on the basis of the history and physical examination
    2. For all patients with **diastolic** or **continuous murmurs**. These murmurs are always abnormal and indicate structural abnormalities of the heart that may require intervention.

IV **TREATMENT.** Once a valve disorder has been definitively diagnosed, the goals of treatment are **symptom reduction** and the **prevention of complications (Table 19-2).**

TABLE 19-2. Valve Disease—Therapeutic Considerations

Therapy	Mitral Stenosis	Mitral Regurgitation	Aortic Stenosis	Aortic Regurgitation	Mitral Valve Prolapse
			Disorder		
Afterload reduction	Not indicated	Consider	Not indicated	Indicated	Not indicated
Surgery	Indicated if symptoms have developed; controversial prior to symptom development*	Indicated if evidence of left ventricular dysfunction or dilation	Indicated when symptoms develop[†]	Indicated if evidence of left ventricular dysfunction or dilation	Not indicated
Endocarditis prophylaxis	Indicated	Indicated	Indicated	Indicated	Consider[‡]
Coagulation prophylaxis	Consider	Not indicated	Not indicated	Not indicated	Not indicated

*In patients with symptomatic mitral valve stenosis, surgery may prevent atrial fibrillation and pulmonary hypertension.
[†]Symptomatic aortic stenosis usually occurs when the aortic valve area reaches 1.0–1.5 cm^2.
[‡]Endocarditis prophylaxis is recommended for patients with mitral valve prolapse only when there is mitral regurgitation or the valve leaflets are thickened and redundant.

A. Endocarditis prophylaxis is indicated for most patients with valve disease and is discussed in Chapter 20.

B. Anticoagulation therapy is indicated for all patients with atrial fibrillation or thromboembolism in the setting of valvular heart disease.

V FOLLOW-UP AND REFERRAL

A. Patients with stenotic or regurgitant murmurs should be followed every 3 months to evaluate for symptoms [e.g., angina, exertional dyspnea, congestive heart failure (CHF), syncope]. Serial echocardiograms should be considered for those with mitral or aortic stenosis, and are necessary for those with mitral or aortic regurgitation.

B. A cardiology consultation should be obtained whenever there is uncertainty about the management of a patient's heart murmur.

References

Chizner MA. The diagnosis of heart disease by clinical assessment alone. *Curr Probl Cardiol* 2001;26(5):285–379.

Etchells E, Bell C, Robb K. Does this patient have an abnormal systolic murmur? *JAMA* 1997; 277(7):564–571.

20. Endocarditis Prophylaxis

I INTRODUCTION

A. Patients with **cardiac structural abnormalities** (e.g., **cardiac valve defects**) have an increased risk of acquiring bacterial endocarditis (Table 20-1). The abnormal structures are thought to be more exposed ("sticky"), and are therefore more susceptible to infection during periods of **bacteremia.**

B. **Sources of bacteremia**
   1. **Certain medical** and **dental procedures** are known to cause transient bacteremia. Patients at risk for the development of bacterial endocarditis may be able to reduce their risk by taking **prophylactic antibiotics** prior to undergoing the procedure.
   2. **Oral inflammation** can predispose to bacteremia. Patients at risk for bacterial endocarditis should be counseled about the importance of **strict dental hygiene.**

II INDICATIONS FOR PROPHYLAXIS.
Certain dental and medical procedures (Tables 20-2 and 20-3) **warrant prophylactic antibiotics**.

A. **High-** and **moderate-risk category** patients should get **prophylactic antibiotics** (see Table 20-1) prior to undergoing certain procedures.

B. Patients in the **negligible-risk category** are not thought to be at higher risk than members of the average population; therefore, prophylactic antibiotics are not routinely recommended for these patients. Nevertheless, prophylaxis should be prescribed according to the patient's individual situation.

III PROPHYLACTIC REGIMENS

A. **Dental, oral,** and **upper respiratory tract procedures.** Oral antibiotics are the recommended form of prophylaxis (Table 20-4). Some practitioners may choose to treat patients at very high risk with intravenous therapy.

TABLE 20-1. Risk of Bacterial Endocarditis Associated with Various Cardiac Conditions

Prophylaxis Recommended

High Risk

Prosthetic cardiac valves (including bioprosthetic and homograft valves)

Previous bacterial endocarditis

Complex cyanotic congenital heart disease (e.g., single ventricle states, transposition of the great arteries, tetralogy of Fallot)

Surgically constructed systemic pulmonary shunts or conduits

Moderate Risk

Most congenital cardiac malformations (other than those specified in the high-risk and negligible risk categories)

Acquired vavular dysfunction (e.g., rheumatic heart disease)

Hypertrophic cardiomyopathy

Mitral valve prolapse with valvular regurgitation, thickened leaflets, or both

Prophylaxis Not Recommended

Negligible risk

Isolated secundum atrial septal defect

Surgical repair of atrial septal defect, ventricular septal defect, or patent ductus arteriosus (without residua beyond 6 months)

Previous coronary artery bypass graft surgery

Mitral valve prolapse without valvular regurgitation

Physiologic, functional, or innocent heart murmurs

Previous Kawasaki disease without valvular dysfunction

Previous rheumatic fever without vavular dysfunction

Cardiac pacemakers (intravascular and epicardial) and implanted defibrillators

Reprinted with permission from Dajani AS, Taubert KA, Wilson W, et al. Prevention of bacterial endocarditis—recommendations by the American Heart Association. JAMA 1997;277(22):1797.

TABLE 20-2. Dental Procedures: Recommendations for Endocarditis Prophylaxis

Prophylaxis Recommended*

Dental extractions

Periodontal procedures, including surgery, scaling and root planning, probing, and recall maintenance

Dental implant placement and reimplantation of avulsed teeth

Endodontic (root canal) instrumentation or surgery only beyond the apex

Subgingival placement of antibiotic fibers or strips

Initial placement of orthodontic bands (but not brackets)

Intraligamentary local anesthetic injections

Prophylactic cleaning of teeth or implants when bleeding is anticipated

Prophylaxis Not Recommended

Restorative denistry† (operative and prosthodontic) with or without re-traction cord‡

Local anesthetic injections (nonintraligamentary)

Intracanal endodontic treatment; post placement and buildup

Placement of rubber dams

Postoperative suture removal

Placement of removable prosthodontic or orthodontic appliances

Taking of oral impressions

Fluoride treatments

Taking of oral radiographys

Orthodontic appliance adjustment

Shedding of primary teeth

Reprinted with permission from Dajani AS, Taubert KA, Wilson W, et al. Prevention of bacterial endocarditis—recommendations by the American Heart Association. *JAMA* 1997;277(22):1797.

*Prophylaxis is recommended for patients with high- and moderate-risk cardiac conditions.

†This includes restoration of decayed teeth (filling cavaties) and replacement of missing teeth.

‡Clinical judgment may indicate antibiotic use in selected circumstances that may create significant bleeding.

TABLE 20-3. Medical Procedures: Recommendations for Endocarditis Prophylaxis

Prophylaxis Recommended

Respiratory tract procedures
   Tonsillectomy or adenoidectomy
   Surgical operations that involve the respiratory mucosa
   Bronchoscopy with a rigid bronchoscope
Gastrointestinal tract procedures*
   Sclerotherapy for esophageal varices
   Esophageal stricture dilation
   Endoscopic retrograde cholangiography with biliary obstruction
   Biliary tract surgery
   Surgical operations that involve the intestinal mucosa
Genitourinary tract procedures
   Prostatic surgery
   Cystoscopy
   Urethral dilation

Prophylaxis Not Recommended

Respiratory tract procedures
   Endotracheal intubation
   Bronchoscopy with a flexible bronchoscope, with or without biopsy[†]
   Tympanostomy tube insertion
Gastrointestinal tract procedures
   Transesophageal echocardiography (TEE)[†]
   Endoscopy with or without gastrointestinal biopsy[†]
Genitourinary tract procedures
   Vaginal hysterectomy[†]
   Vaginal delivery[†]
   Cesarean section
   Urethral catheterization[‡]
   Uterine dilation and curettage[‡]
   Therapeutic abortion[‡]
   Sterilization procedures[‡]
   Insertion or removal of intrauterine devices[‡]
Other procedures
   Cardiac catheterization, including balloon angioplasty
   Implantation of cardiac pacemakers, implanted defibrillators, or
     coronary stents
   Incision or biopsy of surgically scrubbed skin
   Circumcision

Reprinted with permission from Dajani AS, Taubert KA, Wilson W, et al.
Prevention of bacterial endocarditis—recommendations by the American Heart
Association. *JAMA* 1997;277(22):1797.
*Prophylaxis is recommended for high-risk patients; optional for medium-risk patients.
[†]Prophylaxis is optioinal for high-risk patients.
[‡]Unless infection is present, in which case prophylaxis is recommended.

TABLE 20-4. Prophylactic Regimens for Dental, Oral, or Upper Respiratory Tract Procedures

Situation	Agent	Regimen
Standard general prophylaxis	Amoxicillin	**Adults:** 2.0 g orally 1 hour before procedure **Children:** 50 mg/kg orally 1 hour before procedure
Unable to take oral medications	Ampicillin	**Adults:** 2.0 g intramuscularly or intravenously 30 minutes before procedure **Children:** 50 mg/kg intramuscularly or intravenously 30 minutes before procedure
Allergic to penicillin	Clindamycin	**Adults:** 600 mg orally 1 hour before procedure **Children:** 20 mg/kg orally 1 hour before procedure
	OR	
	Azithromycin or clarithromycin	**Adults:** 500 mg orally 1 hour before procedure **Children:** 15 mg/kg orally 1 hour before procedure

Reprinted with permission from Dajani AS, Taubert KA, Wilson W, et al. Prevention of bacterial endocarditis—recommendations by the American Heart Association. *JAMA* 1997;277(22):1797.

B. **Genitourinary** or **gastrointestinal tract procedures.** Intravenous therapy is recommended (Table 20-5), although practitioners may chose to use oral therapy in moderate-risk patients.

C. **Other procedures.** Consultation with a cardiologist is recommended when the situation does not conform to the standard guidelines.

TABLE 20-5. Prophylactic Regimens for Genitourinary and Gastrointestinal Procedures in Adults

Situation	Agent	Regimen
High-risk patient	Ampicillin plus gentamicin	Ampicillin (2.0 g IM or IV) plus gentamicin (1.5 mg/kg, not to exceed 120 mg) within 30 minutes of procedure Ampicillin (1 g IM or IV) or amoxicillin (1 g orally) 6 hours later
High-risk patient with penicillin allergy	Vancomycin plus gentamicin	Vancomycin (1.0 g IV over 1–2 hours) plus gentamicin (1.5 mg/kg IV or IM, not to exceed 120 mg); complete infusion or injection within 30 minutes of starting procedure
Moderate-risk patient	Amoxicillin or ampicillin	Amoxicillin (2.0 g orally 1 hour before procedure) or ampicillin (2.0 g IM or IV within 30 minutes of procedure)
Moderate-risk patient with penicillin allergy	Vancomycin	Vancomycin (1.0 g IV over 1–2 hours); complete infusion within 30 minutes of starting the procedure

IM = intramuscularly; IV = intravenously.
Reprinted with permission from Dajani AS, Taubert KA, Wilson W, et al. Prevention of bacterial endocarditis—recommendations by the American Heart Association. *JAMA* 1997;277(22):1797.

References

Dajani AS, Taubert KA, Wilson W, et al. Prevention of bacterial endocarditis—recommendations by the American Heart Association. *JAMA* 1997;277(22):1794–1801.

Seto TB, Kwiat D, Taira DA, et al. Physicians' recommendations to patients for use of antibiotic prophylaxis to prevent endocarditis. JAMA 2000;284:68–71.

21. Lower Extremity Edema

I INTRODUCTION

A. Edema, the excessive accumulation of interstitial fluid in the tissues, results from alterations in one or more of the following parameters:
  1. Hydrostatic pressure
  2. Oncotic pressure
  3. Capillary permeability
  4. Lymphatic drainage
B. Lower extremity edema presents as swelling of one or both legs.

II APPROACH TO THE PATIENT

A. **Patient history and physical examination.** The clinician can use several pieces of information obtained during the history and examination to shorten the extensive differential diagnosis for lower leg edema (Table 21-1).
  1. **Duration:** acute or chronic?
  2. **Distribution:** unilateral or bilateral?
  3. **Associated signs and symptoms:** dyspnea, pain, skin changes, upper extremity swelling?

HOT
▶
KEY

Lower extremity edema can be a sign of a life-threatening disease, so a diagnosis should be established promptly.

B. **Laboratory and imaging studies.** If the history and physical examination are unrevealing, additional testing may be required. The order of the work-up can be tailored according to any etiologic clues gleaned from the history and physical examination.
  1. **Unilateral edema**
    a. Venous duplex ultrasound with Doppler should be obtained.
    b. A complete blood count (CBC) and a serum creatinine kinase level may also be obtained to evaluate the possibility of infection and compartment syndrome, respectively in the appropriate clinical setting.

TABLE 21-1. Causes of Lower Extremity Edema

Cause	Associated History, Signs, and Symptoms
Unilateral, acute onset*	
DVT	Hypercoagulable stte; age >50 years; bed bound; history of surgery, cancer, or trauma; thigh or calf pain
Cellulitis or abscess	Fever, pain erythema
Ruptured popliteal cyst	Pain, knee swelling
Trauma	History of recent injury
Compartment syndrome	History of trauma (crush injury) or prolonged pressure on the leg
Ruptured muscle or tendon	Forceful ankle dorsiflexion
Erythema nodosum	Fever, pain, patchy erythema
Unilateral, gradual onset	
Chronic venous insufficiency	Painless, edema worse at day's end but improves with elevation, varicose veins
Lymphedema	Painless, edema worse at day's end, dorsum of toes and feet affected first, dry and scaly skin
External venous compression	Painless, localized enlargement
Soft tissue tumor or vascular tumor	Localized tenderness and enlargement
Congenital venous malformation	Leg length discrepancy from childhood
Reflex sympathetic dystrophy	Taut, shiny skin; extreme sensitivity to touch
Bilateral	
CHF	Dyspnea, orthopnea, PND, elevated jugular venous pressure
Nephrotic syndrome	History of diabetes or lupus
Glomerulonephritis	History of recent fever or sore throat
Hepatic cirrhosis	Jaundice, icterus, ascites, history of alcohol abuse or hepatitis
Hypoproteinemia	History of malnutrition or malabsorption
Pretibial myxedema (Graves' disease)	Tachycardia, tremor, weight loss, heat intolerance
Bilateral DVT	Hypercoagulable state; age >50 years; bed-bound; history of surgery, cancer, or trauma; thigh or calf pain

(Continued)

TABLE 21-1. Causes of Lower Extremity Edema (*Continued*)

Cause	Associated History, Signs, and Symptoms
Bilateral cellulitis	Fever, pain, erythema
Chronic venous insufficiency	Painless, edema worse at day's end but improves with elevation, varicose veins
Lymphedema	Inguinal lymphadenopathy, pelvic symptoms, weight loss
Drug reaction	NSAIDs
	Monoamine oxidase (MAO) inhibitors
	Antihypertensive agents
	β Blockers
	Calcium channel blockers
	Clonidine
	Diazoxide
	Guanethidine
	Hydralazine
	Methyldopa
	Minoxidil
	Reserpine
	Hormones
	Corticosteroids
	Estrogen
	Progesterone
	Testosterone

Modified with permission from Ciocon JO, Fernandez BB, Ciocon DG. Leg edema: clinical clues to the differential diagnosis. *Geriatrics* 1993;48(5): 34–40, 45. Copyright by Advanstar Communications, Inc. Advanstar Communications, Inc retains all rights to this article.
CHF = congestive heart failure; DVT = deep venous thrombosis; PND = paroxysmal nocturnal dyspnea; NSAIDs = nonsteroidal anti-inflammatory drugs.
*"Acute" = <72 hours; "gradual" = >72 hours.

2. **Bilateral edema.** Table 21-2 summarizes studies that may be appropriate for the evaluation of bilateral edema.

III TREATMENT

A. **Definitive treatment** involves addressing the underlying disorder [e.g., anticoagulation for deep venous thrombosis (DVT); antibiotics for cellulitis].

TABLE 21-2. Evaluation of Bilateral Edema

Studies	Suspected Cause of the Bilateral Edema
Complete blood count (CBC)	Bilateral cellulitis
Urinalysis and renal panel	Glomerulonephritis, nephritic syndrome
Liver function tests and serum albumin level	Liver disease, malnutrition
Thyroid-stimulating hormone (TSH) level	Thyroid disease
Electrocardiogram (EKG) and chest radiograph, possibly echocardiogram	Congestive heart failure (CHF)
Venous duplex ultrasound with Doppler	Bilateral deep venous thrombosis (DVT), inferior vena cava thrombus
Pelvic ultrasound or pelvic computed tomography (CT) scan	Pelvic malignancy, retroperitoneal fibrosis

B. Symptomatic treatment
  1. **Elevation of the affected limb or limbs** is helpful.
  2. **Discontinuation of medications.** Drugs that may cause or exacerbate the edema should be discontinued, if possible.
  3. **Diuretics** are helpful for patients with bilateral leg edema associated with congestive heart failure (CHF), renal insufficiency, cirrhosis, or venous insufficiency.
  4. **Compression stockings** are most useful for patients with edema caused by CHF or venous insufficiency.

IV FOLLOW-UP AND REFERRAL

A. If infection (e.g., necrotizing fasciitis) or compartment syndrome is the suspected cause of the edema, the patient should be seen by a surgeon immediately.

B. All patients with leg edema should be advised about the importance of meticulous skin care, proper shoes, and early treatment of minor trauma as a means of preventing serious complications, such as venous stasis ulcers, cellulitis, or osteomyelitis.

References

Gorman WP, Davis KR, Donnelly R. ABC of arterial and venous disease. Swollen lower limb-1: general assessment and deep venous thrombosis. *BMJ* 2000;320(7247): 1453–1456.

Topham EJ, Mortimer PS. Chronic lower limb edema. *Clin Med* 2002;2(1):28–31.

PART IV

PULMONOLOGY

22. Chronic Cough

I INTRODUCTION

A. Chronic cough, defined as a **cough of greater than 3 weeks duration,** is a common problem in the outpatient setting. Fortunately, in most patients, a treatable cause of chronic cough can be identified.

B. Chronic cough afflicts 10%–20% of nonsmoking adults, and 80% of adults who smoke.

II CAUSES OF CHRONIC COUGH

A. Common causes. Postnasal drip syndrome, gastroesophageal reflux disease (GERD), and asthma account for more than 90% of cases of chronic cough in non-smoking adults. As many as 60% of patients have more than one of these conditions as the underlying cause.

  1. Postnasal drip syndrome (PND) secondary to allergic or viral rhinitis or sinusitis is the cause in **20%–50%** of non-smoking patients.

  2. GERD is the cause in **10%–40%** of non-smoking patients.

  3. Asthma is the cause in **15%–35%** of non-smoking patients.

  4. Smoking is an extremely common cause of chronic cough.

B. Less common causes include:

  1. Bronchiectasis

  2. Congestive heart failure (CHF)

  3. Angiotensin-converting enzyme (ACE) inhibitor therapy. Up to 15% of patients taking these medications develop a cough, usually within 1 week of starting therapy. However it may occur as late as one year after initiation.

  3 Post-Upper respiratory infection cough—either viral or bacterial.

  4. Malignancy or **chronic infection** (often accompanied by systemic symptoms and weight loss)

> **HOT** ▶ **KEY**
> Bronchogenic cancer should be considered if a current or for-
> mer smoker experiences 1) a new cough or change in chronic
> cough 2) a cough that lasts more than one month after smoking
> cessation 3) hemptysis.

III APPROACH TO THE PATIENT. The approach to evaluation
and treatment of chronic cough is **largely empiric.** There is
no confirmatory diagnostic test for postnasal drip syndrome,
and diagnostic tests for GERD and asthma are relatively expensive relative to treatment measures. As a result, a prag-
matic and cost-effective approach to chronic cough involves
identifying the most likely cause or causes of cough, treating
appropriately, and considering more invasive testing only if
initial therapy is unsuccessful (Figure 22-1).

A. The **history** and **physical examination** should be directed toward
   identifying the underlying cause.
   1. **Postnasal drip syndrome**
      a. In as many as 25% of patients, cough is the only mani-
         festation of postnasal drip, and patients will not report a
         sensation of secretions dripping down the throat.
      b. The physical examination is insensitive for postnasal drip.
         A cobblestone appearance of the posterior pharynx may
         be present in 20% of patients.
   2. **ACE inhibitor therapy.** With discontinuation, cough usually
      resolves in 2–3 weeks. This is a classs effect and other ACE
      inhibitor should not be tried. An angiotensin II receptor an-
      tagonist (e.g., losartan) or another type of antihypertensive
      agent should be used instead.
   3. **Smoking.** All patients who are chronic smokers should be
      encouraged to stop. Smoking-associated cough may be ex-
      acerbated in the first few days after quitting, but generally
      resolves in 1–2 months.
   4. **GERD.** As with postnasal drip syndrome, cough may be the
      only manifestation of reflux.
   5. **Asthma.** So-called "cough variant" asthma may be seen in
      patients who do not complain of more classic asthma symp-
      toms, such as wheezing and dyspnea.
B. **Empiric therapy.** If no obvious cause can be identified, empiric
   therapy should be initiated based on the most likely underlying
   cause, before performing extensive diagnostic tests. (see Figure
   22-1).
C. **Invasive testing** should be used only when patients fail to respond to empiric therapy.

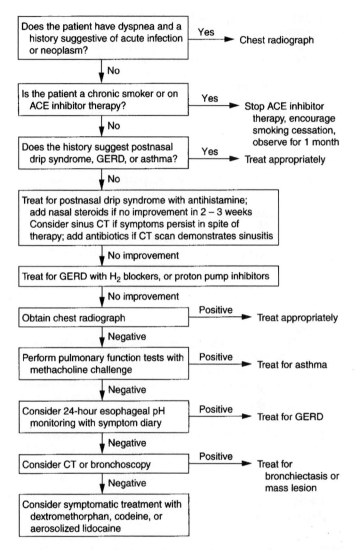

FIGURE 22-1. Algorithm for evaluation and treatment of chronic cough. *ACE* = angiotensin-converting enzyme; *CT* = computed tomography; *GERD* = gastroesophageal reflux disease.

1. **24-Hour esophageal pH monitoring** is useful for diagnosing **GERD-associated cough** and assessing response to therapy. Patients should be asked to keep a **symptom diary.**
2. **Pulmonary function tests** with a **methacholine challenge** are useful for diagnosing **asthma** in patients who fail to respond to empiric therapy for postnasal drip.
   a. A negative result virtually excludes asthma as a cause of cough. Patients with positive results should be treated for asthma.

IV **TREATMENT.** In general, response to treatment may take 2–3 weeks, and full resolution of symptoms may require 1–2 months.

HOT KEY Patients who have only a partial response to treatment may have more than one underlying cause for their cough; these patients may require combination therapy.

A. Postnasal drip syndrome
   1. Antihistamines
      a. Treatment should be initiated with an over the counter **antihistamine,** such as **diphenhydramine** (25–50 mg orally every 6 hours as needed)
      b. If the older antihistamines cause problematic sedation, more selective antihistamines, such as **loratadine** (10 mg orally daily) or **fexofenadine** (60 mg orally daily) may be used during the day.
   2. Nasal steroids, such as **beclomethasone** or **flunisolide** (1–2 sprays per nostril once or twice daily), may be useful for patients with seasonal or allergic rhinitis.
   3. Antibiotics are not helpful unless there are clear signs of sinusitis.
B. GERD treatment is discussed in Chapter 34.
C. Asthma treatment is discussed in Chapter 24.

V **FOLLOW-UP AND REFERRAL**

A. Follow-up. Patients should be seen every 2–4 weeks until symptoms abate or a diagnosis is made.
B. Referral
   1. A pulmonologist should be consulted if bronchoscopy is being considered for patients with persistent symptoms.

2. Consultation with a gastroenterologist is useful if GERD is strongly suspected and the patient remains symptomatic despite maximum therapy.

3. Consultation with an otolaryngologist may be helpful if a patient with suspected postnasal drip syndrome continues to have symptoms despite aggressive therapy.

References

Irwin RS, Madison JM. Primary Care: The Diagnosis and Treatment of Cough. *N Engl J Med* 2000;343:1715–1721.

Pratter MR, Brightling CE, Boulet LP, Irwin RS. An empiric integrative approach to the management of cough: ACCP evidence-based clinical practice guidelines. *Chest* 2006;129(1 Suppl):222S–231S.

23. Dyspnea

I INTRODUCTION. Dyspnea (shortness of breath) refers to discomfort associated with breathing. Many cases of dyspnea present as one of the three main subtypes:

A. Paroxysmal nocturnal dyspnea (PND) is dyspnea that wakes a person from sleep after she has been sleeping for 1–2 hours. PND is usually a manifestation of increased left atrial pressure caused by congestive heart failure (CHF).

B. Orthopnea is dyspnea that begins suddenly when a patient lies down but is immediately relieved when he sits up. Orthopnea implies heart failure or, occasionally, pulmonary disease.

C. Platypnea is the opposite of orthopnea—i.e., the dyspnea occurs when the patient sits up but is relieved when he lies down. Platypnea is caused by right-to-left shunting [e.g., hepatopulmonary syndrome, atrial septal defect (ASD)].

II CAUSES OF DYSPNEA

A. Chronic and subacute dyspnea. The common causes of subacute and chronic dyspnea (the focus of this chapter) are outlined in Table 23-1. The **five most common causes of chronic dyspnea** involve **two cardiac** and **three pulmonary** causes:
1. **Cardiac**
   1) Ischemic heart disease
   2) Congestive heart failure
2. **Pulmonary**
   1) Asthma
   2) COPD
   3) Interstitial lung disease

B. Acute dyspnea. Although this chapter focuses on chronic dyspnea, it is important to be aware of the common causes of acute dyspnea, because many are life-threatening (Table 23-2).

HOT KEY Most patients with acute onset of dyspnea should be referred immediately to an emergency department. The only exceptions are those patients with mild asthma or COPD exacerbations. Occasionally, these patients can be evaluated and treated in the clinic.

TABLE 23-1. Common Causes of Subacute and Chronic Dyspnea	
General Cause	**Specific Disorders**
Pulmonary Disorders	Asthma
	COPD
	Interstitial lung disease (e.g., idiopathic pulmonary fibrosis)
	Pneumonia (primarily caused by an atypical bacterial pathogen, *Mycobacterium tuberculosis*, fungi, or *Pneumocystis carinii*)
	Chronic pulmonary embolism
Cardiac disorders	CHF
	Myocardial ischemia
	Paroxysmal arrythmias
Physiologic conditions	Pregnancy
Metabolic or endocrine disorders	Obesity
	Thyrotoxicosis
Neuromuscular disorders	ALS
	Guillain-Barré syndrome
	Myasthenia gravis
	Severe kyphoscoliosis
Hematologic disorders	Anemia
Psychiatric disorders	Anxiety disorder

ALS = amyotrophic lateral sclerosis; CHF = congestive hear failure; COPD = chronic obstructive pulmonary disease

III APPROACH TO THE PATIENT

HOT KEY When a patient reports a history of dyspnea, a full evaluation is required, even if the patient is not obviously in respiratory distress.

A. Patient history. It is crucial to obtain a complete and detailed history. Be sure to investigate the following:
1. The duration of the dyspnea
2. Exacerbating and alleviating factors
3. Associated symptoms (e.g., chest pain, palpitations, weight loss)
4. The patient's medical history, smoking history, and travel history

TABLE 23-2. Common Causes of Acute Dyspnea	
General Causes	**Specific Disorders**
Pulmonary disorders	Asthma
	COPD
	Pneumonia (usually caused by a typical bacterial pathogen)
	Pulmonary embolism
	Pneumothorax
	Upper airway obstruction
	Aspiration
Cardiac disorders	CHF
	Myocardial infarction
	Myocardial ischemia
	Arrhythmias
	Pericardial tamponade
Metabolic disorders	Sepsis
	Metabolic acidosis
Hematologic disorders	Anemia
Psychiatric disorders	Anxiety disorder
	Panic attack

CHF = congestive heart failure; COPD = chronic obstructive pulmonary disease.

B. Physical examination must also be thorough and should include:
   1. **Vital signs,** including the oxygen saturation
   2. **Lungs.** Are wheezing, rales, or rhonchi present?
   3. **Heart.** Is the jugular venous pressure elevated? Is the point of maximal impulse (PMI) displaced? Can a third heart sound (S_3) or pathologic murmur be detected?
   4. **Neuromuscular system.** Does the patient have obvious weakness or kyphoscoliosis?
   5. **Extremities.** Is there any evidence of clubbing, edema, or cyanosis?
C. Laboratory studies
   1. The following studies should be obtained for most patients with dyspnea:
      a. Chemistry panel including blood urea nitrogen and creatinine level
      b. Complete blood count (CBC)
      c. Chest radiograph
      d. Electrocardiogram (EKG)
   2. The following tests should be considered, depending on the suspected cause of the dyspnea.

a. Pulmonary function tests (PFTs)—obstructive patterns suggest asthma or COPD while restrictive patterns suggest interstitial lung disease.

b. Blood gases—low arterial oxygen concentrations may indicate poor diffusion and damage to lung tissue from COPD or interstital lung disease.

c. Echocardiogram—may show poor contractile function or impaired diastolic relaxation in CHF, regional wall motion abnormalities in ischemic heart disease, or impaired valvular function.

d. Exercise stress testing—may reveal EKG abnormalities in ischemic heart disease.

e. Chest high-resolution computed tomography (HRCT) scan is useful for evaluating the extent of COPD and interstitial lung disease.

f. Brain natriuretic peptide (BNP)—elevated values suggest CHF.

IV THERAPY DEPENDS ON THE UNDERLYING DISORDER

HOT KEY

This is an appropriate time to counsel patients who smoke about health concerns associated with smoking.

V FOLLOW-UP AND REFERRAL

A. **Follow-up.** Initially, patients should be seen in clinic frequently (i.e., **approximately weekly**) until the cause of the dyspnea is diagnosed. During follow-up visits, smoking cessation counseling should be repeated.

B. **Referral.** When a clear cause cannot be determined, consultation with a **pulmonologist** is often appropriate.

References

Karnani NG, Reisfield GM, Wilson GR. Evaluation of chronic dyspnea. *Am Fam Physician* 2005;71(8):1529–1537.

Mahler DA, Fierro-Carrion G, Baird JC. Evaluation of dyspnea in the elderly. *Clin Geriatr Med* 2003;19(1):19–33.

24. Asthma

I. INTRODUCTION

A. Asthma is an **obstructive lung disease** that is most common in children and young adults. Patients generally present with a history of **episodic shortness of breath, chest tightness,** and **wheezing,** often in response to specific stimuli (e.g., exercise, cold air, pollution, allergens).

1. **Asthma has three major components:**
   a. **Airway hyperresponsiveness** to various stimuli
   b. **Airway inflammation**
   c. **Airway obstruction** that is reversible
2. **There are two patterns**
   a. **Acute attacks** usually occur within minutes to hours of exposure to an inhaled stimulus (e.g., pollen, dust, fumes, cold) an ingestion (e.g. aspirin, sulfites), or exercise.
   b. **Subacute attacks** develop over hours to days and are most often caused by viral respiratory infections.

B. Currently, in the United States, asthma affects **3%–5% of the population,** and the morbidity and mortality attributable to the disease is increasing.

II. DIFFERENTIAL DIAGNOSIS

A. Acute shortness of breath. The differential diagnosis for acute shortness of breath is broad, but can be simplified by considering five major categories of disease (see Chapter 23, Table 23-2).

B. Chronic shortness of breath (See Chapter 26, Table 26-1). Remember, **not all that wheezes is asthma.** Patients with apparent chronic asthma may have another condition that causes wheezing, and a physician who "CARES" will consider these alternate diagnoses.

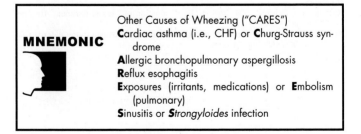

MNEMONIC

Other Causes of Wheezing ("CARES")
Cardiac asthma (i.e., CHF) or **C**hurg-Strauss syndrome
Allergic bronchopulmonary aspergillosis
Reflux esophagitis
Exposures (irritants, medications) or **E**mbolism (pulmonary)
Sinusitis or *Strongyloides* infection

III APPROACH TO THE PATIENT

A. Acute attack. Patients with a moderate to severe attack of asthma should be evaluated in an emergency setting where cardiopulmonary resuscitation (CPR) is readily available.

1. **Patient history.** It is always useful to ask the patient how severe the attack is in comparison with others he has had. Be sure to make the following inquiries:

    a. What is the **time course** of the current attack?

    b. Are there any **known triggers?**

    c. What has been the **frequency** and **severity of past attacks** (e.g., was the patient ever intubated, hospitalized or on oral steroids)?

    d. What **medications** is the patient using?

    e. What is the **peak flow** and how does it compare to baseline measurements?

2. **Physical examination.** Findings vary depending on the severity of the attack, but patients with more severe attacks may have more of the following signs. Importantly, as many as half of patients with severe attacks will have none of these signs:

    a. Tachypnea

    b. Use of the accessory muscles

    c. Intercostal retraction

    d. Wheezing

    e. A prolonged inspiratory-to-expiratory (I:E) ratio

    f. Hyperresonance

    g. Pulsus paradoxus (a fall of systolic blood pressure by >12 mm Hg during inspiration)

3. **Additional studies**

    a. **Pulmonary function tests (PFTs).** Obtain an initial **peak flow** or **forced expiratory volume in 1 second (FEV_1)** as an objective measure of disease severity. This baseline measurement will also enable you to evaluate the patient's response to acute treatment.

    b. A **chest radiograph** should be obtained for most patients with moderate to severe attacks.

    c. **Laboratory studies** are generally not necessary, unless another cause of dyspnea is suspected.

B. Chronic asthma

1. **Patient history.** Inquire about the following:

    a. **History of attacks**

    b. **Triggers**

    c. **Nocturnal symptoms** (wheezing or shortness of breath at night may indicate a trigger, such as cold temperatures or reflux disease, or suggest that current medications are inadequate)

    d. **Medication use**

2. Physical examination. Findings vary, depending on current disease activity. Wheezing, a prolonged I:E ratio, and hyperresonance may be present if the patient is experiencing a mild exacerbation, or if medications are inadequate.

3. Additional studies

    a. Spirometry and **bronchial provocation testing** are useful for diagnosis and monitoring of disease progression. A positive test is defined by a 20% reduction in the FEV_1 in response to methacholine, histamine, hypertonic saline, or other stimulants.

    b. A **chest radiograph** is generally not required for patients younger than 40 years.

    c. Laboratory studies are rarely useful.

IV TREATMENT

A. Acute treatment. Treatment considerations for a patient with an acute asthma attack can be remembered using the mnemonic, "ASTHMA."

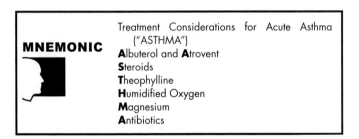

MNEMONIC

Treatment Considerations for Acute Asthma ("ASTHMA")

Albuterol and **A**trovent
Steroids
Theophylline
Humidified Oxygen
Magnesium
Antibiotics

1. Albuterol and **ipratropium bromide (Atrovent)** are both effective **bronchodilators** and are the mainstay of the acute treatment of asthma.

    a. Albuterol (2.5 mg by continuous flow nebulization for 20 minutes, repeating up to three doses) should be the initial treatment in most patients.

    b. Ipratropium bromide (500 mcg by nebulization every twenty minutes, repeating up to three doses) is also recommended by some authorities as a useful adjunct.

2. Steroids. Most patients with an acute attack should be treated with a steroid taper (e.g., prednisone, 3 days each of 60 mg, 40 mg, and 20 mg) to prevent the development of a delayed inflammatory response.

3. Theophylline. The use of theophylline in acute exacerbations of asthma is controversial and rarely used.

4. **Humidified oxygen** should be administered to any patient with moderate to severe shortness of breath until symptoms are controlled.

5. **Magnesium.** The intravenous administration of magnesium is seldom used, but is advocated by some for pediatric patients with severe attacks.

6. **Antibiotics** are generally not indicated for asthma exacerbations because most attacks are caused by allergens or viral infections.

HOT KEY Patients who do not respond rapidly to pharmacologic therapy and those with significant respiratory distress at presentation should be hospitalized for observation. Patients who are not hospitalized should have close home monitoring with a clear plan for return if symptoms worsen.

HOT KEY The peak flow meter is a simple and inexpensive test that can be used both in the emergency department and in the home (after patient instruction) to monitor the severity of attacks and response to treatment. Patients should learn their own peak flow readings when they are doing well and when they are having attacks. Normal values differ with gender, height, and age, but readings less than 200 L/min almost always indicate a severe attack.

B. Chronic treatment

1. **Pharmacologic agents** commonly used for the ongoing treatment of asthma are shown in Table 24-1.

   a. **β agonists.** Therapy should be initiated with a β agonist (e.g., **albuterol)** for patients with mild, intermittent symptoms. Patients with symptoms on more than two days per week (also known as mild, persistent symptoms) or with abnormal pulmonary function tests should be started on inhaled steroids.

HOT KEY Patients with mild asthma who require more than 4 doses per week of a β agonist should begin treatment with inhaled steroids.

   b. **Inhaled steroids** (e.g., **triamcinolone acetonide**) are now considered the treatment of choice in all patients with

TABLE 24-1. Medications for the Chronic Treatment of Asthma		
Class of Drug	**Examples**	**Dose**
β Agonists	Albuterol	2 puffs every 4–6 hours as required
Inhaled steroids	Budesonide	1–2 puffs twice daily (200 μg/puff)
Long-acting β agonists	Salmeterol	2 puffs twice daily
Inhibitors of histamine release	Nedocromil	2 puffs four times daily
Methylxanthines	Theophylline	100–300 mg orally twice daily
Leukotriene antagonists	Zafirlukast	20 mg twice daily

persistent asthma because they reduce morbidity and mortality. Low to medium doses of agents generally provide maximum benefit while reducing the chance of systemic toxicity (e.g., Budesonide 200 mcg twice a day). Patients with persistent symptoms on low to medium dose inhaled steroids should be considered for long-acting β-agonist therapy.

c. **Long-acting β agonists** (e.g., **salmeterol**) provide consistent drug levels and should be considered for patients with persistent symptoms on low to medium dose inhaled steroids.

HOT

▶ Long-acting β agonists cannot be used for acute attacks because they can accumulate, causing toxicity.

KEY

---

d. **Nedocromil,** which is believed to stabilize mast cells, may be useful for prophylaxis prior to animal exposure or exercise.

e. **Theophylline** may be useful in patients with nocturnal symptoms, but is less often used due to frequent side effect profile.

f. **Leukotriene antagonists** are a newer class of medications for asthma that are designed to reduce the inflammatory response by interfering with leukotriene production or binding to cell receptors. **Zafirlukast** (20 mg twice daily) has been shown to improve both symptom scores and objective measures in patients with chronic asthma. It can be considered for use in patients on low-dose inhaled steroids who continue to have symptoms, as an alternative to long-acting β-agonists.

2. Inhaler use. One of the most common causes of inadequate therapy is poor technique when using an inhaler. Patients should be instructed to:

   a. Use a spacer
   b. Shake the canister and exhale completely
   c. Activate the canister and inhale slowly
   d. Hold their breath for 5–10 seconds

3. Monitoring. Patients should be given a peak flow meter and advised to call when their baseline peak flow is worsening (signaling the onset of an attack).

V Follow-up and Referral

A. Patients who have had an acute attack treated in an urgent care setting should be **re-evaluated in 1–5 days.** Those who experience a near-fatal asthma attack are at very high risk for short-term mortality and should be evaluated by a specialist and seen regularly to monitor symptoms.

B. Specialized asthma treatment centers are available and should be considered for patients with difficult to control or severe symptoms.

References

Currie GP, Devereux GS, Lee DK, Ayres JG. Recent developments in asthma management. *BMJ* 2005;330(7491):585–589.

Naureckas ET, Solway J. Clinical practice. Mild asthma. *N Engl J Med* 2001;345(17): 1257–1262.

O'Byrne PM. Related Articles, Pharmacologic interventions to reduce the risk of asthma exacerbations. *Proc Am Thorac Soc* 2004;1(2):105–108.

25. Chronic Obstructive Pulmonary Disease

....

▮ I INTRODUCTION

A. Chronic obstructive pulmonary disease (COPD) is a syndrome characterized by **airflow limitation** that is **not fully reversible.** The limitation in airflow is usually progressive and associated with airway inflammation due to noxious particles or gases. Underlying causes include chronic bronchitis and emphysema; most patients have a combination of both disorders.

    1. Chronic bronchitis is defined as the presence of a cough with sputum production for at least 3 months of the year in 2 consecutive years.

    2. Emphysema is defined pathologically as permanent enlargement of the airspaces distal to the terminal bronchioles and destruction of bronchial walls without fibrosis.

B. Most patients with COPD present in the **fifth to sixth decades** of life, have a **smoking history,** and report some combination of **dyspnea, chronic cough, sputum production,** and **wheezing.**

C. COPD affects more than 15 million Americans and is the **fourth leading cause of death in the United States.**

▮ II DIFFERENTIAL DIAGNOSIS

A. Asthma is differentiated from COPD on the basis of a reversible airway obstruction. This is suggested by the history and confirmed by spirometric improvement in airflow with administration of bronchodilators. Asthma patients often present at a younger age than patients with COPD.

B. Bronchiectasis should be suspected if there is a history of chronic productive cough, frequent pneumonia, and hemoptysis.

C. Cystic fibrosis is an inherited disorder causing chronic productive cough and dyspnea in childhood or early adulthood.

D. Central airway obstruction can be caused by any process that narrows the large central airways (e.g., subglottic stenosis, laryngeal carcinoma). Patients may present with progressive dyspnea. The obstruction can be distinguished from COPD on the basis of spirometry.

E. Congestive Heart Failure (CHF) can be a cause of chronic dyspnea. It is differentaited from COPD based on **spirometry, echocardiography** and **brain natriuretic peptide (BNP)** level. BNP is a hormone released from both the brain (where it was initially discovered) and also from myocardial cells in response to stress, as in CHF.

F. α_1**-Antitrypsin deficiency** is an inherited enzyme deficiency. It should be suspected in patients with severe, early onset COPD without an extensive smoking history.

III APPROACH TO THE PATIENT

A. Initial diagnosis

1. **Patient history.** Answers to the following questions should be sought.

   a. What is the **timing** and **severity** of the **dyspnea** and **cough?**

   b. What is the patient's **smoking history?**

   c. What is the patient's **environmental exposure to pollutants** or **second-hand smoke?**

   d. Is there a **family history of pulmonary disease?**

2. **Physical examination**

   a. Examination of the lungs may reveal **decreased breath sounds,** a **prolonged inspiratory-to-expiratory (I:E) ratio, wheezing,** and **rhonchi.**

   b. Patients with moderate to severe disease may exhibit an increased anteroposterior chest diameter **("barrel chest"), clubbing,** or **central cyanosis.**

3. **Other studies**

   a. A **chest radiograph** is indicated for most patients with suspected COPD. Findings may include **hyperinflation, parenchymal bullae,** and an **enlarged pulmonary artery** (suggestive of pulmonary hypertension).

   b. **Spirometry** is indicated for most patients with suspected COPD. The diagnosis of COPD is suggested by a low **forced expiratory volume in 1 second (FEV$_1$)** and a low **FEV$_1$%.**

HOT KEY In a patient who smokes, has a history, physical, and radiographic findings consistent with COPD, spirometry showing an FEV$_1$ less than 80% predicted or FEV$_1$% less than 70% after bronchodilators confirms a diagnosis of COPD.

---

   c. **Laboratory studies**

      (1) A **complete blood count (CBC)** may show **polycythemia** as a result of chronic hypoxemia.

    (2) **Arterial blood gases (ABGs)** are often useful for determining the **degree of hypoxemia** and **hypercarbia.**

    (3) An α_1-antitrypsin level is indicated for patients with COPD and no history of smoking, and for those who present with the disease at an early age.

B. Acute exacerbations of COPD are common. Most episodes are thought to be caused by **viral infection,** but **bacterial infection** and **inhaled irritants** may also play a role.

HOT
KEY

All patients with COPD should receive a flu vaccination annually and a pneumococcal vaccination every 5–10 years. In addition, they should minimize their exposure to air pollutants, second-hand smoke, and particulate matter.

---

    1. Patients present with an **increase in cough, worsening dyspnea,** or a **change in the color or quantity of sputum.**

    2. Patients with COPD are at risk for a number of other conditions that may cause acute shortness of breath [e.g., pneumonia, pneumothorax, cardiac ischemia, congestive heart failure (CHF), medication side effect]. Always perform a thorough history and physical and **consider all possible causes of shortness of breath in these patients.**

THERAPY

A. Chronic therapy

    1. Smoking cessation has been shown to slow the progression of COPD and is the most important aspect of prevention. Patients with COPD who smoke should be enrolled in a smoking cessation program.

HOT
KEY

Smoking cessation is the single most effective and cost efficient way to slow the progression of COPD.

---

    2. Oxygen therapy. Long-term oxygen therapy has been shown to improve survival and should be considered in patients with either a resting arterial oxygen tension (Pao_2) of less than 55 mm Hg or a resting Pao_2 of 55–59 mm Hg with clinical evidence of cor pulmonale or secondary erythrocytosis.

TABLE 25-1. Agents Used in the Treatment of Chronic Obstructive Pulmonary Disease (COPD)

Drug Class	Examples	Dose	Side Effects and Cautions
Anticholinergics	Ipratropium metered-dose inhaler	4–6 puffs, four times daily	Minimal side effects
β Agonists	Albuterol metered-dose inhaler	2–4 puffs every 4–6 hours* as needed	May cause tremor, agitation, and tachycardia; use with caution in patients with heart disease
Methylxanthines	Theophylline	100–300 mg twice daily†; monitor serum drug levels for range of 8–12 μg/ml	Multipe drugs interact with theophylline
Corticosteroids	Triamcinolane acetonide	2–10 puffs twice daily	Refer to pulmonologist before initiating oral steroids; consider spirometry before and after initiating oral steroids to monitor effect

*Longer-acting agents are available.
†Once-a-day dosing is available.

    3. Pharmacologic therapy. Agents should be used in the order in which they are presented in Table 25-1; add the next medication if the patient remains symptomatic.

B. Acute exacerbations. There are three main treatments that should be considered for patients with acute exacerbations of COPD.

1. **Inhalers.** Both inhaled β agonists and ipratropium are effective in improving symptoms and spirometric measurements. When used properly, metered-dose inhalers are as effective as nebulizers.

2. **Corticosteroids.** Although the role of corticosteroids in the treatment of COPD is controversial, steroid tapers (e.g., prednisone, 3 days each of 60 mg, 40 mg, and 20 mg) appear to be effective in reducing symptoms. Longer tapers may be appropriate for patients with severe disease.

3. **Antibiotics** (e.g. Doxycycline 100 mg bid for 5–10 days) for common respiratory pathogens in patients with increased sputum purulence and volume are likely beneficial.

HOT
▶
KEY

Hospitalization should be considered for all patients with moderate to severe symptoms, hypoxia, or hypercarbia.

V FOLLOW-UP AND REFERRAL

A. **Follow-up.** Stable patients should be seen **every 3–4 months** to monitor symptoms and adjust medications. **Annual spirometry** can be considered to document disease progression, and may help motivate the patient's efforts to stop smoking.

B. **Referral.** Patients with **symptoms that cannot be controlled,** those who require **frequent oral steroids for control,** and those who have α_1**-antitrypsin deficiency** should be referred to a pulmonologist for evaluation.

References

Global Initiative for Chronic Obstructive Lung Disease, Global Strategy for the diagnosis, management and prevention of chronic obstructive pulmonary disease, Executive summary updated 2005.

Sutherland EF, Cherniack RM. Management of chronic obstructive pulmonary disease. *N Engl J Med* 2004;350(26):2689–2697.

26. Pulmonary Function Tests

....

I. INTRODUCTION

A. **Background.** Pulmonary function tests (PFTs) usually evaluate three areas: **expiratory flow rate** (spirometry), **lung volumes,** and **diffusion capacity** (Table 26-1)
B. **Applications.** PFTs can be used to:
   1. Distinguish obstructive lung disease from restrictive lung disease (Table 26-2)
   2. Assess the severity of lung disease
   3. Evaluate the patient's response to therapy

II. OBSTRUCTIVE VERSUS RESTRICTIVE LUNG DISEASE

A. **Flow rate = lung volume/(resistance)(compliance).** The following conclusions can be drawn from examining this equation:
   1. The **flow rate** (as **measured by the forced expiratory volume in one second, or FEV_1) will decrease under any of the following conditions:**
      a. The lung volume decreases (as seen in restrictive disorders)
      b. The resistance increases (as seen in asthma and chronic bronchitis)
      c. The compliance increases (as seen in emphysema)
   2. Therefore, the **flow rate will be decreased in both restrictive and obstructive lung diseases,** and looking at the FEV_1 alone will not enable you to distinguish between these two types of disorders.
B. **FEV_1% = FEV_1/(forced vital capacity, or FVC).** In order to distinguish between obstructive and restrictive lung disorders, the lung volume must be removed from the equation. Dividing by the FVC will accomplish this goal.

III. QUICK APPROACH TO THE INTERPRETATION OF PULMONARY FUNCTION TESTS (PFTs). Interpreting PFTs requires a systematic approach (Figure 26-1).

HOT
▶
KEY

When interpreting PFTs, it is important to note both the observed values and the percent of predicted values.

TABLE 26-1. Abbreviations Associated with Pulmonary Function Tests (PFTs)

Abbreviation	Meaning
Expiratory flow rate	
FEV_1	Forced expiratory volume in 1 second
FVC	Forced vital capacity
$FEV_1\%$	Ratio of the FEV_1 to the FVC
Lung volume	
TLC	Total lung capacity
VC	Vital capacity
RV	Residual volume
Diffusing capacity	
D_{LCO}	Diffusing capacity of the lungs for carbon dioxide

A. **First, look at the FEV_1.**
B. **If the FEV_1 is low, look at the $FEV_1\%$.**
   1. **Obstructive disease.** Both the FEV_1 and the $FEV_1\%$ will be **decreased.**
   2. **Restrictive disease.** The FEV_1 will be **decreased** but the $FEV_1\%$ will be **normal** (or increased). A low TLC supports the diagnosis of a restrictive lung disorder.

TABLE 26-2. Common Diseases Leading to Abnormal Findings on Pulmonary Function Tests (PFTs)

Obstructive disorders
  Asthma
  Chronic obstructive pulmonary disease (COPD)
  Bronchiectasis
  Cystic fibrosis

Restrictive disorders
  Pleural fibrosis or effusion
  Alveolar edema or inflammation
  Interstitial disorders (e.g., sarcoidosis, idiopathic pulmonary
    fibrosis, fungal infection)
  Neuromuscular disorders (e.g., myasthenia gravis, myopathy)
  Thoracic or extrathoracic disorders (e.g., kyphoscoliosis,
    pregnancy, obesity)

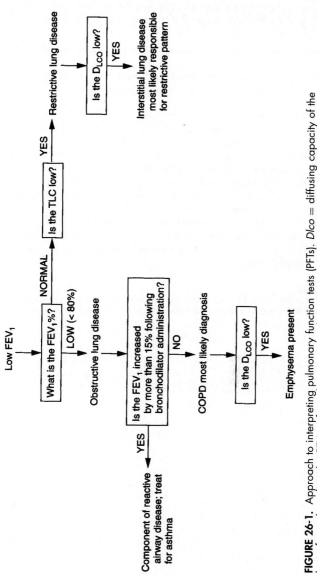

FIGURE 26-1. Approach to interpreting pulmonary function tests (PFTs). D_{LCO} = diffusing capacity of the lungs for carbon dioxide; FEV_1 = forced expiratory volume in 1 second; $FEV_1\%$ = ratio of the FEV_1 to the forced vital capacity (FVC); TLC = total lung capacity.

HOT KEY The incidence of postoperative complications tends to increase if the FEV₁ is less than 2.0 L/sec and the FEV₁% is less than 50%.

C. **If the patient has obstructive lung disease, determine if the obstruction is reversible** by administering bronchodilators and re-evaluating the FEV₁.
   1. **Improvement** of the FEV₁ by more than 12% following bronchodilator administration implies reversible airway obstruction (i.e., **asthma**).
   2. If there is **no improvement,** the patient probably has **chronic obstructive pulmonary disease (COPD).**
D. **Look at the D$_{LCO}$.** A decreased D$_{LCO}$ is seen whenever there is an inability to transfer gas across the alveolar–capillary interface.
   1. If the patient has **restrictive disease,** a low D$_{LCO}$ implies that **interstitial lung disease** is the cause of the restrictive pattern.
   2. If the patient has **obstructive lung disease,** a low D$_{LCO}$ implies **emphysema.**

Reference
Al-Ashkar F, Mehra R, Mazzone PJ. Interpreting pulmonary functions test: recognize the pattern, and the diagnosis will follow. *Clev Clin J Med* 2003;70:866–873.

27. Acute Bronchitis

I INTRODUCTION

A. Acute bronchitis is the **acute onset of cough** and **sputum production** in a patient with **no history of chronic pulmonary disease** and **no evidence of pneumonia or sinusitis.**
   1. **Sputum production** is the **hallmark** of the disorder.
   2. Fever may or may not be present.
B. Acute bronchitis **accounts for more than 10 million annual office visits** in the United States; direct costs are in the hundreds of millions of dollars.

II CAUSES OF ACUTE BRONCHITIS

A. **Viral infections** cause **most cases** of acute bronchitis.
B. **Atypical bacteria** (e.g., *Mycoplasma pneumoniae, Chlamydia pneumoniae, Legionella*) may cause as many as **10% of cases.**
C. **Typical bacteria** (e.g., *Streptococcus pneumoniae, Haemophilus influenzae*) are rarely involved.
D. **Allergic reactions** and **air pollutants** may be responsible for some cases.

III DIFFERENTIAL DIAGNOSIS

A. **Acute, productive cough.** Acute bronchitis must be distinguished from the other common causes of an acute productive cough in otherwise healthy individuals: **pneumonia** and **sinusitis** (in sinusitis, the cough is stimulated by postnasal drip).
B. **Nonproductive cough.** Acute bronchitis must also be distinguished from the many causes of a nonproductive cough in healthy patients, including **upper respiratory tract infections, asthma,** GERD and post-nasal drip.

IV APPROACH TO THE PATIENT

A. **Patient history.** Focus on three questions:
   1. **Is the cough productive?** If not, consider upper respiratory tract infections and other causes of nonproductive cough.
   2. **Does the patient have a history of pulmonary disease?** A history of asthma, chronic obstructive pulmonary disease (COPD), or another pulmonary disorder suggests an exacerbation of the underlying condition.

3. How severe are the symptoms?
  a. A productive cough accompanied by fever, shortness of breath, or pleuritic pain suggests pneumonia.
  b. Sinus pain and purulent nasal discharge in combination with fever suggests sinusitis.
B. Physical examination. The examination should be focused to exclude pneumonia and sinusitis.
  1. Pneumonia is suggested by focal crackles or bronchial breath sounds.
  2. Sinusitis is suggested by fever, purulent nasal discharge, and pain with palpation of sinuses.
C. Imaging studies
  1. A **chest radiograph** is usually indicated for patients with abnormal findings on lung examination or abnormal vitals.
  2. A **sinus computed tomography (CT) scan** is occasionally necessary to rule out sinusitis.
D. Laboratory studies [e.g., a complete blood count (CBC), sputum Gram stain or culture] are usually not necessary.

 V   TREATMENT. Symptoms should improve gradually over 1–2 weeks.

> **HOT KEY**
> Antibiotics for the treatment of acute bronchitis in healthy adults is not recommended and is one the most common causes of antibiotic overuse.

A. Cough suppressants, throat lozenges, and **decongestants** may relieve symptoms but have not been shown to alter the course of the illness.
B. Antiviral medications, oseltamivir or **amantadine,** may benefit patients with acute bronchitis due to **influenza** infection if given within the first 48 hours of illness, and are typically only given in known disease outbreaks.
C. Antibiotics for pertussis infection is recommended when there is a strong clinical suspicion of pertussis, based on prolonged paroxysms of cough (> 2 weeks), inspiratory "whooping" sound, post-tussive emesis, or known disease outbreak. Confirmatory testing with nasopharyngeal bacterial culture or PCR is useful, though clinical availability of these tests is limited. Patients should be treated with azithromycin for 3 days or clarithromycin for 7 days, and they should avoid contact with children and infants for 5 days after initiating treatment.

VI **FOLLOW-UP AND REFERRAL.** Otherwise healthy patients do not need to have scheduled follow-up, unless their symptoms do not improve within 3 weeks.

References

Aagaard E, Gonzales R. Management of acute bronchitis in healthy adults. *Infect Dis Clin North Am* 2004;18(4):919–937.

Braman SS. Chronic cough due to acute bronchitis: ACCP evidence-based clinical practice guidelines. *Chest* 2006;129(1 Suppl):95S–103S.

28. Community-Acquired Pneumonia

I INTRODUCTION

A. Community-acquired pneumonia is a **leading cause of death** and the **number one cause of infectious disease–related mortality in the United States.**

B. Approximately **80% of patients** with community-acquired pneumonia **are treated entirely as outpatients.**

II CLINICAL MANIFESTATIONS OF COMMUNITY ACQUIRED PNEUMONIA.

Community-acquired pneumonia may be classified as "typical" or "atypical" on the basis of the causative organism. Practitioners often attempt to classify community-acquired pneumonia as "typical" or "atypical" on the basis of the patient's signs and symptoms; however, this approach may only partially predict the underlying pathogen and has fallen out of favor.

A. **Typical community-acquired pneumonia**
   1. **Symptoms** commonly include subjective fever, cough, sputum production, pleuritic chest pain, and dyspnea.
   2. **Signs** commonly include fever, tachypnea (> 20 respirations/min), and signs of lobar consolidation (bronchial breath sounds, egophony, dullness to percussion, crackles).

B. **Atypical community-acquired pneumonia** classically is characterized by the **gradual onset of disease,** a **dry cough** (or cough productive of only scant sputum), and **prominent extrapulmonary symptoms** (e.g., headache, myalgia, diarrhea, hepatosplenomegaly, elevated aminotransferase levels). However, "atypical" organsims can presents with clinical syptoms of "typical" pneumonia.

III CAUSES OF COMMUNITY-ACQUIRED PNEUMONIA

A. **Typical community-acquired pneumonia** is usually caused by *Streptococcus pneumoniae, Haemophilus influenzae, Staphylococcus aureus,* or Gram-negative bacilli (e.g., *Klebsiella*).
   1. *S. pneumoniae* is one of the most common organisms responsible for community-acquired pneumonia.

HOT KEY Usually, pneumococcal pneumonia presents abruptly; however, an indolent presentation is common when pneumococcal disease follows a viral respiratory tract infection.

2. *H. influenzae* is an especially common cause of community-acquired pneumonia in patients with **chronic obstructive pulmonary disease (COPD).**

3. *S. aureus* infection may be seen in patients who have **influenza,** are **immunocompromised,** or live in **nursing homes.**

4. **Aerobic Gram-negative rods.** Infection caused by aerobic Gram-negative rods is more common in **patients older than 60 years** and in **alcoholic patients.**

B. **Atypical community-acquired pneumonia** is usually caused by *Mycoplasma pneumoniae, Chlamydia pneumoniae, Legionella pneumophila,* or *Moraxella catarrhalis.*

1. *M. pneumoniae* usually causes a **mild pneumonia** in adults. *M. pneumoniae* infection has been associated with even more **prominent extrapulmonary involvement** than other atypical causes of community-acquired pneumonia, including **hemolytic anemia, erythema multiforme, myocarditis, erythema nodosum, bullous myringitis,** and **several neurologic abnormalities.**

2. *C. pneumoniae* also usually causes a **mild pneumonia.** Although the clinical manifestations are generally similar to those of other causes of atypical pneumonia, **hoarseness with severe pharyngitis** is considered a distinguishing feature of pneumonia caused by *C. pneumoniae.*

HOT KEY *M. pneumoniae* and *C. pneumoniae* together account for 25% of all cases of community-acquired pneumonia managed by primary care providers.

3. *Legionella* species can cause **severe pneumonia. Gram-staining** usually reveals **numerous polymorphonuclear neutrophils (PMNs) but no organisms.** *Legionella* **urinary antigen testing is positive in the majority of cases.**

4. *M. catarrhalis, Mycobacterium tuberculosis, Pneumocystis carinii,* respiratory **viruses** (e.g., influenza virus) and **fungi** can also cause an atypical community-acquired pneumonia.

IV APPROACH TO THE PATIENT

HOT KEY

The causative organism is identified in less than 50% of community acquired pneumonia cases.

A. Diagnostic tests

1. **Chest radiograph.** Posterior-anterior (PA) and lateral views are indicated for most patients with suspected community-acquired pneumonia. In young, otherwise healthy patients who will be treated as outpatients, a chest radiograph may be all that is needed for patient evaluation.

HOT KEY

Chest radiographs cannot distinguish between pneumonia due to "atypical" or "typical" organisms.

2. **Laboratory studies.** The following tests may be appropriate for some patients:
   a. **Complete blood count (CBC)**
   b. **Serum electrolyte panel**
   c. **Blood urea nitrogen (BUN)** and **creatinine levels**
   d. **Peripheral blood cultures,** on samples drawn from two separate sites
   e. **Arterial blood gases (ABGs),** especially appropriate if the room air oxygen saturation is <92%
   f. **Sputum analysis**
      (1) Gram-staining and culture of even a properly expectorated sputum sample may not yield the responsible organism; therefore, it is reasonable to omit this test if it cannot be readily obtained.
      (2) If *M. tuberculosis* or *P. carinii* infection is suspected, sputum analysis using special stains should always be done.
   g. **Influenza DFA** during the correct season may be helpful and can guide antiviral treatment.
   h. **Thoracentesis.** If a pleural effusion is present and the patient has clinical evidence of empyema (e.g., hypotension, toxic appearance), thoracentesis should be performed promptly and the pleural fluid should be sent for a cell

count and differential, Gram staining, culture, total protein, lactate dehydrogenase (LDH), glucose, pH, and if indicated acid-fast stain and culture for fungi and mycobacteria.

B. Criteria for hospital admission. There are no absolute criteria for hospital admission, but specific factors place the patient at greater risk for a complicated clinical course, mortality, or both. The following mnemonic can help you remember some of the most important criteria for admitting a patient: "ADMIT NOW." Several prediction rules, including the pneumonia severity index (PSI), can aid in predicting mortality and the need for admission.

MNEMONIC

Criteria for Hospital Admission of Patients with Community-Acquired Pneumonia ("ADMIT NOW")

Age > 65 years (depending on individual situation)

Decreased immunity (e.g., cancer, diabetes, AIDS, splenectomy, COPD)

Mental status changes

Increased A-a gradient or increased respiratory rate

Two or more lobes involved

No home (i.e., homeless patients)

Organ system failure (increased creatinine, bone marrow suppression, systolic blood pressure $\leq$ 90 mm Hg, liver failure, CHF)

WBC count greater than 30,000/mm^3 or less than 4000/ mm^3

In general, if a patient meets more than one of these criteria, hospitalization is reasonable. Sometimes the most important criterion is the **"eyeball" test** (i.e., how sick a person looks to an experienced physician).

V TREATMENT. When a patient does not meet the criteria for hospital admission and has passed the "eyeball" test, **outpatient management** is usually indicated.

A. Empiric therapy. Patients should be treated with a first-line agent unless they have been exposed to one of these antibiotics in the last three months (in which case they are at higher risk for resistant organisms, and should be given a second-line agent). Dosages in Table 28-1.

TABLE 28-1. Dosages for First- and Second-Line Agents Used Empirically in the Outpatient Treatment of Community-Acquired Pneumonia

Agent	Dose
Clarithromycin	500 mg orally, twice daily for 10–14 days
Azithromycin	500 mg orally on the first day, 250 mg orally daily on days 2–5
Doxycycline	100 mg orally, twice daily for 10–14 days
Levofloxacin	750 mg daily for 7–10 days

1. **First-line agents:**
   a. An advanced generation macrolide **(azithromycin or clarithromycin)** covers both "typical" and "atypical" organisms. **Doxycycline** is a reasonable alternative if patients are intolerant or allergic to macrolides. **Erythromycin** therapy has fallen out of favor due to frequency of dosing, stomach upset and QT prolongation.
2. **Second-line agents** for patients **with exposure to macrolides in the previous 3 months.**
   a. Anti-pneumoccocal quinolones **(levofloxacin, gatifloxacin, moxifloxacin)** provide broad-spectrum coverage for suspected pathogens and are dosed once a day. The combination of an **oral β-lactam (cefuroxime or amoxacillin/clavulanate)** with **doxycycline** or a **macrolide** is a reasonable alternative. β-lactams alone do not cover "atypical" organisms.
3. **Duration of therapy** typically ranges from 7–14 days. Recent evidence suggests that shorter therapy is as effective as longer therapy.

B. **Specific therapy.** If the causative organism is identified and the patient has not shown expected clinical improvement, antibiotic susceptibility testing should be done to direct further therapy.

VI FOLLOW-UP AND REFERRAL

A. **Follow-up**
   1. All patients treated in the ambulatory setting should be instructed to call if their symptoms worsen, dyspnea develops, or they are unable to continue taking medication orally.
   2. Most outpatients should experience subjective improvement and decreased fever within 2–4 days of initiating antibiotic therapy.

    a. Office follow-up within 4–7 days to assess response to treatment is reasonable in older patients and in those with comorbid conditions, such as COPD or diabetes.

    b. All patients who smoke or who used to smoke, and any patient with a lingering cough despite resolution of other symptoms should have a follow-up chest radiograph at 4–6 weeks.

  3. Immunizations against pneumococcus (every 5 years) and influenza (yearly) should be given to appropriately selected patients.

B. Referral. Consultation with a pulmonologist or an infectious disease specialist may be helpful for patients who do not respond to standard therapy or have severe symptoms. In general, however, most patients with community-acquired pneumonia can be adequately managed by primary care physicians.

References

Ewig S, de Roux A, Bauer T, et al. Validation of predictive rules and indices of severity for community acquired pneumonia. *Thorax* 2004;59(5):421–427.

Niederman MS. Review of treatment guidelines for community-acquired pneumonia. *Am J Med* 2004;117 Suppl 3A:51S–57S.

29. Solitary Pulmonary Nodule

I INTRODUCTION

A. Solitary pulmonary nodules are **asymptomatic, spherical densities** within the lung parenchyma discovered on chest radiographs or computed tomography (CT) scans.

B. These nodules are **relatively common,** occurring in approximately **one in every five hundred chest radiographs.** They present a problem for the primary care provider, because it is often difficult to determine whether the nodule is malignant or benign.

II DIFFERENTIAL DIAGNOSIS (TABLE 29-1)

A. Malignant tumors account for approximately 40% of all solitary pulmonary nodules. Most malignant solitary pulmonary nodules are **primary lung tumors.**

B. Non-malignant lesions. Most benign pulmonary nodules are **healed granulomas** caused by tuberculosis or fungal infections (e.g., histoplasmosis, coccidioidomycosis) or hamartomas.

III APPROACH TO THE PATIENT.
The goal of evaluation is to determine the likelihood of malignancy so that an informed decision can be made about the risks and benefits of surgery.

A. Patient history. Older patients and patients with a **history of smoking** are more likely to have malignant nodules.

B. Imaging studies
1. **Comparison of recent and old chest films** is a crucial part of the evaluation.
   a. **Growth rate.** If the nodule is present on an old film and has shown no growth for 500 days or more, then malignancy is unlikely. However, lesions that have shown growth, especially those with a volumetric doubling time of less than 500 days, are more likely to be malignant.
   b. **Nodule size** is also important. The likelihood of malignancy increases with size. Nodules greater than 3 cm have a greater than 80% chance of being malignant.
2. **Computed Tomography (CT).** All patients should have a chest CT scan to allow better evaluation of the nodule. CT characteristics that increase the likelihood of malignancy

TABLE 29-1. Differential Diagnosis of Solitary Pulmonary Nodule

Malignancy
  Primary lung tumor (e.g., bronchogenic carcinoma, carcinoid)
  Metastatic cancer

Non-malignant lesion
  Healed granuloma
  Hamartoma
  Arteriovenous malformation
  Rheumatoid nodule
  Pseudolymphoma
  Hydatid cyst
  Wegener's granulomatosis

include an **uncalcified nodule,** an **irregular (spiculated) border,** and a **nodular cavity with a thick wall.**

3. **Positron Emission Tomography** scanning can define the metabolic activity of nodules and is up to 95% sensitive for malignancy. PET positive lesions should be biopsied or excised.

IV TREATMENT

A. The treatment strategy depends on the likelihood of malignancy and the desires of the patient. Some patients may prefer to have nodules resected that have only a remote possibility of malignancy. Others, such as those with multiple medical problems, may be reluctant to undergo surgery because of the associated risks.

B. There are no precise "cutoffs" where the probability of malignancy dictates treatment strategy. The following treatment options should be discussed with each patient.

1. **Observation** entails obtaining serial chest radiographs over an extended period of time to see if the nodule is growing. Nodules that exhibit no growth or have a doubling time greater than 500 days are less likely to be malignant.

   a. Generally, this approach is not recommended unless the probability of malignancy is very low.

   b. Patients who have chosen the observation strategy should be followed in consultation with a pulmonologist.

2. **Biopsy** can be **transbronchial** (i.e., performed during bronchoscopy) or **transthoracic** (i.e., CT-guided).

   a. A positive diagnosis is helpful for ruling in cancer, but a negative biopsy does not rule out malignant disease.

      b. Transthoracic biopsy carries a risk of pneumothorax; transbronchial biopsy has a low yield but carries less risk of pneumothorax.

   3. Resection can be the first step for high risk nodules.

      a. Video-assisted thoracoscopy (VAT) with resection, has largely replaced thoracotmy for the management of peripheral nodules. It is less morbid than thoracotomy and can be used in place of fine needle aspiration (FNA) in many circumstances.

   4. Thoracotomy with resection is occasionally used for central lesion that cannot be removed by VAT.

V FOLLOW-UP AND REFERRAL. Consultation with a radiologist, a pulmonologist, and a surgeon is always helpful in determining the best strategy.

References

Detterbeck FC, Falen S, Rivera MP, Halle JS, Socinski MA. Seeking a home for a PET, part 1: Defining the appropriate place for positron emission tomography imaging in the diagnosis of pulmonary nodules or masses. *Chest* 2004;125(6):2294–2299.

Ost D, Fein AM, Feinsilver SH. Clinical practice. The solitary pulmonary nodule. *N Engl J Med* 2003;348(25):2535–2542.

30. Sleep Apnea Syndrome

I INTRODUCTION

A. Recurrent cessation of breathing (i.e., apnea) during sleep leads to a syndrome marked by daytime hypersomnolence.

  1. **Apnea is defined as cessation of airflow at the mouth for at least 10 seconds.** More than five apneic episodes an hour suggests the presence of sleep apnea syndrome.

  2. The **apnea** can be **obstructive, central,** or **mixed.**

   a. Obstructive apnea is the most common type; airflow limitation is caused by upper airway obstruction (usually from the tongue, uvula, tonsils, or nasopharynx).

   b. Central apnea is rare. In these patients, ventilatory effort is absent during the apneic episode.

   c. Mixed apnea is a combination of the obstructive and central types.

B. Sleep apnea syndrome is **common,** affecting approximately 4% and 9% of middle-aged women and men, respectively.

II CLINICAL MANIFESTATIONS OF SLEEP APNEA

A. Symptoms may include the following:

  1. **Snoring**
  2. **Daytime hypersomnolence,** which may lead to accidents, poor work performance, depression, or personality changes
  3. **Morning headache, confusion and dry mouth**
  4. **Impotence**
  5. **Nocturia** and sometimes **enuresis**
  6. **Pedal edema** or **exercise fatigue** (as a result of right-sided heart failure caused by pulmonary hypertension)

HOT

KEY

Often, a history of snoring is noted only if you ask the patient's spouse.

B. Signs. Physical examination may reveal the following:

  1. **Systemic hypertension**
  2. **Characteristic body habitus** (i.e., obese; large neck; red, florid complexion)

3. **Evidence of right-sided heart failure** (e.g., **elevated jugular venous pressure, lower extremity edema, ascites, hepatosplenomegaly**), if pulmonary hypertension has developed.

C. Laboratory abnormalities
1. A **complete blood count (CBC)** may reveal **polycythemia.**
2. Waking **arterial blood gases (ABGs)** are **usually normal,** although in some obese patients with sleep apnea syndrome, **hypoxemia** will be apparent (a syndrome known as **obesity–hypoventilation, or Pickwickian syndrome).**
3. The **electrocardiogram (EKG)** may reveal evidence of systemic or pulmonary **hypertension.**

III DIFFERENTIAL DIAGNOSIS. Sleep apnea syndrome should be distinguished from:

A. Narcolepsy, which is characterized by sudden sleep attacks during any type of activity, cataplexy, sleep paralysis, and auditory or visual hallucinations either preceding or occurring during the sleep attacks
B. Kleine-Levin syndrome, which is usually seen in young men and consists of sleep attacks a few times a year, characterized by a combination of hypersexuality, hyperphagia, and confusion.

IV APPROACH TO THE PATIENT

A. Exclude hypothyroidism and **acromegaly** as causes of the apnea. Thyroid-stimulating hormone (TSH) levels should be obtained for all patients.
B. Consider sleep studies.
1. **Indications.** Sleep studies are appropriate for chronic snorers with daytime somnolence and those with observed periods of apnea (even if daytime sleepiness is not a complaint).
2. **Types.** Sleep studies are generally of two types.
   a. **Nocturnal polysomnography,** the gold standard test, is performed in a specialized sleep center.
   b. **Portable nocturnal oximetry** is less expensive and easier to perform than nocturnal polysomnography, and is useful for ruling out significant sleep apnea.

V TREATMENT

A. Behavioral modifications include:
1. **Weight loss**
2. **Avoidance of alcohol** and **sedatives**

   3. **Establishment of regular sleeping hours** (in order to avoid sleep deprivation)

   4. **Adoption of the lateral position for sleep**

B. Medical management

   1. **Continuous positive airway pressure (CPAP)** should be guided by polysomnography.

   2. **Oral devices** (e.g., tongue-retaining devices, mandible-forward devices) should be considered for those with mild sleep apnea who do not tolerate CPAP.

   3. **Medical therapy** (protriptyline and acetazolamide) have largely fallen out of favor.

C. Surgical intervention should only be considered in consultation with a sleep apnea expert. Procedures include:

   1. **Uvulopalatopharyngoplasty**

   2. **Genioglossal** or **maxillomandibular advancement**

   3. **Tracheostomy** (the definitive therapy for obstructive sleep apnea)

VI FOLLOW-UP AND REFERRAL

A. Follow-up. Initially, patients should be seen frequently (e.g., every 2–4 weeks) in order to monitor adherence with treatment.

B. Referral

   1. Consultation with a **nutritionist** may be required to help the patient lose weight.

   2. The patient should be referred to a **sleep center** or **pulmonologist specializing in sleep apnea** if the diagnosis remains unclear or formal polysomnography or surgery is being considered.

References

Flemons WW. Clinical practice: Obstructive sleep apnea. *N Engl J Med* 2002;347: 498–504.

Piccirillo JF, Duntley S, Schotland H. Obstructive sleep apnea. *JAMA* 2002;284: 1492–1494.

PART V

GASTROENTEROLOGY

31. Abdominal Pain

 INTRODUCTION

A. The following factors complicate evaluation of abdominal pain:
1. Multiple potential diagnoses
2. Nonspecific signs and symptoms
3. Limited usefulness of radiographic studies

B. Life-threatening conditions can easily "hide" in the abdomen, initially causing few, if any, symptoms. The consequences of wrongly attributing the pain to a benign condition (e.g., gastritis) can be catastrophic.

HOT

KEY
    Patients older than 65 years with acute abdominal pain frequently have an illness requiring surgery.

II **CAUSES OF ABDOMINAL PAIN**

A. Pain of abdominal origin. A broad differential diagnosis can be formed by remembering that **infection, obstruction,** or **ischemia** can cause pain in any intra-abdominal organ.

B. Referred pain. Disorders of the **thoracic region** (e.g., myocardial ischemia or infarction, pneumonia) and **pelvic region** [e.g., testicular torsion, pelvic inflammatory disease (PID)] can present with abdominal pain.

C. Systemic and metabolic causes of abdominal pain can be remembered with the following mnemonic:

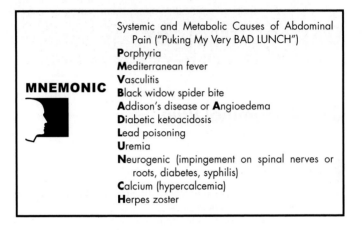

MNEMONIC

Systemic and Metabolic Causes of Abdominal Pain ("Puking My Very BAD LUNCH")
Porphyria
Mediterranean fever
Vasculitis
Black widow spider bite
Addison's disease or **A**ngioedema
Diabetic ketoacidosis
Lead poisoning
Uremia
Neurogenic (impingement on spinal nerves or roots, diabetes, syphilis)
Calcium (hypercalcemia)
Herpes zoster

III APPROACH TO THE PATIENT

A. Patient history

1. **Past medical history.** Knowledge of epidemiologic factors and the patient's past medical history can help narrow the differential diagnosis. For example, a history of intravenous drug abuse may suggest hepatitis; alcohol abuse may suggest pancreatitis or alcoholic hepatitis; and hypertension may suggest myocardial ischemia or abdominal aneurysm.

2. **Time course**
   a. Discern whether the pain is **acute** or **chronic.** Chronic pain is more likely than acute pain to have a benign cause (e.g., irritable bowel syndrome).
   b. The **progression of certain symptom complexes** can also provide important clues. For instance, appendicitis begins with pain (usually periumbilical) that almost always precedes nausea and vomiting; the pain may later move to the right lower quadrant.

3. **Symptoms**
   a. **Pain.** An effort should be made to characterize the pain:
      (1) **Quality.** Judgements regarding the quality of the pain are often not helpful in narrowing the differential diagnosis.
      (2) **Location.** Defining the location of the pain may help determine the likely cause (Table 31-1).
   b. **Other symptoms.** Always question the patient about cardiac, pulmonary, and pelvic symptoms, associated gastrointestinal symptoms (Table 31-2), as well as exacerbating or remitting factors such as food.

TABLE 31-1. Differential Diagnosis for Abdominal Pain as Suggested by Location

Location of Pain	Associated Organs	Common Diseases
Right upper quadrant	Liver, gallbladder, lung	Choledocholithiasis, cholecystitis, ascending cholangitis, hepatitis, hepatic tumor or abcess, AIDS cholangiopathy, pneumonia, pleural effusion
Epigastric region	Stomach, esophagus, pancreas, duodenum, abdominal aorta	Peptic ulcer disease, gastroesophageal reflux, pancreatitis, gastritis, food impaction, abdominal aortic aneurysm, cardiac disease
Left upper quadrant	Spleen, lung	Splenic enlargement, infarct or abcess, pneumonia, pleural effusion
Right or left lower quadrant	Appendix, ovary, colon, small intestine, kidney, testes, ureter	Appendicitis,* diverticulitis, ovarian cyst or torsion, ectopic pregnancy, pelvic inflammatory disease, intestinal ischemia, incarcerated hernia, nephrolithiasis, pyleonephritis, epididymitis, testicular torsion
Periumbilical region	Small intestine, appendix, abdominal aorta	Small bowel obstruction, gastroenteritis, early appendicitis, abdominal aortic aneurysm, ischemic bowel[†]
Suprapubic region	Bladder, uterus, ovaries, fallopian tubes	Urinary tract infection, pelivic inflammatory disease, endometriosis, ovarian cyst, ectopic pregnancy

*Pain of appendicitis may start periumbilical, and then localize to the right lower quadrant.
[†]The location of pain from ischemic bowel is variable.

TABLE 31-2. Symptoms and Associated Organ Systems	
Symptom	**Likely Site of Pathology**
Dysuria, frequency	Kidney, bladder
Nausea, vomiting, diarrhea	Gastrointestinal tract
Jaundice, pruritus	Liver, gallbladder
Pain that decreases on sitting up	Pancreas
Abrupt onset of midline pain that is out of proportion to the exam	Mesenteric vessels

B. Physical examination
   1. **Auscultation** is usually not helpful because the presence or absence of bowel sounds usually does not narrow the differential diagnosis.
   2. **Palpation.** Always start away from the area of the patient's complaint and move gently toward it. The presence or absence of guarding and rebound (suggestive of peritonitis) should be noted.
   3. **Rectal and pelvic examinations** should always be performed. Pain during rectal or pelvic examination may indicate pelvic pathology, or a disorder involving a lower intra-abdominal structure (e.g., a retrocolic appendix).
C. Laboratory and imaging studies
   1. **Basic tests.** These tests can help to narrow the differential diagnosis.
      a. **Complete blood count (CBC).** Look for leukocytosis or anemia. These findings may indicate a serious disorder.
      b. **Renal panel.** Electrolyte disturbances can be the cause or a result of the illness. Elevated blood urea nitrogen (BUN) and creatinine levels may suggest volume depletion or renal pathology. An anion gap can indicate severe infection or bowel ischemia induced acidemia.
      c. **Liver chemistry tests** screen for liver or biliary pathology.
      d. **Amylase level.** The addition of a lipase level may increase the sensitivity and specificity of this test for pancreatitis.
      e. **Urinalysis** is helpful to evaluate for diabetic ketoacidosis and renal pathology.
      f. **Urine pregnancy test.** Any woman of childbearing age should have a urine pregnancy test, regardless of how probable pregnancy seems to her.
   2. **Ancillary tests** should be ordered on the basis of your initial diagnostic impressions.
      a. A **serum calcium level** can rule out hypercalcemia.

    b. A **fecal white blood cell (WBC) count** may be ordered to screen for bowel inflammation in a patient with diarrhea.

    c. **Abdominal radiographs** are useful to evaluate bowel obstruction and kidney stones.

       (1) Layering air-fluid levels are seen in small bowel obstruction.

       (2) Abdominal radiographs have a sensitivity of approximately 50% for detecting kidney stones.

    d. **Thoracic radiographs**

       (1) **Posterior-anterior (PA)** and **lateral views** are indicated for patients with upper abdominal pain (to rule out a lower lobe pneumonia) and when there is suspicion of peritonitis (to rule out free air). Lateral views may demonstrate free air that is not visible on a PA film.

HOT KEY The patient must be maintained upright for at least 5 minutes prior to taking the film to increase the test's sensitivity for detecting air beneath the diaphragm. Left lateral decubitus views can be used to evaluate possible free air in a patient who cannot be maintained upright (e.g., as a result of pain or hypotension).

---

    e. **Abdominal ultrasound** is often the best study when gallbladder, biliary, or renal disease is suspected.

    f. **Abdominal computed tomography (CT)** is better than ultrasound for evaluating most intra-abdominal structures, except for the biliary tree and perhaps the kidney. **Triple-contrast studies** (i.e., intravenous, oral, and rectal) are usually performed and yield much finer detail. For patients with elevated creatinine, intravenous contrast can sometimes be avoided if the bowel is of primary concern; however, abscesses may be missed unless intravenous contrast is used.

    g. **Paracentesis.** If the patient has ascites, spontaneous bacterial peritonitis should always be ruled out.

    h. **Electrocardiogram (EKG).** Every patient with abdominal pain (especially upper abdominal pain) and a history of, or risk factors for, cardiac disease should have an EKG to rule out myocardial ischemia.

IV **TREATMENT DEPENDS ON THE CAUSE OF THE ABDOMINAL PAIN.** When the cause of the pain is not apparent but the patient appears ill (e.g., fever, diaphoresis, resting tachycardia, abdominal tenderness), observation in the hospital is usually necessary. In these situations, there is no substitute for frequent follow-up examinations.

V FOLLOW-UP AND REFERRAL

A. When appendicitis, cholecystitis, peritonitis, or another disorder requiring surgical observation or intervention is suspected, a **surgeon** should be consulted early in the course of evaluation.

B. Consultation with a **gastroenterologist** may be necessary when a diagnosis cannot be determined, even after performing an extensive and thorough work-up.

Reference

Glasgow RE, Mulvihil SJ. Abdominal pain including the acute abdomen. In: Sleisenger and Fordtran's Gastrointestinal and Liver Disease, 7th ed. Feldman M, Friedman LS, Sleisenger MH, eds. Philadelphia: WB Saunders, 2002:71–81.

32. Diarrhea

I INTRODUCTION

A. Diarrhea is a common presenting complaint in the outpatient setting.

B. **Diarrhea may be best characterized as loose and/or more frequent stools.** In addition, stool weight of more than 200 grams/24 hour period is consistent with diarrhea. A patient's perception of diarrhea may not always herald a pathologic process, but warrants attention as it may affect quality of life.

C. To aid in diagnosis and management, diarrhea should be generally characterized as acute or chronic:

    1. **Acute diarrhea** is present for less than 3 to 4 weeks.

    2. **Chronic diarrhea** is present for more than 3 to 4 weeks.

II CAUSES OF ACUTE DIARRHEA

A. **Acute diarrhea** generally can be characterized as infectious or non-infectious. Common causes are listed in Table 32-1.

B. **Chronic diarrhea.** There are several major types of chronic diarrhea, which can be remembered using the mnemonic, "SOME MD FUNCTION."

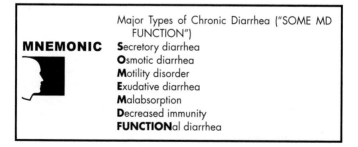

MNEMONIC	Major Types of Chronic Diarrhea ("SOME MD FUNCTION")
	Secretory diarrhea
	Osmotic diarrhea
	Motility disorder
	Exudative diarrhea
	Malabsorption
	Decreased immunity
	FUNCTIONal diarrhea

    1. **Secretory diarrhea** occurs following active intestinal secretion of electrolytes and water into the bowel lumen. Secretory diarrhea often persists despite fasting. Causes include:

        a. **Hyperthyroidism**

        b. **Bile salt diarrhea (after cholecystectomy)**

        c. **Colon cancer**

TABLE 32-1. Common Causes of Acute Diarrhea			
Infectious Causes		**Noninfectious Causes**	
Environ-mental:	Campylobacter species Shigella species Salmonella species *Clostridium difficile* *Entamoeba histolytica* *Giardia lamblia* Rotavirus Norovirus Cryptosporidium	**Medications:**	Antibiotics Laxatives Antacids Colchicine Metformin
Food poisoning:	Salmonella species Campylobacter species E. coli species *Staphylococus aureus* *Bacillus cereus* *Clostridium botulinum* *Clostridium perfringens*	**Ischemic colitis** **Inflammatory bowel disease**	
Nosocomial:	*Clostridium difficile*	**Radiation enteritis**	

    d. Colonic polyps
    e. Drugs (cholinergic drugs)
    f. Carcinoid syndrome
    g. Hypersecretion of vasointestinal polypeptide
  2. Osmotic diarrhea is often due to **malabsorption.** The stool osmolality commonly exceeds that of the serum. Causes include:
    a. Lactase deficiency (i.e., **lactose intolerance**)
    b. Excessive "sugar-free" product intake.
    c. Celiac disease
    d. Drugs (e.g. Magnesium containing antacid, lactulose)
    e. Pancreatic insufficiency (steatorrhea)
    f. Ileal resection ($\geq$**100cm resection**)
    g. Enteric fistula
    h. Radiation enteritis
    i. Bacterial overgrowth
    j. Short bowel syndrome

3. **Exudative diarrhea,** including protein-losing enteropathy, is characterized by the release of protein, blood, and mucus from an inflamed gut wall. The **stools may contain leukocytes and blood.** Causes of exudative diarrhea include:
   a. **Ulcerative colitis**
   b. **Crohn's disease**
   c. **Lymphoma**
   d. **Ischemic colitis**
   e. **Whipple's disease**
   f. **Collagenous colitis**

HOT

Hypoalbuminemia in the absence of hepatic or renal disease may be suggestive of a protein-losing enteropathy.

KEY

---

4. **Motility disorders,** including anorectal dysfunction. Causes include:
   a. **Accentuated gastro-colic reflex**
   b. **Poor anal sphincter tone**
   c. **Diabetes mellitus**
   d. **Scleroderma**
   e. **Surgically induced** (i.e., postgastrectomy syndrome, post-vagotomy syndrome)
5. **Decreased immunity.** Transplant recepients and HIV-positive patients are susceptible to organisms that generally do not cause disease in immunocompetent hosts. Consider:
   a. *Cryptosporidium parvum*
   b. *Microsporidia species*
   c. *Isospora belli*
   d. *Giardia lamblia*
   e. *Strongyloides stercoralis*
   f. *Entamoeba histolytica*
   g. *Mycobacterium avium-intracellulare* **complex**
   h. *Clostridium difficile*
   i. **Cytomegalovirus (CMV)**
6. **Functional diarrhea,** including **irritable bowel syndrome** has no identifiable organic cause. While irritable bowel syndrome can be confidently diagnosed by the presence of abominal pain or discomfort in conjunction with improvement with defection, change in frequency of defection and/or change in form of stool, "functional diarrhea" not consistent with irritable bowel syndrome should remain a diagnosis of exclusion after extensive work-up.

	The causes of acute and chronic diarrhea overlap to some
HOT	degree. In general, infections (including food poisoning) are
▶	more commonly a cause of acute diarrhea, whereas medica-
	tions, systemic disorders, and noninfectious gastrointestinal dis-
KEY	orders are more commonly causes of chronic diarrhea.

III APPROACH TO THE PATIENT

A. Patient history. Patients should be asked about the duration of diarrhea and the character of stools (volume, color, consistency, presence of blood, constant or intermittent, association with foods or eating), as well as their medical and travel history (diabetes, HIV risk factors, recent travel).

B. Physical examination

1. **Volume status.** Orthostatic hypotension and resting tachycardia indicate volume depletion.
2. **Abdominal examination.** Check for masses or focal tenderness.
3. **Rectal examination.** Evaluate for sphincter tone, masses, fecal impaction, anal pain or fissures, and blood in the stool.
4. **General examination.** Extraintestinal manifestations may provide clues to the underlying cause:
   a. Spondyloarthritis and pyoderma gangrenosum—inflammatory bowel disease
   b. Lower extremity edema—protein-losing enteropathy
   c. Dermatitis herpetiformis—celiac disease

C. Laboratory studies are ordered according to the duration of the diarrhea and the patient's clinical manifestations.

   If the patient's history suggests that lactase deficiency or a medication is the cause of the diarrhea, a trial with a lactose-exclusion diet or medication withdrawal is reasonable prior to more extensive investigations.

1. **Acute diarrhea**
   a. **Acute diarrhea lasting less than 3 days.** No laboratory work-up is usually necessary unless gross blood is present in the stool or the patient appears systemically ill.
   b. **Acute diarrhea lasting more than 3 days,** or **gross blood in the stool**
      (1) A stool sample should be sent for **bacterial culture,** to look for *Campylobacter, Shigella, Salmonella, E. coli,* and *Yersinia* species. Depending on the patient's history, it may be appropriate to send a stool sample for *C. difficile* **toxin assay, stool ova and parasites (O&P),** or *Giardia* **antigen assay.**

(2) A stool sample may be collected to screen for fecal leukocytes, which can suggest an infectious/inflammatory diarrhea, though sensitivity and specificity are sub-optimal.

HOT
KEY

When testing for *C. difficile* take note of the type of test sent, as ELISA testing for toxin A and B, and testing with a cytotoxic assay are most sensitive.

---

(3) If the patient has bloody diarrhea, fever, or volume depletion, a **complete blood count (CBC) and differential, serum electrolyte panel, albumin, blood urea nitrogen (BUN) and creatinine level** should be ordered.

2. Chronic diarrhea

a. General screening tests. Initially, a stool sample should be submitted for the following tests:

(1) Stool osmolar gap

(2) Stool guaiac (to evaluate for occult blood associated with inflammatory bowel disease or celiac sprue)

(3) Sudan staining (to evaluate for fat malabsorption)

(4) *C. difficile* **toxin assay**

(5) *Giardia* **antigen assay**

(6) Stool O&P

HOT
KEY

Stool osmolar gap may effectively distinguish between osmotic and secretory diarrhea: *serum* **osmolarity—2([*stool* sodium] + [*stool* potassium]). A gap of <50 mOsm/ kg is consistent with secretory diarrhea; a gap of >125 mOsm/kg is consistent with osmotic diarrhea.**

---

b. Specific tests may be appropriate depending on the patient's history and physical examination findings (Table 32-2)

(1) stool and/or urine **laxative screen** for **laxative abuse**

(2) endoscopy for suspected **celiac sprue, inflammatory bowel disease,** or **ischemic colitis**

(3) If **immunodeficiency** is the suspected cause of the diarrhea, the laboratory evaluation should include tests to identify the most likely causative organisms.

(4) If an **osmotic diarrhea** is suspected, a **quantitative fecal fat collection** should be performed, and testing for bacterial overgrowth may be considered

TABLE 32-2. Common Tests for Diarrhea and Interpretations		
Test	Result	Possible Diagnosis
Stool osmolar gap	>125 mOsM/kg	Osmotic diarrhea
	<50 mOSM/kg	Secretory diarrhea
Stool osmolality	<290 mOSM/kg	Contamination with urine or water
Fecal occult blood	Positive	Celiac sprue, ischemic colitis
Serum C-reactive protein	Elevated	Inflammatory bowel disease or other inflammatory condition
Fecal Sudan stain	Positive	Pancreatic insufficiency
Fecal elastase	Low	Pancreatic insufficiency
Quantitative fecal fat	>14 gm/d	Fat malabsorption
Fecal pH	<5.3	Carbohydrate malabsorption (e.g. lactase deficiency)
Lactose breath H_2 test	Positive	Lactose deficiency or bacterial overgrowth
Glucose H_2 breath test	Positive	Bacterial overgrowth
Lactulose H_2 breath test	Positive	Bacterial overgrowth
Fecal α-1 antitrypsin	Elevated	Protein-losing enteropathy
Serum albumin	Low	Protein-losing enteropathy

c. **Blood studies** should include a **CBC and differential;** a **serum electrolyte panel; BUN, creatinine, albumin,** and **thyroid-stimulating hormone (TSH) levels.**

IV TREATMENT

A. Most patients in the outpatient setting can be treated with **diet** or **medication adjustments, oral rehydration,** and **antidiarrheal agents** (Table 32-3).

HOT KEY Antidiarrheal agents are safe to use in patients with mild to moderate diarrhea. However, they should be avoided in those with bloody diarrhea or severe systemic illness. If the patient's symptoms deteriorate despite therapy, antidiarrheal agents should be discontinued.

B. Antibiotic therapy
  1. Empiric therapy. Patients who are systemically ill, older than age 50, have a history of cancer, are immunosuppressed, or who have a potential nidus for infection should be considered for empiric therapy. Treatment for lower-risk with blood and/or pus in the stool must be considered on a case by

TABLE 32-3. Antidiarrheal Agents

Generic Name	Brand Name	Dosage
Loperamide	Imodium	2 tablets orally initially, followed by 1 tablet after each loose stool (to a maximum of 8 tablets per day)
Diphenoxylate	Lomotil	2 tablets orally 4 times daily
Bismuth subsalicylate	Pepto-Bismol	2 tablets or 30 ml initally; repeat every 30–60 minutes as needed
Kaolin	Kaopectate	30 ml or 1.5–2 tablets (1200–1500 mg) orally after each loose stool
Tincture of opium	—	15–30 ml orally after each loose stool, up to 4 times daily

TABLE 32-4. Selected Antibiotic Regimens for the Specific Treatment of Infectious Diarrhea*

Pathogen	Antimicrobial Agent	Dose	Duration
Shigella species	Ciprofloxacin	500 mg BID	3 days
	Trimethoprim-sulfamethoxazole	Double-Strength BID	3 days
Salmonella typhi	Ciprofloxacin	500 mg BID	10 days
	Azithromycin	1 gm once, then 500 mg Q day	6 days
Campylobacter jejuni	Azithromycin	500 mg Q day	3 days
	Ciprofloxacin	500 mg BID	3 days
Clostridium difficile	Metronidazole	500 mg TID	10 to 14 days
	Vancomycin[†]	125 mg QID	10 to 14 days
Giardia lamblia	Tinidazole	2 gm	Once
	Nitazoxanide	500 mg BID	3 days
Yersinia enterocolitica (if severe)	Doxycycline AND Gentamycin OR Tobramycin	100 mg BID 5 mg/kg Q day	Variable
Entamoeba histolytica	Metronidazole[‡]	500–750mg TID	10 days
	Tinidazole[‡]	2 gm Q day	3 days
Vibrio cholerae	Ciprofloxacin	1 gm	Once
	Doxycycline	300 mg	Once

*Resistance patterns based on recent travel, local factors should be considered prior to prescription, particularly with regard to fluoroquinolone use
[†]Regimen for severe case
[‡]Initial therapy should be followed by paromycin 500 mg TID for 7 days or iodoquinol 650 mg TID for 20 days

case basis, as those with suspected non-typhi salmonella or Shiga toxin-producing E. coli generally should not be treated. Knowledge of the suspected pathogen and associated resistance patterns should guide choice of empiric therapy. For patients with an increased risk of *C. difficile* infection (e.g., those who have recently had antibiotic therapy) or parasitic infection (e.g., travelers to endemic regions), **metronidazole** is is frequently employed.

2. Specific therapy. Once a specific pathogen is identified, one of the regimens described in Table 32-4 can be used.

> **HOT KEY**
>
> Antibiotic therapy may not shorten symptom duration when the causative agent is non-typhoidal *Salmonella, Yersinia,* or *E. coli.*

V FOLLOW-UP AND REFERRAL

A. Referral to a gastroenterologist is appropriate when:
  1. A thorough evaluation has been performed and the cause of the diarrhea still cannot be identified
  2. Neoplasia or malabsorption is the suspected cause
  3. Toxic megacolon or ischemic bowel is the suspected cause
  4. Inflammatory bowel disease is diagnosed or suspected.

References

Gilbert DN, Moellering RC, Biopoulos GM, Sande MA, eds. The Sanford Guide to Antimicrobial Therapy 2006. Hyde Park, VT: Antimicrobial Therapy Inc., 2006.

Guerrant RL, Van Gilder T, Steiner TS, et al. Practice guidelines for the management of infectious diarrhea. *Clin Infect Dis* 2001;32(3):331–351.

Longstreth GF, Thompson WG, Chey WD, et al. Functional bowel disorders. *Gastroenterology* 2006;130(5):1480–1491.

33. Constipation

I. INTRODUCTION

A. Constipation is the most common gastrointestinal complaint in the United States. Approximately 30% of people older than 60 years use laxatives routinely.

B. Constipation is diagnosed when a patient reports fewer than three bowel movements per week, straining with defecation, hard stools, or sensation of incomplete stool evacuation.

II. CAUSES OF CONSTIPATION.
The most common causes of constipation can be remembered with the mnemonic, "Obstructed AMID Stool."

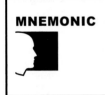

MNEMONIC	**O**bstruction
	Anorectal dysfunction
	Motility disorders
	Irritable bowel syndrome
	Diet & **D**rugs
	S(Ps)ych

A. Obstruction

    1. Neoplasia. Colon cancer must always be considered in an adult patient with changes in bowel habits, though the rate of colorectal cancer detected on colonoscopy may be similar to those undergoing routine asymptomatic screening. Other types of malignant masses in the abdomen can compress the sigmoid colon or rectum, leading to constipation.

    2. Strictures may result from diverticuli, ischemic bowel, or radiation therapy.

    3. Surgical adhesions or **rectoceles** can also cause mechanical obstruction.

B. Anorectal dysfunction, particularly due to **pelvic floor dysfunction** with difficulty in stool expulsion is a common cause of constipation.

C. Motility disturbances are most commonly **idiopathic** in nature and can cause slow transit constipation. Known causes include hypothyroidism, hypercalcemia, diabetes mellitus, hypokalemia, hypomagnesemia, uremia, spinal cord injury, and Parkinson's disease. Low motility constipation may be exacerbated by a **low-fiber diet** or **low water intake.**

D. **Irritable bowel syndrome** is a common cause of constipation, particularly if bloating and abdominal pain are prominent complaints.

E. **Drugs** such as opiates, iron supplements, calcium channel blockers, anticholinergic medicines, tricyclic antidepressants, antihistamines, neuroleptics, and diuretics, and antacids often cause constipation.

F. **Diet** with poor water intake or low fiber intake may contribute to constipation.

G. **Psychiatric conditions,** such as **depression, somatization disorders,** and **obsessive-compulsive disorders,** may be associated with constipation.

III APPROACH TO THE PATIENT

A. **Patient history**
1. **Exclude colon cancer in adults.** Assess the patient's **risk factors** for colon cancer.
   a. Have the patient's **bowel habits changed** recently after a long period of "normality"?
   b. Has the patient **lost weight?**
   c. Has the patient observed **blood** in the stools, or stools that have **changed in shape or form?**
   d. Does the patient have a **family history** of colon cancer?
2. **Evaluate the patient for other causes of constipation**
   a. Does the patient have a history consistent with **anorectal dysfunction**? Sensation of incomplete evacuation of stool, or difficulty in expelling soft stool may suggest pelvic floor dysfunction, particularly in patients with a history of traumatic childbirth.
   b. Is abdominal pain and/or bloating a prominent symptom? This may signify **irritable bowel syndrome**.
   c. Does the patient have any **symptoms suggestive of hypothyroidism, hypercalcemia, diabetes,** or **uremia?**
   d. Has the patient ever had **abdominal surgery?**
   e. What **medications,** including laxatives and over-the-counter drugs, is the patient currently taking?
   f. What is the patient's **dietary** and **exercise history?**

B. **Physical examination.** Perform abdominal and rectal examinations to detect possible masses. The rectal exam is critical in evaluating for signs of rectal dysfunction. The inability to relax the external anal sphincter on instruction to "expel my finger," or the obvious presence of rectal prolapse may indicate a mechanical cause for constipation.

C. Diagnostic Testing

   1. **Colonoscopy** should be considered for adult patients with new-onset constipation.
   2. **Laboratory studies.** Depending on the patient's history, it may be appropriate to order certain laboratory studies, such as:
      a. Thyroid function tests
      b. Serum electrolyte panel, including blood urea nitrogen, creatinine, glucose, calcium and magnesium levels
   3. **Imaging studies.** Abdominal plain films (flat and upright) should be obtained in patients with abdominal pain or distention. A Sitz marker study can evaluate the speed of colonic transit.

IV TREATMENT takes a step-wise approach, and is dependent on suspected etiology.

For constipation due to slow transit:

A. Perform fecal disimpaction in patients with impacted stool in the rectal vault.

B. Discontinue constipation-causing medications, if possible.

C. Correct metabolic abnormalities such as hypothyroidism.

D. Recommend lifestyle changes. The patient should be advised to **increase exercise, water intake** (to at least 1.5–2 liters daily), and **fiber intake** (preferably to at least 10–20 grams daily). Sources of fiber include:

   1. **Wheat bran** or **high-bran cereals**
   2. **Psyllium (Metamucil),** 1 tablespoon 2–3 times per day, mixed with water or juice.
   3. **Methylcellulose (Citrucel)** or **calcium polycarbophil (Fibercon),** which are often associated with less intestinal gas, but are significantly more expensive than psyllium

E. Consider laxatives if the patient continues to experience constipation despite implementing dietary changes and increasing the amount of exercise.

HOT
▶
KEY

Side effects of prolonged laxative therapy include laxative-dependent stooling, incontinence, and abdominal cramping.

1. **Oral laxatives** (in order of increasing potency)
   a. **Milk of magnesia,** 15–30 ml twice daily, has few side effects, is cheap, and often effective
   b. **Docusate sodium (Colace),** 100 mg once or twice daily may be effective
   c. **Sorbitol,** 15–30 ml once or twice daily or **Lactulose** 15-60 ml daily although effective, are often associated with uncomfortable bloating
   d. **Magnesium citrate,** 15–30 ml daily
   e. **Tegaserod 2 mg or 6 mg twice daily can increase the number of bowel movements per week**
   f. **Polyethylene glycol 3350 powder, 17 gm per day or more, titrated to effect, mixed in water or juice.**
2. **Rectal suppositories** [e.g., **bisacodyl (Dulcolax),** 1 suppository 3 times per week] can be used as an alternative or an adjunct to oral laxatives.
3. **Tap water enema, 500 ml, or mineral oil enema, 100–250 ml can be effective as rescue therapy, but are generally not convenient for daily use.**

HOT **KEY**   Initiate treatment with an oral agent, unless the patient has been constipated for more than 5–7 days; it is then preferable to initiate therapy with an enema because oral laxatives may be ineffective and result in worsening abdominal distention.

For constipation due to suspected anorectal dysfunction:

A. Referral for **biofeedback therapy** may be indicated.

V FOLLOW-UP AND REFERRAL

A. Follow-up. Patients with constipation often must implement significant lifestyle changes in order to achieve lasting relief. The importance of careful patient education and continual reinforcement cannot be overemphasized.

B. Referral. The primary indications for referral to a gastroenterologist are to rule out colon cancer, and if anorectal dysfunction and/or irritable bowel syndrome are suspected. Those with chronic constipation unresponsive to conservative measures may also benefit from consultation.

References
Jost WH, Eckardt VF. Constipation in idiopathic Parkinson's disease. *Scand J Gastroenterol* 2003;38(7):681–686.

Kamm MA, Muller-Lissner S, Talley NJ et al. Tegaserod for the treatment of chronic constipation: a randomized, double-blind, placebo-controlled multinational study. *Am J Gastro* 2005;100(2):362–372.

Locke GR, Pemberton JH, Phillips SF. American Gastroenterological Association medical position statement: guidelines on constipation. *Gastroenterology* 2000;119(6):1761–1766.

Locke GR, Pemberton JH, Phillips SF. American Gastroenterological Association technical review on constipation. *Gastroenterology* 2000;119(6):1766–1778.

34. Heartburn and Gastroesophageal Reflux Disease

··

I INTRODUCTION

A. **Gastroesophageal reflux disease (GERD)**, most commonly manifested by **heartburn** (a retrosternal burning sensation), is believed to be caused by the abnormal reflux of acid from the stomach into the esophagus. GERD has four underlying mechanisms:

1. Recurrent, abnormal relaxation of the lower esophageal sphincter, which allows reflux of gastric acid into the esophagus
2. Impaired clearance of the acid from the esophagus (inadequate peristalsis and swallowing of saliva)
3. Susceptibility of the esophageal mucosa to the acid
4. Increased pain sensitivity to esophageal acid exposure

B. Heartburn is experienced daily by approximately 5%–10% of American adults, and at least once a month by approximately 40% of the adult population.

II COMPLICATIONS OF GASTROESOPHAGEAL REFLUX DISEASE

A. **Esophageal complications**

1. **Esophagitis** results from prolonged exposure of the esophageal mucosa to gastric acid. The severity of the pain does not correlate well with the severity of the esophagitis.

HOT KEY

Dysphagia may be a sign of reflux esophagitis

2. **Esophageal ulcer** (i.e., erosion of the mucosa) can result from persistent esophagitis. Patients usually have more severe pain than that experienced with esophagitis and may present with bleeding or anemia.

3. **Esophageal stricture,** which may result from chronic inflammation or ulceration, causes luminal narrowing and often presents as dysphagia, particularly to solid foods.
4. **Barrett's esophagus** results when columnar epithelium replaces the normal squamous epithelium in the distal esophagus after prolonged exposure to gastric acid. Barrett's esophagus is a strong risk factor for esophageal adenocarcinoma.

B. **Extraesophageal complications**
1. **Asthma.** Symptoms of asthma may be worsened or even caused by GERD. Bronchoconstriction is thought to be caused by either aspiration of small amounts of gastric acid or stimulation of a vagal reflex arc by esophageal acid.
2. **Otolarnygologic complications.** Persistent acid reflux can irritate any structure in the pharynx or larynx, possibly leading to chronic cough, hoarseness, laryngitis, difficulty clearing the throat, and dental decay.

III APPROACH TO THE PATIENT

> **HOT KEY**
> All patients with retrosternal pain should be evaluated for other causes of chest pain, especially those with risk factors for coronary artery disease (CAD; see Chapter 16).

A. **Patient history**
1. Patients with GERD typically complain of **heartburn** (which is relieved by antacids and exacerbated by eating, lying down, or bending over) and a **feeling of regurgitation.** These symptoms are approximately 90% specific for GERD. Epigastric pain may also be a symptom of GERD.
2. Patients may present with symptoms resulting from complications of GERD, including **dysphagia, odynophagia, worsening asthma, chronic coughing, hoarseness, laryngitis, difficulty clearing the throat,** and **dental decay.**

> **HOT KEY**
> A history of exercise-induced symptoms, or of new symptoms in a patient with risk factors for heart disease, should prompt an evaluation for CAD.

B. **Physical examination** should focus on identifying **signs of conditions that can exacerbate GERD** (e.g., Raynaud's disease as a sign of scleroderma; palmar erythema or spider angioma as a sign of chronic alcohol use). Use the mnemonic "ACIDS" to remember the conditions that can exacerbate GERD:

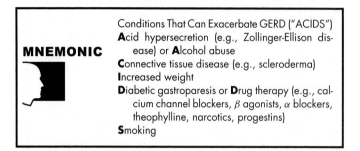

MNEMONIC

Conditions That Can Exacerbate GERD ("ACIDS")
Acid hypersecretion (e.g., Zollinger-Ellison disease) or **A**lcohol abuse
Connective tissue disease (e.g., scleroderma)
Increased weight
Diabetic gastroparesis or **D**rug therapy (e.g., calcium channel blockers, β agonists, α blockers, theophylline, narcotics, progestins)
Smoking

C. Other studies
  1. **Endoscopy.** Patients with a history suggestive of complications (e.g., dysphagia, odynophagia, early satiety, weight loss, anemia, asthma exacerbations, oropharyngeal pathology), or who do not respond to emperic therapy, should be referred to a gastroenterologist promptly for endoscopy.
  2. **Esophageal biopsy** may be indicated, depending on the endoscopy findings. Patients with **esophageal ulcer** or **stricture** should have esophageal biopsies to rule out dysplastic changes and adenocarcinoma. Patients with changes suspicious for Barrett's esophagus should have biopsies to rule out dysplasia.

IV TREATMENT

A. Mild GERD is treated with diet and lifestyle changes. Antacids or over-the-counter histamine-2 (H_2) antagonists can be used on an as-needed basis for intermittent symptoms. For more persistent symptoms, an over-the counter omeprazole may be beneficial.
  1. **Diet.** Patients should be advised to avoid smoking. Avoidance of coffee, alcohol, chocolate, high-fat meals, and acidic or spicy foods may help, though rigorous data are not available to support benefit. Smaller, more frequent meals and avoidance of lying supine within 3 hours after eating may also be beneficial.
  2. **Lifestyle changes.** Weight loss and smoking cessation are indicated for obese patients and those who smoke, respectively. Tight-fitting garments should be avoided. Elevating the head of the bed may help alleviate symptoms at night.

TABLE 34-1. Pharmacologic Therapy for Gastrointestinal Reflux Disease (GERD)

Generic Name	Brand Name	Dose Range
Histamine-2 (H₂) antagonists*		
Cimetidine	Tagamet	400–800 mg up to twice daily
Ranitidine	Zantac	150–300 mg up to twice daily
Nizatidine	Axid	150–300 mg up to twice daily
Famotidine	Pepcid	20–40 mg up to twice daily
Proton-pump inhibitors†		
Omeprazole	Prilosec, Prilosec OTC	20–40 mg up to twice daily
Esomeprazole	Nexium	20–40 mg up to twice daily
Lansoprazole	Prevacid	15–30 mg up to twice daily
Rabeprazole	Aciphex	20–40 mg up to twice daily
Pantoprazole	Protonix	20–40 mg up to twice daily

*H_2 antagonists and antacids can be used for intermittent symptoms, H_2 antagonists or over-the-counter omeprazole can be used for mild persistent symptoms
†Proton pump inhibitors can be used for moderate to severe or refractory symptoms, and are first-line therapy for esophagitis

3. **Antisecretory therapy** (Table 34-1). If the patient's symptoms do not improve with conservative methods, or persist or recur after over-the-coutner therapy, a 4 week trial of a **proton-pump inhibitor (PPI)** is indicated. Failure of pharmacologic therapy should prompt referral to a gastroenterologist.

HOT KEY

Different formulations of PPIs are generally not believed to differ in efficacy in a clinically signficant manner.

B. **Moderate to severe GERD**, defined as daily or debilitating symptoms, should prompt empiric therapy with a **PPI** for a 4- to 8-week trial followed by widthdrawal of the medicine and reassessment. Incomplete symptom relief can be managed by increasing the dose and/or twice-a-day administration of **PPI** therapy. Consultation with a gastroenterologist for early endoscopy is also an appropriate option.

C. Complications of GERD

1. Esophagitis

a. **Antisecretory therapy.** An 8-week course of therapy with a **PPI** is the treatment of choice. Many patients experience a relapse after initial therapy; therefore, long-term PPI therapy is often required.

   (1) Although an H_2 antagonist may be used instead, PPIs are much more effective.

   (2) Clinically signficant adverse effects of long term PPI therapy have not been identified.

b. **Surgery** (e.g., laparoscopic Nissen fundoplication) may be an option, particularly for young patients who do not want to take medicines for life, but only 40% of patients who undergo therapy will not be on medical therapy for GERD on follow-up. In addition, surgery can be associated with signficant morbidity, including dysphagia and the gas-bloat syndrome.

HOT KEY

Evidence suggests that surgery does not reduce the rate of esophageal adenocarcinoma in patients with GERD.

---

2. Esophageal ulcer
is treated with a **PPI** for at least 8 weeks, and then **repeat endoscopy** is performed to document ulcer healing and rule out cancer. Long-term pharmacologic treatment is often necessary.

3. Esophageal stricture

a. Most patients have dramatic improvement with **serial dilatation** of the stricture, which can be repeated periodically.

b. Long-term **PPI** prevents recurrence of strictures.

c. **Surgery** may be considered for patients with severe symptoms or frequent recurrence.

4. Barrett's esophagus

a. If it is identified on endoscopy, biopsies should be taken to rule out dysplasia.

b. high-grade dysplasia requires confirmation by an expert pathologist, and surgery in suitable risk candidates.

c. low-grade dysplasia requires follow up endoscopy at 6 and 12 months.

d. absence of dyplasia may allow for follow up endoscopy in 3 to 5 years.

HOT KEY

Caucasian males with long-standing GERD are at highest risk for Barrett's esophagus and esophageal adenocarcinoma

    e. Long-term **PPI therapy** theoretically may reduce progression to dysplasia.

  5. **Asthma.** It is difficult to know which patients with asthma will benefit from treatment of GERD.

    a. Patients with symptoms of both diseases can be given a trial of **PPIs.**

    b. **Surgery** may be more effective than medical therapy for relieving asthmatic symptoms in these patients.

  6. **Otolaryngologic complications.** A trial of **PPIs** is indicated when symptoms are believed to be caused by GERD.

V FOLLOW-UP AND REFERRAL

A. Follow-up

  1. Patients with mild GERD should be followed monthly until symptoms are controlled. Patients with more severe symptoms require closer follow-up.

  2. All patients with documented esophageal disease should be followed in consultation with a gastroenterologist.

B. Referral to a gastroenterologist is useful when GERD is the suspected cause of asthmatic or otolaryngological disease.

References

Fox M, Forgacs I. Gastro-oesophageal reflux disease. *BMJ* 2006;332(7533):88–93.

Peterson WL, ed. American Gastroenterological Association consensus opinion: Improving the management of GERD: evidence-based therapeutic strategies. Retrieved March 2006, from www.gastro.org/phys-sci/edu-cme/GERDmonograph.pdf.

35. Dyspepsia

....

I INTRODUCTION

A. Dyspepsia is an imprecise term that refers to **chronic** or **recurrent epigastric** or **upper abdominal pain,** often accompanied by bloating, nausea, or postprandial fullness (i.e., "indigestion").

B. Approximately 25% of Americans complain of dyspepsia, one of the leading causes of office visits to primary care providers.

II CAUSES OF DYSPEPSIA.

The differential diagnosis list for dyspepsia is long, encompassing pathology in all of the abdominal organs (Table 35-1). Fortunately, the list of common causes is short.

A. **Peptic ulcer disease** is diagnosed in **5 to 15% of patients** with dyspepsia. Duodenal and gastric ulcers are approximately equal in incidence; the vast majority are associated with *Helicobacter pylori* (*H. pylori*) infection.

1. *H. pylori* **infection** in absence of peptic ulcer disease may be associated with dyspepsia in 20 to 60% of patients.

2. **Nonsteroidal anti-inflammatory drug (NSAID) use** is responsible for most ulcers not caused by *H. pylori* infection.

B. **GERD,** including **Esophagitis.** As many as **20% of patients** with dyspepsia have GERD. Most patients with GERD have symptoms of "heartburn" or a sensation of acid reflux, but exceptions are common, as some may have only a vague sensation of abdominal pain. Esophagitis is may be found in 5 to 15% of patients with dyspepsia referred for endoscopy.

C. **Non-ulcer, or "functional" dyspepsia** is dyspepsia that is not associated with any structural defects based on endoscopy. As many as 60% of patients with dyspepsia have functional dyspepsia—the exact cause of pain is usually unclear.

D. **Medication side effect.** A number of commonly prescribed medications, such as NSAIDs, theophylline, and iron, may induce dyspepsia.

III APPROACH TO THE PATIENT

A. **Patient history** is not a reliable predictor of the cause of dyspepsia.

TABLE 35-1. Selected Causes of Dyspepsia

Common Causes
  Non-ulcer dyspepsia
  Peptic ulcer disease
  Gastroesophageal reflux disease (GERD)
  Helicobacter pylori
  Medication side effect (particularly non-steroidal,
    anti-inflammatory drugs)
Less common causes
  Gastric cancer
  Gastroparesis
  Biliary tract disease (e.g., cholelithiasis, hepatobiliary
    neoplasm)
  Pancreatic disease (e.g., chronic pancreatitis, pancreatic
    cancer)
  Bacterial overgrowth
  Chronic intestinal ischemia
  Parasitic infection (e.g. *Giardia, Strongyloides*)
  Systemic conditions (e.g., hypercalcemia, thyroid
    disease, diabetes, pregnancy, collagen vascular
    disease)
  Crohn's disease involving the stomach

1. Always ask about **NSAID** use.
2. Ask about **GERD** associated symptoms, as patients with such symptoms should be treated as if they have GERD (see Chapter 34).

B. **Physical examination** should be thorough in all patients. The abdomen should be palpated for masses, organomegaly, and ascites.

C. **Laboratory studies**
   1. **Standard work-up.** A complete blood count (CBC), serum electrolyte panel, calcium, amylase, lipase, and glucose levels, as well as a liver panel are often ordered for all patients with unexplained abdominal pain, though the utility of such testing in every patient is unproven.
   2. *H. pylori* **testing.** Because *H. pylori* is responsible for most cases of peptic ulcer disease, it makes a signficant contribution to functional dyspepsia, and is considered a modifiable risk factor for gastric cancer. A "test and treat" strategy for *H. pylori* is believed to be efficient and cost-effective, particularly if the local prevalence of *H. pylori* exceeds 12%.
      a. Noninvasive testing methods for *H. pylori* include **stool antigen** and the **urease breath test,** which both have high

TABLE 35-2. Antisecretory Therapy for Peptic Ulcer Disease

Generic Name	Brand Name	Dose
Histamine-2 (H$_2$) antagonists		
Cimetidine	Tagamet	400 mg twice daily
Ranitidine	Zantac	150 mg twice daily
Nizatidine	Axid	150 mg twice daily
Famotidine	Pepcid	20 mg twice daily
Proton-pump inhibitors (PPI)		
Omeprazole	Prilosec	20 to 40 mg up to twice daily
Lansoprazole	Prevacid	15 to 30 mg up to twice daily
Pantoprazole	Protonix	20 to 40 mg up to twice daily
Esomeprazole	Nexium	20 to 40 mg up to twice daily
Rabeprazole	Aciphex	20 mg up to twice daily

     sensitvity and specificity. Because of insufficient sensitivity and specificity, blood serologic testing is no longer recommended.

    b. For patients who undergo endoscopy, **biopsy specimens** can be tested for *H. pylori* using a **urease test or histologic stains.**

D. Endoscopy and Imaging studies

    1. Though the specificity of alarm symptoms for gastric cancer is limited, **Upper endoscopy** should be performed in patients with severe symptoms or any of the following "DANGER" signs:

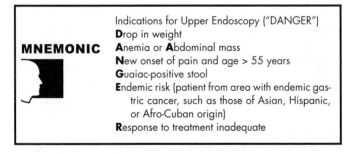

MNEMONIC

Indications for Upper Endoscopy ("DANGER")
Drop in weight
Anemia or **A**bdominal mass
New onset of pain and age > 55 years
Guaiac-positive stool
Endemic risk (patient from area with endemic gastric cancer, such as those of Asian, Hispanic, or Afro-Cuban origin)
Response to treatment inadequate

HOT KEY

Patients less than 55 years old are very unlikely to have gastric cancer as an etiology for dyspepsia.

2. An **upper gastrointestinal series** is less accurate than endoscopy and does not allow biopsy of suspicious lesions. This study is generally used only when patients cannot tolerate endoscopy.
3. **Abdominal ultrasound** is useful if biliary or pancreatic disease is suspected, though should not be ordered routinely.
4. **Computed tomography (CT)** and **magnetic resonance imaging (MRI)** are rarely indicated; they may be useful when an intra-abdominal malignancy is suspected.

IV TREATMENT

HOT KEY
Advise patients, with dyspepsia, who are taking NSAIDs to discontinue the medication, change formulation, consider dose reduction, or add a proton pump inhibitor (PPI).

A. Peptic ulcer disease
1. *H. pylori* positive patients should receive "triple therapy;" the PPI should be continued for 8 weeks. Because treatment failures can approximate 10%, re-testing for *H. pylori*, particularly if symptoms persist, may be warranted. Two effective regimens for *H. pylori* eradication are given in Table 35-3 (both are approximately 90% effective).
2. *H. pylori* **negative** patients should receive **PPI therapy** for 8 weeks.

HOT KEY
Patients with a documented duodenal ulcer should receive anti-*H. pylori* therapy regardless of the results of *H. pylori* testing (due to the high prevalence of the infection in these patients).

B. GERD. Therapy is described in Chapter 34 IV.
C. Non-ulcer dyspepsia and/or dyspepsia in patients < age 55.
1. A "test and treat" strategy for *H. pylori* may improve symptoms and induce a cure in some patients, and is the recommended initial strategy. If treatment fails, empiric PPI for 4 weeks should be implemented, and if the patient continues to be symptomatic, endoscopy should be conducted in those who have not had prior endoscopy.

TABLE 35-3. Selected Regimens for the Eradication of *Helicobacter pylori*

	Regimen
Option 1	**FOR 10 to 14 DAYS:** **Amoxicillin:** 1 gm bid **Clarithromycin:** 500 mg bid **Proton-pump inhibitor*** before meal(s)
Option 2	**FOR 10 to 14 DAYS:** **Bismuth subsalicylate:** 2 tablets (525 mg) four times daily **Metronidazole:** 250 mg four times daily **Tetracycline:** 500 mg four times daily **Proton pump inhibitor*** before meal(s)

***Omeprazole** 20 mg, **Rabeprazole** 20 mg, **Lansoprazole** 30 mg, or **Pantoprazole** 40 mg twice daily, or **Esomeprazole** 40 mg once daily may be used interchangeably

HOT KEY

PPIs are most effective if taken 30 minutes prior to a meal.

D. NSAID-associated dyspepsia.

1. If an ulcer is present, a PPI, H$_2$ antagonist, or misoprostol can promote healing with 4–8 weeks of therapy even if the NSAID is continued; the PPI is the most potent agent. The healing agent should be continued for the duration of NSAID use.

HOT KEY

Ideally, NSAIDs should be stopped if associated with a peptic ulcer, as this will maximize healing and relief of symptoms.

2. If an ulcer is absent, PPI's, and to a lesser degree H$_2$ antagonists, may offer symptom relief. Alternatively the patient can be switched to a different NSAID, or a non-NSAID agent such as acetaminophen.

HOT KEY   COX-2 inhibitors, which are sometimes used as alternatives to NSAIDs should be used with caution, particularly in patients with risk factors for cardiovascular disease because of potential toxicity.

3. Patients with suspected or documented NSAID-induced ulcers who are *H. pylori*-positive should be treated for the infection.

V FOLLOW-UP AND REFERRAL

A. **Follow-up**
   1. Patients who are tested and treated for *H. pylori* and/or given empiric PPI therapy should be followed up within 4 weeks to assess symptoms. If initial emperic therapy has been unsuccesful, dose increase in PPI, or endoscopy for further investigation can be considered.
   2. Patients who have documented gastric ulcers who did not have biopsies taken from the ulcer at initial endoscopy should have a follow up endoscopy to document ulcer healing and rule out gastric cancer.
B. **Referral** to a gastroenterologist is warranted if any of the danger signs are present or if the patient has severe or persistent symptoms.

References

Canga C, Vakil N. Upper GI malignancy, uncomplicated dyspepsia, and the age threshold for early endoscopy. *Am J Gastro* 2002;97(3):600–603.

Gupta S, McQuaid K. Management of nonsteroidal, anti-inflammatory drug-associated dyspepsia. *Gastroenterology* 2005;129(5):1711–1719.

Laine L, Hunt R, El-Zimaity H, Nguyen B, Osato M, Spenard J. Bismuth-based quadruple therapy using a single capsue of bismuth biskalcitrate, metronidazole, and tetracycline given with omeprazole versus omeprazole, amoxicillin, and clarithromycin for eradictaion of *Helicobacter pylori* in duodenal ulcer patients: a prospective, randomized, multicenter, North American trial. *Am J Gastro* 2003;98(3):562–567.

Talley NJ, Vakil NB, Moayyedi P. American Gastroenterological Association technical review on the evaluation of dyspepsia. *Gastroenterology* 2005;129(5):1756–1780.

36. Involuntary Weight Loss

I **INTRODUCTION.** Weight loss is a common outpatient complaint with important prognostic significance. Weight loss of 5%–10% of the body mass index (BMI) is a predictor of increased mortality for patients older than 60 years.

$$BMI = weight\ (kg)/height\ (m^2)$$

II **CAUSES OF WEIGHT LOSS.** There are many causes of involuntary weight loss. The most common are presented here.

A. Cancer. Gastrointestinal cancers (e.g., colon, pancreatic, gastric) are a primary cause of neoplasia-associated weight loss. Ovarian cancer, lung cancer, prostate cancer, lymphoma, and myeloma also should be considered.

B. Gastrointestinal disorders. Think about the entire gastrointestinal tract, from the mouth to the anus. Loss of teeth, oral ulcers, mechanical or functional esophageal obstruction, peptic ulcer disease, pancreatic insufficiency, cholelithiasis, liver disease, and diseases of the small bowel or colon (infectious, inflammatory, ischemic, and malabsorptive) should be considered.

C. Psychiatric disorders that can be associated with weight loss include **depression**, **dementia**, anxiety, anorexia nervosa, and bipolar disorder.

MNEMONIC

Common causes of weight loss ("Can't Get Phat")
Cancer
Gastrointestinal disorders
Psychiatric disorders

D. Other causes of involuntary weight loss include:
1. **Congestive heart failure (CHF)**
2. **Chronic obstructive pulmonary disease (COPD)**
3. **Alcohol abuse** and **illicit drug use**
4. **Therapeutic drug use** (particularly any that cause abdominal discomfort or xerostomia)
5. **Chronic infections,** such as AIDS, tuberculosis, abscess, endocarditis, and osteomyelitis
6. **Endocrine disorders,** such as hyperthyroidism, diabetes, hypercalcemia, and adrenal insufficiency

7. **Metabolic disorders,** such as uremia and cirrhosis
8. **Collagen vascular disorders,** such as systemic lupus erythematosus (SLE) and rheumatoid arthritis

III APPROACH TO THE PATIENT (FIGURE 36-1)

A. Patient history. Patients will usually volunteer that they think they have lost weight. Often, they will have associated complaints, such as pain, weakness, or gastrointestinal symptoms

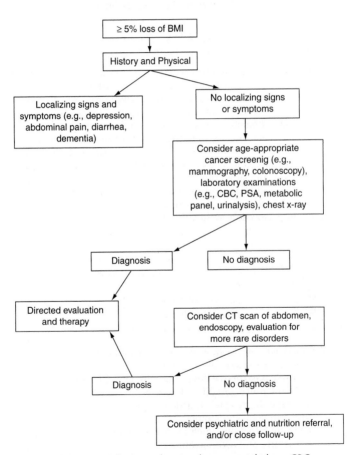

FIGURE 36-1. Directed approach to involuntary weight loss. *CBC* = complete blood count, *PSA* = prostate specific antigen.

that should guide the initial work up. Your job is to identify those who really have lost weight and figure out why.

HOT KEY

As many as 50% of patients who claim to have lost weight have not actually lost any weight.

1. **Patient records.** Obtaining the patient's weight should be a routine part of every patient visit, making it possible to document weight loss by using the weights recorded in the patient's chart as a basis for comparison with his current weight.

   a. Like sphygmomanometers, scales can vary greatly in accuracy, so it is best to use hospital scales and follow trends instead of individual readings.

   b. Weight loss can be corroborated by noting a change in clothing size (e.g., pants, belts, shirt collar). Family members may also be able to give an objective opinion. Driver's licence photographs are often useful.

2. **Questions** should be designed to identify symptoms of and risk factors for the common causes of involuntary weight loss. Do not forget to screen patients for evidence of depression (depressed mood and anhedonia), limited access to food, abuse, and dementia (use the mini-mental state examination; see Chapter 65, Table 65-1).

B. **Physical examination.** A complete examination should be performed.

   1. The major **lymph node groups** (i.e., the cervical,-supraclavicular, axillary, and inguinal nodes) should be palpated.

   2. A careful **abdominal examination** should be performed.

   3. A **prostate examination** should be performed in men and a **breast** and **pelvic examination** are required for women.

C. **Laboratory and imaging studies.** When the cause of the weight loss remains unclear despite a detailed history and physical examination, the following tests are usually obtained. Age appropriate cancer screening should be conducted.

   1. **Laboratory tests**

      a. Complete blood count

      b. Serum electrolyte panel

      c. Glucose and calcium levels

      d. Liver panel

      e. Thyroid-stimulating hormone level

      f. Erythrocyte sedimentation rate

      g. Urinalysis

      h. Prostate-specific antigen in men

HOT

KEY

Obtain an HIV test in any patient with weight loss and risk factors for HIV disease.

2. **Imaging and Invasive studies**
   a. A **chest radiograph** should be obtained.
   b. **Mammography** is indicated for women older than 50 years and should also be considered for younger women with weight loss.
   c. **Colonoscopy** is usually recommended for patients older than 50 years and should be considered for younger patients with weight loss.
   d. **Upper endoscopy** may be performed if symptoms suggest an upper gastrointestinal tract disorder, if the patient comes from an area with endemic gastric cancer, or if colonoscopy is unremarkable.
   e. An **abdominal computed tomography scan** may be obtained if symptoms, signs, or laboratory test results suggest an abdominal disorder or if no other cause has been identified.

IV TREATMENT

A. **Definitive treatment** entails treating the underlying cause.
B. **Symptomatic treatment**
   1. Consider the use of **megestrol acetate** (800 mg orally daily) or **dronabinol** (5–10 mg orally twice daily) to stimulate the appetite and quell nausea in patients with cancer- or AIDS-related cachexia. The utility of these drugs in the treatment of other causes of involuntary weight loss is unproven.
   2. **Testosterone, growth hormone,** or **thalidomide** may be useful for those with AIDS-associated weight loss.

V FOLLOW-UP AND REFERRAL

A. Patients with documented involuntary weight loss that has eluded diagnosis after 1 month should be referred to a gastroenterologist for endoscopy.
B. Psychiatric consultation should be considered for patients with persistent weight loss that remains unexplained despite a complete evaluation.
C. Referral to a nutritionist may aid in optimizing caloric intake.

Reference
Bouras E, Lange S, Scolapio J. Rational approach to patients with unintentional weight loss. *Mayo Clin Proc* 2001;76:923–929.

37. Abnormal Liver Chemistry Tests

I. INTRODUCTION

A. Liver chemistry tests may be ordered on suspicion of liver disease (e.g., jaundice, abdominal pain) or as part of a screening laboratory examination. In the outpatient setting, as many as one third of all screening liver chemistry tests are abnormal. Of these, only about 1% represent clinically significant yet unsuspected liver disease. Clinicians must place these biochemical abnormalities in context of physical exam findings and risk factor history to determine what they mean and how far to pursue them. In general, if initial evaluations are non-diagnostic and the patient is asymptomatic, more extensive evaluations can be reserved for those with persistent primary liver chemistry test abnormalities on repeat examination.

HOT KEY

Normal liver chemistry tests do not rule out the possiblity of liver disease, including cirrhosis and viral hepatitis.

B. A primary liver profile most often includes **total bilirubin, alkaline phosphatase (AP), aspartate aminotransferase (AST), and alanine aminotransferase (ALT) levels,** as well as a **prothrombin time (PT).** Ancillary tests, such as conjugated and unconjugated bilirubin, γ-glutamyl transferase (GGT) level, and platelet count can aid in narrowing the differential diagnosis of primary liver chemistry test elevations.

II. APPROACH TO THE PATIENT

A. Consider the possibility that the abnormality could represent an extrahepatic disorder. Table 37-1 summarizes some of the common extrahepatic disorders that could lead to abnormal liver chemistry test results.

B. Categorize the abnormality as either cholestatic or hepatocellular.

TABLE 37-1. Extrahepatic Causes of Abnormal Liver Function Tests

Abnormality	Potential Extrahepatic Cause
Elevated AST	Myocardial infarction, muscle disorder
Elevated AP	Bone disease, pregnancy, hyperthyroidism
Elevated bilirubin	Hemolysis, sepsis
Increased PT	Malaborption, anticoagulant or antibiotic use, vitamin K deficiency
Decreased albumin	Malnutrition, protein-losing enteropathy, nephrotic syndrome, congestive heart failure (CHF)

AP – alkaline phosphatase; AST = aspartate aminotransferase; PT = prothombin time.

1. The **cholestatic pattern** is characterized by **increased AP** and **bilirubin levels.** Aminotransferase levels may be elevated, but not as markedly as the AP and bilirubin levels.

HOT KEY The differential diagnosis for an isolated elevated AP level can be narrowed by obtaining a GGT level, which will commonly be concurrently elevated in patients with liver but not bone disease.

2. The **hepatocellular pattern** is characterized primarily by **increased AST** and **ALT levels.** The bilirubin level and the PT can also be increased in patients with chronic hepatocellular disease; in later stages, the serum albumin level may decrease.

   a. AST is a sensitive but not a specific marker of hepatocyte necrosis.

   b. ALT is found primarily in the liver and is thus more specific for hepatocellular injury.

HOT KEY Distinguishing a cholestatic pattern from a hepatocellular pattern can be difficult because elevated transaminase levels can occur in both. Elevations in the AP level out of proportion to the AST and ALT levels imply a cholestatic pattern, whereas elevation of AST and ALT levels out of proportion to the AP level implies a hepatocellular pattern.

C. Narrow the differential diagnosis.

1. Cholestatic pattern. Figure 37-1 presents an algorithm for narrowing the differential diagnosis in patients with liver function test results suggestive of cholestasis.

HOT KEY

Infiltrative liver disease often presents with a markedly elevated AP level that is out of proportion to the elevated bilirubin level.

2. Hepatocellular pattern. Elevated transaminases are the most common liver function test abnormality. Figure 37-2 presents an algorithm for narrowing the differential diagnosis in patients with liver chemistry test results suggestive of a hepatocellular disorder.

   a. The **most common causes** of elevated transaminases in the United States include the following.

      (1) Nonalcoholic steatohepatitis (NASH) is a clinical and biochemical diagnosis made after excluding significant alcohol consumption and other identifiable liver diseases. It is associated with obesity, possibly diabetes, and hypertriglyceridemia. The natural history is poorly understood but suggests that as many as 15% of patients with NASH will progress to end-stage liver disease.

        (a) NASH presents with mild to moderate AST elevations. Characteristically, the AST:ALT ratio is less than 1.

        (b) Ultrasound often reveals the hyperechoic texture of fatty infiltration.

        (c) If NASH is suspected, liver biopsy may be considered for prognostic information (i.e. degree of inflammation, presence of cirrhosis); no specific therapies for NASH are available at this time.

HOT KEY

The most common diagnosis in patients with abnormal liver function tests and normal viral serologies is NASH or hepatic steatosis.

      (2) Viral hepatitis. Patients with chronic hepatitis B or C are often asymptomatic. Infection leads to end-stage liver disease in approximately 20% of infected

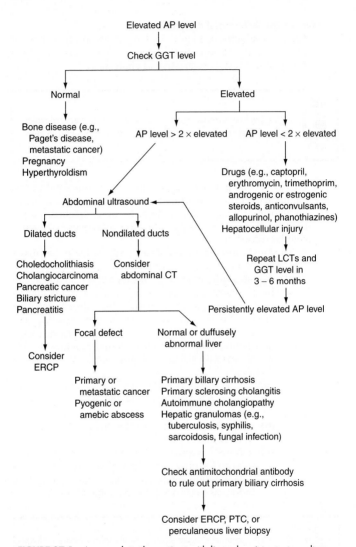

FIGURE 37-1. Approach to the patient with liver chemistry test results suggestive of cholestasis. *AP* = alkaline phosphatase; *CT* = computed tomography; *ERCP* = endoscopic retrograde cholangiopancreatography; *GGT* = γ-glutamyl transferase; *LCTs* = liver chemistry tests; *PTC* = percutaneous transhepatic cholangiogram. (Modified with permission from Moseley RH: Evaluation of abnormal liver function tests. *Med Clin North Am* 80(5):887–906, 1996.)

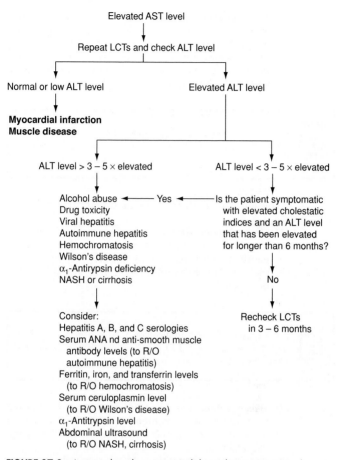

FIGURE 37-2. Approach to the patient with liver chemistry test results suggestive of a hepatocellular disorder. *ALT* = alanine aminotransferase; *ANA* = antinuclear antibody; *AST* = aspartate aminotransferase; *LCTs* = liver chemistry tests; *NASH* = nonalcoholic steatohepatitis; *R/O* = rule out. (Modified with permission from Kamath PS: Clinical approach to the patient with abnormal liver test results. *Mayo Clin Proc* 71(11):1089–1095, 1996.)

        patients and may be associated with the development of hepatocellular carcinoma.

(3) Alcohol-induced hepatitis is associated with high morbidity and mortality rates. Patients usually have an AST level of less than 500 U/L and an AST:ALT ratio that is greater than or equal to two.

      (4) Drug-induced hepatitis. Common offenders include acetaminophen, nonsteroidal anti–inflammatory drugs (NSAIDs), vitamin A, sulfonamides, isoniazid, tetracyclines, 3-hydroxy-3-methylglutaryl coenzyme A (HMG-CoA) reductase inhibitors, valproic acid, and propylthiouracil.

HOT KEY Inquire about use of herbal and other alternative medications, which may be associated with liver chemistry test abnormalities.

---

  b. Rarer but potentially treatable causes include the following:

    (1) Hemochromatosis (clinical iron overload) is an autosomal recessive multisystemic disease that predominantly affects Caucasian men. Early recognition and therapy with phlebotomy is crucial in preventing complications.

HOT KEY A transferrin saturation greater than 55%, or a ferritin of >200 mcg/L in women or >300 mcg/L in men is concerning for hemochromatosis.

---

    (2) Wilson's disease results from copper overload in the liver and is most common in patients younger than 30 years. A low serum ceruloplasmin level suggests the diagnosis.

    (3) Autoimmune hepatitis is found primarily in young women. Positive results on antinuclear antibody (ANA) or anti-smooth muscle antibody testing suggest the diagnosis.

    (4) α_1-Antitrypsin deficiency. Patients may also have emphysema. A serum α_1-antitrypsin level can be obtained to evaluate possible deficiency.

III FOLLOW-UP AND REFERRAL

A. Cholestasis. Patients with bile duct dilatation require referral to a gastroenterologist.

  1. Extrahepatic biliary dilatation

a. Consider **endoscopic retrograde cholagiopancreatography (ERCP),** which can be both diagnostic and therapeutic, particularly in the setting of choledocholithiasis.

b. If pancreatic cancer or cholangiocarcinoma suspected, consider staging computed tomography or magnetic resonance imaging prior to ERCP, as presence of metastatic disease may guide decision to undertake palliative endoscopic therapy.

HOT

KEY

Patients with bile duct dilation and fever in setting of cholestatic liver chemistry tests require urgent referral for ERCP.

---

2. **Intrahepatic biliary obstruction. ERCP, percutaneous transhepatic cholangiography (PTC), or magnetic resonance cholagiopancreatography (MRCP)** should be performed to confirm the suspicion of intrahepatic biliary obstruction. A **percutaneous liver biopsy** may be needed to further clarify the diagnosis.

B. Hepatocellular Disorders

1. Referral to a gastroenterologist for percutaneous liver biopsy may be indicated for the following patients:

   a. Chronic carriers of either the hepatitis B or C virus

   b. Patients with elevated transferrin saturations

   c. Patients with low serum ceruloplasmin levels

   d. Patients with persistent evaluation of AST or ALT of unclear etiology.

2. Patients with suspected autoimmune hepatitis or α_1-antitrypsin deficiency should be referred to a gastroenterologist for evaluation and treatment.

3. Patient with suspected cirrhosis should be referred to a gastroenterologist for further evaluation and consideration for liver transplantation.

HOT

KEY

Patients with cirrhosis, including those with compensated cirrosis, should be carefully evaluated and considered for liver transplantation listing prior to elective surgery, as the risk for decompensation postoperatively is signficant.

References

Green RM, Flamm S. AGA technical review on the evaluation of liver chemistry tests. *Gastroenterology* 2002;123(4):1367–1384.

Qaseem A, Aronson M, Fitterman N, Snow V, Weiss KB, Owens DK. Screening for
    hereditary hemochromatosis: a clinical practice guideline from the American Col-
    lege of Physicians. *Ann Intern Med* 2005;143(7):517–521.
Ziser A, Plevak DJ, Wiesner RH, Rakela J, Offord KP, Brown DL. Morbidity and
    mortality in cirrhotic patients undergoing anesthesia and surgery. *Anesthesiology*
    1999;90(1):42–53.

PART VI

NEPHROLOGY AND UROLOGY

38. Renal Failure

I INTRODUCTION

A. Elevated serum creatinine levels (greater than 0.8–1.4 mg/dL, depending on age and muscle mass) are often detected on a chemistry panel done for other reasons; patients can be asymptomatic.

B. Evidence shows that patients with severe chronic kidney disease (CKD) are often referred late to a nephrologist, resulting in increased complications and mortality.

C. Over 18 million Americans have CKD, and the incidence is increasing.

II DIFFERENTIAL DIAGNOSIS

A. **Acute renal failure (ARF).** A helpful guide is to separate the causes into prerenal, intrarenal, and postrenal disease.

1. **Prerenal** causes involve inadequate blood flow to the kidneys; this can be caused by hypovolemia (dehydration, blood loss) or by decreased effective arterial volume (congestive heart failure, cirrhosis).

2. **Intrarenal** causes occur at the level of the blood vessels (e.g., bilateral renal artery stenosis), glomerulus (glomerulonephritis), interstitium (acute interstitial nephritis), or tubules (acute tubular necrosis)

3. **Postrenal** causes involve obstruction of the urinary tract. Prostatic hyperplasia, external masses (tumors, lymphadenopathy) and nephrolithasis can result in renal failure.

HOT
▶
KEY

In patients with normal anatomy and no pre-existing renal disease, obstructions above the bladder generally must involve both ureters to cause elevations in creatinine.

---

4. Multiple medications can cause ARF, especially non-steroidal anti-inflammatory drugs (NSAIDs) and antibiotics, including penicillins and aminoglycosides.

B. Chronic kidney disease. In the United States, **diabetes** is the most common causes of chronic kidney disease, followed by hypertension, glomerulonephritis, and polycystic kidney disease.

III APPROACH TO THE PATIENT

A. The first step is to consider **rechecking the creatinine** and to look through the chart for prior evidence of an elevated creatinine.

B. Use the **history and physical findings** to determine if the elevated creatinine is due to acute renal failure or chronic kidney disease.
  1. Patients with **no evidence of previous kidney disease** should be presumed to have ARF.
  2. Patients with an **acute illness** (dehydration, exacerbation of congestive heart failure), fever, or new hematuria are more likely to have ARF.
  3. Patients with evidence of normocytic anemia with normal iron levels, abnormal serum calcium, or high phosphorous levels are more likely to have chronic disease.
  4. Note that an important risk factor for ARF is pre-existing chronic kidney disease.

C. Estimation of glomerular filtration rate (GFR). Serum creatinine is not a reliable estimate of GFR due to variations with muscle mass and age. Severity of renal failure in patients with elevated creatinines should be further characterized by estimating GFR. While GFR can be estimated by urine creatinine collection, a simple alternative is the Cockroft-Gault formula:

$$\text{Estimated GFR (mL/min)} = \frac{(140 - \text{age}) \times \text{weight(kg)} \times 0.85(\text{if female})}{\text{serum creatinine(mg/dL)} \times 72}$$

  1. Estimated GFR **may not be reliable in patients with ARF** because these patients may have rapidly changing creatinine levels.
  2. Table 38-1 shows the current classification of chronic kidney disease by estimated GFR.

D. Basic studies and imaging.
  1. Laboratory studies.
    a. Initial labs may include a full chemistry panel (including potassium, calcium, and phosphorous), glucose level (for diabetes), and urinalysis with microscopy (for sediment analysis).

TABLE 38-1. Classification of Chronic Kidney Disease		
Stage	Estimated GFR (mL/min)	U.S. Prevalence (%)
1	≥90	3.3
2 (Mild)	60–89	3.0
3 (Moderate)	30–59	4.3
4 (Severe)	15–29	0.2
5 (Kidney Failure)	<15	0.1

    b. Proteinuria should also be quantified. Recent data suggests that a spot urine protein to creatinine ratio is a reliable alternative to a 24-hour urine collection for protein. (See Chapter 40 for evaluation of Proteinuria).

    c. Other labs, including antinuclear antibodies (ANA), complement studies, tests for hepatitis B and C, an HIV antibody test, serum and urine protein electrophoreses, anti-neutrophil cytoplasmic antibodies (ANCA), and anti-glomerular basement membrane antibodies should be considered in patients with suspected intrarenal pathology.

  2. Imaging

    a. The initial imaging test should be a **renal ultrasound.** Ultrasound can be used to assess kidney size or urinary obstruction; doppler ultrasound can detect vascular thrombosis.

HOT KEY

Severe chronic kidney disease is usually characterized by small, atrophic kidneys. If enlarged kidneys are detected on ultrasound, consider diabetes, multiple myeloma, HIV, polycystic kidney disease, sarcoid, and amyloidosis as causes of CKD.

    b. A plain film of the abdomen is not generally helpful, but may demonstrate **nephrolithasis. Computed tomography (CT) of the abdomen** is useful for evaluating nephrolithasis and can also detect vascular thrombosis or polycystic kidney disease.

HOT KEY

A plain film of the abdomen will not detect uric acid stones, which are radiolucent.

    c. Magnetic resonance imaging is a sensitive test for detecting renal artery stenosis and does not use iodinated contrast. It is used today as an alternative to **renal angiography.**

IV FOLLOW-UP AND REFERRAL

A. If the disease is believed to be acute, steps to reverse the cause of ARF should be taken immediately (e.g, stopping any offending medications, optimizing volume status). The patient will require very close followup with serial chemistry panels; hospitalization should be considered early.

B. If the disease is chronic, steps to optimize comorbid conditions should be taken, including glucose control in diabetics, as well as aggressive blood pressure and lipid control. Multiple other interventions, such as the use of angiotensin converting enzyme inhibitors, may slow the progression of CKD.

C. Referral to a nephrologist. In general, patients benefit from early referral to nephrology. Indications for referral for CKD include:

    1. An estimated GFR less than 60 mL/min. Consider referral early given that it takes up to a year to secure permanent access for hemodialysis (e.g., placement of an arteriovenous fistula).

    2. An inability to identify the cause of renal failure

    3. Nephrotic range proteinuria (>3.5 g/day)

    4. Difficulty in managing the renal failure

    5. Progressively rising serum creatinine levels. While patients with CKD may have a decline in GFR over the course of years, patients with creatinines rising over weeks to months should be seen immediately by a nephrologist.

References

Snyder S, Pendergraph B. Detection and evaluation of chronic kidney disease. *Am Fam Physician* 2005;72:1733–1734.

Tremblay R. Approach to managing elevated creatinine. *Can Fam Physician* 2004;50: 735–740.

39. Hematuria

....

I INTRODUCTION

A. Hematuria is defined as **3 or more red blood cells (RBCs) per high-power field** in a centrifuged urine sample. Hematuria may be **gross** (i.e., visible blood in the urine) or **microscopic**.

B. The most important reason for understanding hematuria is that **hematuria is a presenting sign of certain malignancies.**

C. Hematuria is **rarely emergent:** hemodynamic instability due to urinary blood loss is unusual. However, significant anemia is possible, and bladder outlet obstruction from clots can occur with gross hematuria, necessitating immediate catheterization.

II DIFFERENTIAL DIAGNOSIS

A. **Pseudohematuria.** It is important to confirm that hematuria is truly present. "Pseudohematuria" refers to discolored urine that is mistaken for bloody urine. Causes include certain foods (beets), drugs (phenazopyridine, rifampin), hyperbilirubinemia, myoglobinuria (from rhabdomyolysis), and hemoglobinuria (from hemolysis).

> **HOT KEY**
> If a patient has a urinary dipstick positive for heme but no RBCs are seen on microscopic examination, consider the diagnosis of rhabdomyolysis.

B. **Hematuria.** The differential diagnoses for gross and microscopic hematuria are the same, although urologic cancer is more frequently found in patients with gross hematuria. On most urine dipsticks, the presence of heme causes a color change from yellow to green. Think, "GREEN PIS," to remember the causes of hematuria:

	Causes of Hematuria ("GREEN PIS")
MNEMONIC	**G**lomerulonephritis
	Renal cyst or trauma
	Exercise
	Embolism or infarction
	Neoplasm
	Prostate hypertrophy
	Infection
	Stones

1. **Glomerulonephritis** (e.g., IgA nephropathy, poststreptococcal glomerulonephritis, vasculitis) can cause hematuria.
2. **Renal cysts** or **trauma.** Hemorrhage into cysts (usually in polycystic kidney disease) or blunt kidney trauma can cause hematuria.
3. **Exercise-induced hematuria** usually occurs within 24–48 hours of vigorous exercise. The hematuria may be microscopic or gross.
4. **Embolism** or **infarction.** Renal infarction may occur as a result of emboli (e.g., endocarditis, aortic atherosclerosis) or other arteriolar pathologies [e.g., sickle cell disease, malignant hypertension).
5. **Neoplasm. Transitional cell carcinoma, renal cell carcinoma,** and **prostate carcinoma** are important to consider in patients with hematuria.
6. **Prostate hypertrophy.** Benign prostatic hypertrophy (BPH) may cause hematuria.
7. **Infection** of the urinary or seminal tract can lead to hematuria. Infections include urethritis (in association with sexually transmitted diseases), cystitis, prostatitis, epididymitis, pyelonephritis, tuberculosis, and schistosomiasis.
8. **Stones** in the urogenital tract can lead to hematuria. Ureteral calculi are usually associated with pain.

III APPROACH TO THE PATIENT

A. **Verify hematuria using urinalysis with microscopy.**
B. **Try to determine the cause** by obtaining a careful history, performing a physical examination, and ordering selected laboratory tests.
   1. **Patient history.** Be sure to ask:
      a. Does the patient have **risk factors for malignancy?** Risk factors include history of urologic cancer, smoking, age greater than 40 years, chemical exposures (benzenes and aromatic amines), and pelvic irradiation.

    b. Does the patient have **pain with urination or flank or groin pain?** Pain suggests the presence of infection or stones.

    c. What is the patient's **medication and travel history?** Is there a history of **vigorous exercise, sexual activity,** or **trauma**?

2. Physical examination should include palpation of the flank and abdomen, genital inspection, and a digital rectal examination.

3. Standard laboratory studies

    a. Urinalysis

        (1) Proteinuria (1+ or greater) on the urine dipstick suggests glomerular pathology in the setting of microscopic hematuria. Proteinuria should be confirmed with a spot urine protein to creatinine ratio or a 24-hour urine collection. With gross hematuria, proteinuria is a less reliable marker.

        (2) Pyuria. White blood cells (WBCs) in the urine suggest infection but may be seen with nephritis, especially tubulointerstitial nephritis. As with protein, small numbers of WBCs may be a "normal" finding with gross hematuria. WBC casts suggest a renal source.

        (3) RBC casts are nearly pathognomonic for glomerulonephritis. Dysmorphic RBCs are also associated with glomerular disease.

    b. Blood urea nitrogen (BUN) and **creatinine levels** should be assessed.

    c. A **complete blood count (CBC), prothrombin time (PT),** and **partial thromboplastin time (PTT)** are indicated for patients with gross hematuria.

C. Initiate a diagnostic work-up if the cause of the hematuria is not evident from the history, physical examination, and initial laboratory studies. Patients meeting any of the criteria in Table 39-1 should undergo further evaluation.

    1. Intravenous urography (IVU) has traditionally been considered the first test in the work-up of hematuria. IVU is less expensive than computed tomography (CT) and has long-established data on efficacy. IVU may miss some renal malignancies and requires intravenous contrast, which may be contraindicated in patients with renal insufficiency.

    2. Computed tomography (CT) of the kidneys and urinary tract is also an acceptable first imaging study. Non-contrast CTs are used to identify stones, while intravenous contrast is used to evaluate cysts, masses, and some infections. Although more expensive than IVU, it can identify a wider range of pathology. The risk of contrast may not be acceptable in patients with elevated creatinine.

TABLE 39-1. Criteria for Diagnostic Work-Up of Hematuria

1. Risk factors for malignancy: history of urologic cancer, smoking, age >40, chemical exposure, and pelvic irradiation
2. Evidence of intrarenal disease: red cell casts or dysmorphic RBCs, elevated creatinine, microscopic hematuria with proteinuria
3. Previous urologic disease
4. Abdominal/flank pain or pain with urination
5. Any gross hematuria without a clear reason for benign, transient hematuria (e.g., vigorous exercise, minor trauma, bladder catheterization, sexual activity)

RBCs = red blood cells

---

3. **Ultrasound of the kidneys and upper urinary tract.** Ultrasound does not use intravenous contrast and can identify renal cysts or upper urinary tract pathology.
4. **Cystoscopy** is the test of choice for bladder pathology. Cystoscopy should be performed in patients with persistent gross hematuria or risk factors for malignancy (Table 39-1).
5. **Urine cytology** may detect bladder carcinoma when other tests are negative, but the sensitivity is low (40 to 76%). Urine cytology is recommended in patients with risk factors for malignancy. The test is performed on the first morning specimen to ensure prolonged urine exposure to the bladder wall, and is often repeated 3 times.
6. **Other tests** (e.g., serologic studies, renal or prostate biopsy, magnetic resonance imaging [MRI]) may be indicated, depending on the patient's history and physical examination findings.

IV FOLLOW-UP AND REFERRAL

A. **Active, gross hematuria or risk factors for malignancy.** A urologist should be consulted promptly.
B. **Signs of intrarenal disease** (Table 39-1). These patients should be referred to a nephrologist.
C. **Negative initial work-up.** In patients with negative evaluations, follow-up includes urinalysis with urine cytology every 6 months. Repeat imaging and/or cystoscopy yearly should be considered, especially if the patient has risk factors for malignancy.

References

Grossfeld GD, Wolf JS, Litwin MS, Hricak H, Shuler C, Agerter DC, Carroll PR. Asymptomatic microscopic hematuria in adults: summary of the AUA best practice policy recommendations. *Am Fam Physician* 2001;63:1145–1154.

Yun EJ, Meng MV, Carroll PR. Evaluation of the patient with hematuria. *Med Clin N Am* 2004;88:329–343.

40. Proteinuria and Nephrotic Syndrome

I INTRODUCTION

A. Proteinuria is significant when over 150 mg of protein is excreted in a 24-hour period. Proteinuria is classified as either **nonrenal ("benign")** or **renal.**

   1. Nonrenal (benign) proteinuria is proteinuria without known renal disease and with an otherwise normal urinary sediment. These patients usually do not develop progressive kidney disease.

   2. Renal proteinuria is caused by a renal disorder. A significant percentage of these patients develop chronic kidney disease.

B. Nephrotic syndrome. The hallmark of nephrotic syndrome is **heavy proteinuria (>3.5 grams/24 hours).** Patients also have **hypoalbuminemia, hyperlipidemia,** and **peripheral edema.** These patients may look "PALE" because of protein excretion.

MNEMONIC

Characteristics of the Nephrotic Syndrome ("PALE")
Proteinuria (>3.5 grams/24 hours)
Albumin (low)
Lipids (elevated)
Edema

II CAUSES OF PROTEINURIA

A. Nonrenal (benign) proteinuria. Benign proteinuria tends to be transient and mild (<1 gram/day). It is caused by acute illness, fever, stress, or strenuous exercise. Orthostatic proteinuria is a benign condition in which proteinuria is present when standing, but absent when lying down.

B. Renal proteinuria. Several renal disorders are associated with proteinuria.

   1. Nephrotic syndrome. Causes of nephrotic syndrome include:

      a. Renal disease. Nephrotic syndrome is caused by primary renal disease in two-thirds of patients. Glomerular diseases associated with nephrotic syndrome include:

         (1) Membranous nephropathy

         (2) Minimal change disease

      (3) **Focal glomerulosclerosis**
      (4) **Membranoproliferative glomerulonephritis**
      (5) **Rapidly progressive glomerulonephritis**
  b. **Systemic disease.** Nephrotic syndrome also occurs secondary to systemic disease. These causes can be remembered using the mnemonic, "THIS LAD HAS nephrotic syndrome."

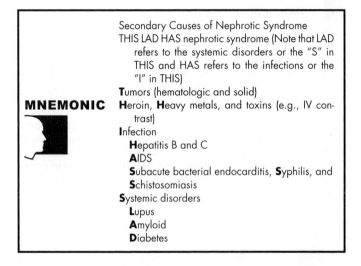

MNEMONIC

Secondary Causes of Nephrotic Syndrome
THIS LAD HAS nephrotic syndrome (Note that LAD refers to the systemic disorders or the "S" in THIS and HAS refers to the infections or the "I" in THIS)
Tumors (hematologic and solid)
Heroin, **H**eavy metals, and toxins (e.g., IV contrast)
Infection
  Hepatitis B and C
  AIDS
  Subacute bacterial endocarditis, **S**yphilis, and **S**chistosomiasis
Systemic disorders
  Lupus
  Amyloid
  Diabetes

HOT KEY

The disorders that can cause nephrotic syndrome can also lead to non-nephrotic range proteinuria.

  2. **Other causes** of renal proteinuria include **nephritic syndrome,** acute and chronic **renal failure, urinary tract infection (UTI), hypertension,** and **nephrolithiasis.**

III **APPROACH TO THE PATIENT.** Proteinuria is often detected from a urinalysis done for other reasons. When confronted with a patient with proteinuria on urinalysis, take the following approach:

A. First, **confirm the presence of proteinuria** on two more dipstick urine samples.

B. If the proteinuria is still present, **consider both nonrenal and renal causes.**

1. If the patient has a condition associated with benign proteinuria (e.g., fever, acute illness), **consider repeating the urinalysis** after the condition has resolved.

2. If the proteinuria is persistent, obtain **either a spot protein/creatinine ratio or a 24-hour urine collection to quantify the proteinuria.** A protein/creatinine ratio is obtained from a single urine sample; the ratio of protein to creatinine estimates the milligrams of protein excreted over a 24-hour period. If the 24-hour urine collection or protein/creatinine ratio reveals an abnormal amount of protein (i.e., more than 150 mg), the following studies should be performed:

   a. Initial studies

   (1) Complete urinalysis with microscopy. If the patient has evidence of a UTI, treatment with antibiotics may precede further evaluation.

   (2) Electrolyte panel, including blood urea nitrogen (BUN), creatinine, and glucose values.

   b. Specific studies. In patients with **suspected nephrotic syndrome,** the following tests may be indicated:

   (1) Antinuclear antibody (ANA) assays

   (2) Hepatitis serologies

   (3) Rapid plasma reagin (RPR) (for syphilis)

   (4) HIV test

   (5) Blood cultures (for endocarditis)

   (6) Fat pad biopsy (for amyloidosis)

   c. Renal biopsy is performed in those with a suspected renal cause after consultation with a nephrologist.

IV TREATMENT AND FOLLOW-UP OF PROTEINURIA FOCUSES ON THE UNDERLYING DISORDER

A. Nonrenal (benign) proteinuria. If asymptomatic and transient, reassurance is usually all that is needed, with no scheduled follow-up.

B. Renal proteinuria

1. Refer to a nephrologist for evaluation, a possible renal biopsy, and treatment recommendations.

2. General management strategies for the nephrotic syndrome include:

   a. A diet low in sodium and saturated fat

   b. Adequate protein intake (approximately 1 g/kg/d)

   c. Diuretics for edema

   d. Fluid restriction (if hyponatremia is present)

References
Carroll MF, Temte JL. Proteinuria in adults: a diagnostic approach. *Am Fam Physician* 2000;62(6):1333–1340.
Kashif W, Siddiqi N, Dincer AP, Dincer HE, Hirsch S. Proteinuria: how to evaluate an important finding. *Cleve Clin J Med* 2003;70(6):535–537, 541–544, 546–547.

41. Dysuria

I. INTRODUCTION

A. Dysuria (i.e., **pain** or **burning with urination**) is a common complaint in the outpatient setting.

B. Dysuria suggests inflammation of the urethra and is usually associated with **other irritative symptoms: frequency, urgency, nocturia,** and/or **hematuria.** The duration and severity of the symptoms do not always correlate with the degree of pathology.

II. DIFFERENTIAL DIAGNOSIS

A. Women

1. **Urinary tract infections (UTIs)** are more common in women. Predisposing factors include failure to void after intercourse, diaphragm use, and postmenopausal status.

   a. **Etiology.** Eighty percent of UTIs in women are caused by *Escherichia coli;* the rest are caused by *Staphylococcus saprophyticus, Proteus mirabilis, Staphylococcus aureus, Enterococcus,* and *Klebsiella.*

   b. **Clinical manifestations.** Patients report acute onset of dysuria with frequency and urgency. Examination may reveal suprapubic or costovertebral angle tenderness.

2. **Vaginal infections** (e.g., **candidiasis, trichomoniasis**). Patients often report vaginal discharge and external genital discomfort. Examination usually reveals a discharge and erythema of the external genitalia.

3. **Sexually transmitted urethritis.** Infections include *Chlamydia trachomatis, Neisseria gonorrhoeae,* or herpes simplex virus (HSV).

4. **Urethral syndrome without clear etiology.** In 5% of patients, no cause is found for symptoms. A history of postcoital voiding dysfunction and dyspareunia is suggestive of an idiopathic urethral syndrome.

5. **Interstitial cystitis** is chronic, idiopathic, and most often affects middle-aged women. Cystoscopic examination reveals inflammation of the bladder wall. A history of nocturia is almost universal; hematuria and dyspareunia can be present as well. Examination may reveal suprapubic tenderness.

B. Men

1. **UTIs** are much less common in men. The most common

causative organisms are *E. coli, Staphylococcus* species, *Enterococcus, Proteus,* and *Klebsiella.*

2. **Bladder stones** and **tumors** are more common in men and may present with pain or hematuria.

3. **Prostatic disorders**
   a. **Prostatitis** may be acute bacterial, chronic bacterial, or chronic nonbacterial.
      (1) **Acute bacterial:** Characterized by a positive urine culture, a tender, boggy prostate, and often signs of systemic toxicity. Causes include *Pseudomonas, E. coli,* and *Enterococcus.*
      (2) **Chronic bacterial:** Characterized by a tender prostate, a lack of systemic findings, and persistently positive urine cultures despite treatment. Gram-negative rods are often the causal organisms.
      (3) **Chronic nonbacterial:** Characterized by a tender prostate, white blood cells on urinalysis after prostatic massage, and negative urine cultures. Causal organisms include *Chlamydia, Ureaplasma,* and *Trichomonas.*
      (4) **Prostatodynia:** A diagnosis of exclusion characterized by a tender prostate but negative urine cultures and no white blood cells on urinalysis.

4. **Urethritis** may be gonococcal (35% of cases, caused by ***Neisseria gonorrhoeae***) or nongonococcal (usually unknown etiology, but can be caused by ***Chlamydia trachomatis*** or ***Ureaplasma urealyticum***). Patients may have a history of penile discharge, but asymptomatic infection is common. A history of multiple sex partners or a new sex partner increases the likelihood of urethritis.

5. **Epididymitis** is the most common intrascrotal infection in men.
   a. **Etiology**
      (1) In **young men, *C. trachomatis*** and ***N. gonorrhoeae*** are the most common causes.
      (2) In **older men, coliform bacteria** are more often responsible.
   b. **Clinical manifestations** include scrotal pain and an enlarged or tender epididymis on examination.

 APPROACH TO THE PATIENT. Algorithms for women and men are given in Figures 41-1 and 41-2, respectively.

 TREATMENT. Selected therapies for common causes of dysuria in women and men are summarized in Tables 41-1 and 41-2, respectively.

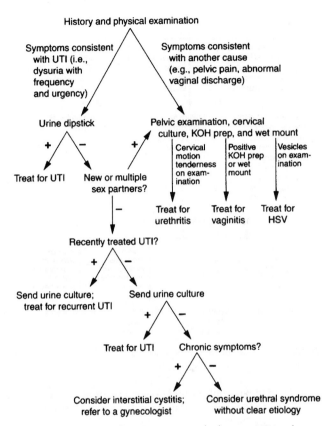

FIGURE 41-1. Approach to a woman with dysuria. *HSV* = herpes simplex virus; *KOH prep* = potassium hydroxide preparation; *UTI* = urinary tract infection.

V FOLLOW-UP AND REFERRAL

A. Women

   1. UTI

   a. Symptoms should be markedly reduced within 72 hours of initiating antimicrobial treatment.

   (1) If symptoms persist, urine should be cultured (or recultured). If bacteriuria is present, consider the possibility of nonadherence, an underlying structural abnormality, or a resistant organism.

   (2) In women with persistent or recurrent UTIs (i.e., more than 3 episodes per year), a work-up should be done

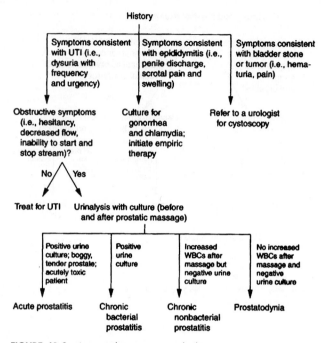

FIGURE 41-2. Approach to a man with dysuria. *UTI* = urinary tract infection; *WBCs* = white blood cells.

to rule out an underlying structural abnormality. If pathology is found, the patient should be referred to a urologist.

  b. Avoiding diaphragm use and urinating after intercourse can help patients prevent future infections. Women with dysuria without clear etiology should take similar precautions.

 2. Vaginitis. These patients do not need follow-up, provided there is an adequate response to therapy.

 3. Sexually transmitted urethritis. These patients should be counseled about using barrier protection. Follow-up tests for HIV and syphilis are usually performed and partners should also be treated. The disease should be reported to the local health department.

 4. Interstitial cystitis. Patients should be referred to a urologist. Patients may obtain support through national support groups.

B. Men

 1. UTI. In men, any UTI warrants an investigation to rule out an underlying structural abnormality.

TABLE 41-1. Selected Therapies for the Common Causes of Dysuria in Women*

Diagnosis	Therapy
Uncomplicated UTI	**Ciprofloxacin** (250 mg PO twice daily for 3 days), or **nitrofurantoin sustained release** (100 mg PO twice daily for 3 days)[†] **Phenazopyridine** (200 mg three times daily for 2 days) to relieve symptoms
Recurrent UTI or pyelonephritis	Use culture to guide treatment, which should be given for 7–14 days; admit for IV antibiotics if toxicity is present. Therapy may be initiated with **ciprofloxacin** (500 mg PO twice daily)
Urethritis	Treat for both *N. gonorrhoeae* and *C. trachomatis*: **ceftriaxone** (125 mg IM, one dose) and **doxycycline** (100 mg PO, twice daily for 7 days)
Vaginitis	*Candida albicans*: **fluconazole** (150 mg PO, one dose) *Trichomonas vaginalis* or *Gardnerella vaginalis*: **metronidazole** (2 g PO, one dose)
HSV infection	**Acyclovir** (200 mg PO, five times daily for 7 days)
Interstitial cystitis	**Refer to urologist**
Urethral syndrome of unclear etiology	**Sitz baths** and **phenazopyridine** (200 mg orally, three times daily for 3 days)

HSV = herpes simplex virus; IM = intramuscularly; PO = orally; UTI = urinary tract infection.

*Regional resistance to certain antibiotics has been observed; check your local antibiotic guide for resistance patterns.

[†]Trimethoprim-sulfamethoxazole may also be used in selected regions with less than 20% *E. Coli* resistance.

2. **Urethritis** or **epididymitis.** These patients should be counseled about using barrier protection and partners should be treated. Follow-up tests for HIV and syphilis are usually performed.

3. **Prostatitis.** Patients with acute bacterial prostatitis should be seen expeditiously by a urologist. Patients with chronic prostatitis or prostatodynia may also benefit from urology consultation.

TABLE 41-2. Selected Therapies for the Common Causes of Dysuria in Men[*]

Diagnosis	Therapy
UTI	Use culture to guide treatment, which should be given for 7–14 days Therapy may be initiated with **ciprofloxacin** (500 mg PO twice daily)
Acute bacterial prostatitis	**Ciprofloxacin** (500 mg PO twice daily until culture results are available); therapy (based on culture results) given for 30 days; admit for IV antibiotics if toxicity is present
Chronic bacterial prostatitis	**Ciprofloxacin** (500 mg PO twice daily for 4–16 weeks)[†]
Chronic nonbacterial prostatitis	**Doxycycline** (100 mg PO, twice daily for 7 days) or **azithromycin** (1 g PO, one dose)
Young man with urethritis or epididymitis	Treat for both *N. gonorrhoeae* and *C. trachomatis*: **ceftriaxone** (125 mg IM, one dose) and **doxycycline** (100 mg PO, twice daily for 7 days)
Older man with epididymitis	Use culture to guide treatment, which should be given for 7–14 days Therapy may be initiated with **ciprofloxacin** (500 mg PO twice daily)
Prostatodynia	May respond to α **blockers**
Bladder stone or tumor	**Refer to urologist** for cystoscopy

HSV = herpes simplex virus; IM = intramuscularly; PO = orally; UTI = urinary tract infection.
[*]Regional resistance to certain antibiotics has been observed; check your local antibiotic guide for resistance patterns.
[†]Cure rates for chronic bacterial prostatitis are reported to be less than 50%. If a patient does not show improvement in 14 days, changing therapies should be considered.

4. Bladder stone or **tumor.** Patients with suspected bladder pathology need to be seen by a urologist.

References
Bent S, Nallamothu BK, Simel D, Fihn SD, Saint S. Does this woman have an acute uncomplicated urinary tract infection? *JAMA* 2002;287:2701–2710.
Bremnor JD, Sadovsky R. Evaluation of dysuria in adults. *Am Fam Physician* 2002;65: 1589–1597.

42. Scrotal Mass

I **DIFFERENTIAL DIAGNOSIS.** Scrotal masses can be classified as painful or painless (Table 42-1).

A. Painful masses. The main concerns are **epididymitis** and **testicular torsion.** Other causes include **orchitis, cellulitis,** and **trauma.**

1. **Epididymitis** is ten times more common than testicular torsion.

   a. In **heterosexual men younger than 35 years,** the infection is often sexually transmitted and caused by *Chlamydia trachomatis* or *Neisseria gonorrhoeae.*

   b. In **homosexual men** and **men older than 35 years,** the infection is usually caused by **Enterobacteriaceae.**

2. **Testicular torsion** occurs in young adults and is rare over the age of 40. The pain and swelling result from rotation of the testicle around the spermatic cord, which leads to venous occlusion, edema, and ischemia.

3. **Orchitis** occurs in association with mumps and develops 7–10 days after parotitis. Involvement is usually unilateral with swelling, pain, and tenderness.

4. **Cellulitis** of the groin is usually caused by mixed bacteria. It is more common in patients with serious comorbid disease (e.g., diabetes, chronic renal failure, alcoholism). **Fournier's gangrene** is a necrotizing fasciitis of the genitalia, and is a surgical emergency.

B. Painless masses. Most painless lesions are discovered incidentally.

1. **Tumor.** Testicular tumors are usually malignant germ cell tumors (seminoma and nonseminoma). The peak incidence is between the ages of 20 and 40 years.

2. **Hydrocele** is a fluid collection between two layers of the tunica vaginalis, a potential space created by the descent of the testicle. Hydrocele usually occurs in men older than 40 years.

3. **Spermatocele** is a sperm-filled cyst on the testis caused by blockage of an efferent ductule.

4. **Varicocele** is a venous dilatation above the testis in the spermatic cord. This lesion is more common in young men and on the left side.

TABLE 42-1. Differential Diagnosis of a Scrotal Mass

Painful Scrotal Mass	Painless Scrotal Mass
Infection (e.g., epididymitis, orchitis, Fornier's gangrene)	Tumor
Torsion	Hydrocele, spermatocele, varicocele
Trauma	Inguinal hernia
Referred pain (e.g., kidney stone, appendicitis, abdominal aortic aneurysm, prostatitis, retroperitoneal cancer)	Tuberculous mass
	Sperm granuloma

5. **Inguinal hernia** presents with the sudden onset of a groin mass following the herniation of bowel through the inguinal canal.

6. **Sperm granulomas** occur in patients post-vasectomy and present as tender nodules at the surgical site.

7. **Tuberculous mass.** *Mycobacterium tuberculosis* can cause infections in the testicle. Infection may present as a firm mass or a draining sinus.

II APPROACH TO THE PATIENT

A. **Painful mass**
  1. **Patient history**
     a. **Epididymitis** presents in hours to days as scrotal pain that may radiate to the flank. Fever, swelling of the epididymis, urethral discharge, and dysuria are common.
     b. **Testicular torsion.** Patients often have nausea but rarely have fever or irritative voiding symptoms. There is often a history of pain episodes that resolved spontaneously. A history of trauma does not exclude the possibility of torsion.
  2. **Physical examination** should include careful inspection and palpation of the scrotum.
     a. **Epididymitis.** The epididymis, which is located posterior to the testicle, is swollen and painful. In advanced cases, the swelling may involve the entire testicle.

HOT KEY

Unlike testicular torsion, the pain of epididymitis may improve with testicular elevation (Prehn's sign).

b. Testicular torsion results in a painful, swollen testicle that may be elevated in the scrotum.

c. Cellulitis presents with painful swelling of the scrotum, perineum, or penis. In **Fournier's gangrene**, evidence of necrosis may be noted.

HOT KEY

Referred pain from the retroperitoneum (as in ureterolithiasis or abdominal aortic aneurysm) or prostate should be suspected if the testicular examination is normal.

3. Laboratory studies
  a. Urinalysis and **urine culture.** Pyuria suggests the diagnosis of epididymitis.
  b. Urethral culture should be performed if a sexually transmitted disease is suspected.

B. Painless mass
  1. Patient history. Certain aspects may provide clues to the diagnosis:
    a. A sudden onset suggests an inguinal hernia.
    b. Patients who have undergone vasectomy are at risk for sperm granuloma.
    c. Fluid or discharge from a sinus may suggest a tuberculous mass.
  2. Physical examination
    a. Determine by palpation if the mass is within the testicle or external to it. Masses external to the testicle and masses that transilluminate are more likely benign. All intratesticular masses are cancer until proven otherwise.
    b. A varicocele often increases in size when the patient performs a Valsalva maneuver and decreases in size when the patient lies down. When palpated, a varicocele may feel like a "bag of worms."

HOT KEY

A right-sided or a rapidly enlarging left-sided varicocele should lead to an evaluation for a retroperitoneal tumor with venous obstruction.

  3. Imaging studies. An **ultrasound** and **urologic consultation** should be obtained for patients with intratesticular masses. Most extratesticular masses should be evaluated with ultrasound because many can occur in association with cancer.

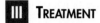 **Treatment**

A. Painful mass

1. **Epididymitis.** Antibiotic therapy should be directed at the likely cause.
   a. For heterosexual patients younger than 35 years, treat for both *C. trachomatis* and *N. gonorrhoeae* (a suitable regimen is ceftriaxone 125 mg IM, one dose, and doxycycline 100 mg PO twice daily for 7 days)
   b. For homosexual men or men older than 35 years, treat for Enterobacteriaceae with ciprofloxacin (500 mg orally twice daily for 10–14 days).

2. **Testicular torsion** is a **surgical emergency.** Surgical consultation should be immediate because salvage of the testicle is more likely when the condition is corrected within 6 hours.

3. **Fournier's gangrene** is also a **surgical emergency,** requiring immediate debridement.

4. **Trauma** can be managed with oral analgesics unless rupture of the testicle is suspected, in which case surgery is required.

B. Painless masses

1. **Testicular cancer** is treated with excision; radiation and chemotherapy are sometimes required.

2. **Hydroceles** can be aspirated with a needle, but the fluid often reaccumulates.

HOT

KEY
Needle aspiration of a hydrocele should be performed only after cancer has been excluded because malignant cells can seed the needle tract.

---

4. **Other painless swellings** can be left alone once cancer has been excluded. For conditions that remain uncomfortable, surgery can be considered.

IV Follow-up and Referral

A. Patients with epididymitis must be reevaluated after treatment to ensure that there are no remaining masses, because patients with testicular cancer can initially present with epididymitis.

B. All patients with masses suspicious for malignancy should be referred to a urologist.

References
Albers P, Albrecht W, Algaba F, Bokemeyer C, Cohn-Cedermark G, Horwich A, Klepp O, Laguna MP, Pizzocaro G. Guidelines on testicular cancer. *Eur Urol* 2005;48(6):885–894.
Sandlow J. Pathogenesis and treatment of varicoceles. *BMJ* 2004;328:967–968.

43. Erectile Dysfunction

I INTRODUCTION

A. Erectile dysfunction (ED) is the **consistent inability to maintain an erection sufficient for sexual intercourse.** Male erection relies on **sufficient libido,** an **intact nerve supply** to the penis, and proper **vascular function.**

B. Approximately 20 to 30 million men in the United States are affected by ED.

C. Often, men will not report this complaint; thus, it is important to ask **during routine health screenings.** Men who experience occasional erectile dysfunction should be reassured that this is common.

II CAUSES OF ERECTILE DYSFUNCTION. ED is either **organic** (i.e., neurogenic, vascular, hormonal, or pharmacologic in origin) or **psychogenic.** Table 43-1 lists the most common causes of erectile dysfunction.

III APPROACH TO THE PATIENT

A. Patient history. Ask about:
1. The presence of disorders that lead to ED (e.g., hypertension, atherosclerosis, diabetes)
2. The use of drugs that commonly lead to ED
3. Any surgeries involving the pelvic area
4. The time course of the ED
5. The presence of occasional erections during sleep or early morning (absence suggests an organic cause)

B. Physical examination
1. Note any absence of secondary sexual characteristics.
2. Evaluate the peripheral pulses of the lower extremities.
3. Note testicular size and consistency.

> **HOT**
> **KEY**
> In most patents with impotence, the physical exam is relatively normal.

TABLE 43-1. Causes of Erectile Dysfunction

Classification of Disease	Specific Examples	Approximate Incidence
Neurogenic	Diabetic neuropathy, surgical damage to pelvic nerves	30%
Vascular	Related to arteriosclerosis, hypertension, or smoking	20%
Pharmacologic	Alcohol, narcotics, selective serotonin reuptake inhibitors (SSRIs), clonidine	15%
Psychogenic	Generalized anxiety, depression, performance anxiety	10%
Hormonal	Hypogonadism, thyroid disease	5%
Multifactorial	Combination of the above	20%

C. Laboratory studies should include a **fasting glucose** for diabetes and a **total testosterone level.**

  1. If the testosterone level is decreased, follicle–stimulating hormone (FSH), luteinizing hormone (LH), and prolactin levels should be determined.

  2. Additional tests [e.g., a thyroid-stimulating hormone (TSH) level] should be ordered according to clinical suspicion.

IV TREATMENT

A. Definitive therapy depends on the cause, which is often difficult to ascertain in many patients.

  1. Psychogenic impotence. Consultation with a psychiatrist and **psychosexual therapy** are often helpful.

  2. Hypogonadism with documented androgen deficiency. Patients can be treated with **intramuscular testosterone injections** or testosterone patches.

HOT KEY

Before prescribing exogenous testosterone to any man, screen for prostate cancer by obtaining a prostate-specific antigen (PSA) level and performing a digital rectal examination.

---

  3. Vascular dysfunction. Patients with vascular disorders who fail more conventional therapy may be eligible for **vascular reconstruction.**

B. Symptomatic therapy

  1. First-line oral medications that inhibit phosphodiesterase type 5 and induce temporary erections are sildenafil, vardenafil, and tadalafil. A tablet is taken 1 hour prior to sexual intercourse; depending on the drug, the ability to maintain normal erections can last for 24 to 72 hours. These medications should not be given to men receiving nitrate therapy, and caution should be exercised when prescribing to patients on α-blockers.

  2. Injection therapy entails the injection of prostaglandins into the penis and may be considered after consultation with a urologist. Intraurethral prostaglandin suppositories are also available.

  3. Penile prostheses may be considered in consultation with a urologist.

V FOLLOW-UP AND REFERRAL

A. Referral to a psychiatrist is appropriate for those with psychogenic impotence.

B. Referral to a urologist or an impotence clinic is usually indicated when the patient:

  1. Fails oral medications, has a normal testosterone level, and the impotence is not obviously psychogenic in origin

  2. Desires injection or surgical therapy

References

Lue TF. Erectile dysfunction. *N Engl J Med* 2000;342(24):1802–1813.

Mikhail N. Management of erectile dysfunction by the primary care physician. *Cleve Clin J Med* 2005;72(4):293–294, 296–297, 301–305.

44. Benign Prostatic Hyperplasia

I **INTRODUCTION.** Benign prostatic hyperplasia (BPH) is characterized by proliferation of epithelial and stromal elements of the prostate.

II **CLINICAL MANIFESTATIONS.** Patients often present with both obstructive and irritative symptoms.

A. **Obstructive symptoms,** caused by blockade of the prostatic urethra, include a decreased urinary stream, hesitancy, and a feeling of incomplete emptying.

B. **Irritative symptoms,** caused by incomplete emptying and bladder hypersensitivity, include frequency, urgency, nocturia, and dysuria.

III **DIFFERENTIAL DIAGNOSIS.** It is important to rule out other medical conditions that mimic the symptoms of BPH (Table 44-1).

IV **APPROACH TO THE PATIENT**

A. **Patient history**
  1. Does the patient have a **medical history** of or symptoms suggestive of **diabetes, congestive heart failure (CHF), alcoholism,** or **neurologic disease?**
  2. What is the patient's **past urologic history?** Has the patient had strictures, a sexually transmitted disease, a urinary tract infection, or urethral instrumentation?
  3. What is the patient's **medication history?** Decongestants, anticholinergic agents, and diuretics can worsen the symptoms of BPH.

B. **Physical examination**
  1. Palpate the abdomen. A palpable bladder suggests severe obstruction.
  2. Examine the prostate for size, tenderness (suggestive of prostatitis), and nodularity (suggestive of prostate cancer).
  3. Focus the rest of the examination on signs suggestive of CHF, diabetes, or alcoholism.

TABLE 44-1. Differential Diagnosis of Benign Prostatic Hyperplasia (BPH)

Differential Diagnosis	Symptoms or Signs Similar to Those of BPH
Systemic Disorders	
Congestive heart failure (CHF)	Nocturia
Diabetes	Frequency and nocturia
Alcoholism	Frequency and nocturia
Neurologic disease	Incontinence, frequency, incomplete emptying
Medication side effects	Frequency and obstructive symptoms
Genitourinary Disorders	
Infection	Frequency, urgency, nocturia, dysuria
Prostatitis	
STDs	
UTIs	
Renal, bladder, or prostate cancer	Dysuria
Strictures	Incomplete emptying, irritative symptoms

STDs = sexually transmitted diseases; UTIs = urinary tract infections.

C. Laboratory studies
1. A **urinalysis** and **urine culture** should be ordered to rule out infection, hematuria, and glycosuria.
2. **Serum creatinine level.** If elevated, upper tract imaging (e.g., ultrasound) to rule out obstruction is indicated.
3. **Serum prostate-specific antigen (PSA)** may be ordered to screen for prostate cancer.

D. Other studies
1. A **post-void residual (PVR) study** is ordered when severe obstruction is suspected. If the PVR is greater than approximately 200 ml, the obstruction may be severe, and urology referral is warranted.

HOT KEY In a patient with severe urinary symptoms or suprapubic tenderness/fullness, a PVR can be performed with a foley catheter. If the PVR is >250, the foley should be left in place to drain to a leg bag while urology is consulted.

2. The **maximum urine flow rate** is used as a marker of severity. For total voided volumes of 150 ml or more, a maximum flow rate of less than 10 ml/sec is considered low.

V **TREATMENT.** There are three major treatment options: watchful waiting, medical therapy, and surgery.

A. **Watchful waiting** is appropriate for patients with mild symptoms. Approximately 50% of patients report improvement without treatment.
B. **Medical therapy**
  1. α **Antagonists** decrease the tone of the prostatic smooth muscle and are the first-line treatment for BPH. **Terazosin** is commonly used (initiate therapy with 1 mg orally at bedtime and advance weekly; maximum dose is 20 mg). Patients should be warned that postural hypotension may occur.
  2. **5α-Reductase inhibitors** should be considered for patients with an enlarged prostate who do not respond to therapy with α **antagonists**. **Finasteride** (5 mg daily) is commonly used.
C. **Surgery** should be considered for severe symptoms and for those who remain symptomatic despite medical therapy. **Transurethral resection of the prostate, transurethral incision,** and **laser, microwave, balloon,** and **stenting procedures** are all effective.

VI **FOLLOW-UP AND REFERRAL**

A. Patients with mild symptoms who choose watchful waiting can be followed at 3- to 6-month intervals.
B. Treatment with an α antagonist necessitates that the patient be seen several times over 2 months to assess treatment effect and medication side effects.
C. Patients with signs of impending obstruction (e.g., a large postvoid residual or severe symptoms) and those considering surgical treatment should be referred to a urologist.

References
Dull P, Reagan RW, Bahnson RR. Managing benign prostatic hyperplasia. *Am Fam Physician* 2002;66:77–84, 87–88.
Thorpe A, Neal D. Benign prostatic hyperplasia. *Lancet* 2003;361:1359–1367.

PART VII

GYNECOLOGY

• •

45. Amenorrhea

I INTRODUCTION

A. **Primary amenorrhea** is the failure of menses to begin (menarche) in a patient 16 years or older. An evaluation is started at age 14 if a patient has no signs of secondary sexual characteristics.

B. **Secondary amenorrhea** is the absence of menstrual periods for three consecutive cycles or for 6 months in a woman who had experienced menarche.

II CAUSES OF AMENORRHEA

A. **Primary amenorrhea**

1. **Congenital abnormalities** of the uterus, cervix, or vagina can cause primary amenorrhea.

2. **Pseudohermaphroditism**

   a. **Female pseudohermaphroditism** is the presence of ovarian tissue in a patient with some male morphologic features. **Congenital adrenal hyperplasia** is a common example. In this condition, adrenal hormone (e.g., 21-hydroxylase, 11β-hydroxylase) deficiencies decrease adrenal hydrocortisone production. In response, more adrenocorticotropic hormone (ACTH) is released, causing adrenal hyperplasia and excess androgen production.

   b. **Male pseudohermaphroditism** is the presence of testicular tissue in a patient with female morphologic features. **Testosterone resistance (testicular feminization)** and **testosterone deficiency** are examples.

3. **Hypothalamic** or **pituitary abnormalities**

   a. Genetic deficiencies of GnRH such as Kallmann's syndrome occurs when a deficiency of luteinizing hormone-releasing hormone (LHRH) leads to low luteinizing hormone (LH) and follicle-stimulating hormone (FSH) levels, resulting in primary amenorrhea.

   b. Other causes of abnormal pulsatile LHRH or gonadotropin release (e.g., hypothalamic or pituitary tumors,

Cushing's syndrome, hypothyroidism, excessive dieting or exercise, stress) can cause primary or secondary amenorrhea.

4. Ovarian failure

  a. Primary ovarian failure can be caused by abnormal gonadal development or ovarian dysgenesis. Examples include Turner's syndrome (45,XO karyotype) and chromosomal mosaicism (e.g., 45X/46X,X). A Y chromosome can be present, and is associated with an increased risk for gonadal neoplasm.

  b. Other causes of ovarian failure, which can lead to primary or secondary amenorrhea, include autoimmune destruction and idiopathic ovarian failure.

B. Secondary amenorrhea

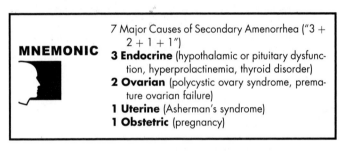

MNEMONIC

7 Major Causes of Secondary Amenorrhea ("3 + 2 + 1 + 1")

3 Endocrine (hypothalamic or pituitary dysfunction, hyperprolactinemia, thyroid disorder)

2 Ovarian (polycystic ovary syndrome, premature ovarian failure)

1 Uterine (Asherman's syndrome)

1 Obstetric (pregnancy)

1. Endocrine causes

  a. Hypothalamic or pituitary dysfunction

   (1) Hypothalamic dysfunction, with loss of the normal LHRH pulsatile release, can be caused by stress, heavy exercise, or extreme weight loss (e.g., anorexia nervosa). Hypothalamic masses are rare.

   (2) A pituitary tumor or Sheehan's syndrome (i.e., pituitary necrosis that typically results from postpartum hemorrhage and hypotension) can lead to secondary amenorrhea. Patients with pituitary tumors may also experience headache or visual disturbances.

  b. Hyperprolactinemia of any cause leads to both pituitary and ovarian dysfunction by disrupting the pulsatile release of FSH and LH. Medications (e.g., tricyclic antidepressants, phenothiazines) or a pituitary tumor can cause hyperprolactinemia. Galactorrhea is often present.

  c. Thyroid disorders. Hypothyroidism (and less commonly, hyperthyroidism) can lead to secondary amenorrhea.

2. Ovarian causes

  a. Polycystic ovary syndrome results in amenorrhea due to chronic anovulation. It is due at least in part to insulin resistance. Common features include irregular or absent menses, obesity, hirsutism, glucose intolerance, infertility, and an LH:FSH ratio greater than 2.

   b. Premature ovarian failure is ovarian failure prior to age 40 years accompanied by elevated gonadotropin levels. Approximately 0.1% of women are affected by age 30, and 1% by age 40. Autoimmunity, chemotherapy, and radiation are common causes. In women younger than 30 years, a karyotype is necessary to exclude the presence of a Y chromosome (which increases the risk for gonadal neoplasm).

   c. Menopause is due to physiologic decline in ovarian function, resulting in anovulation and eventual amenorrhea. The average age of menopause in the United States is about 51 years.

3. Uterine cause. Asherman's syndrome (i.e., intrauterine adhesions, usually caused by dilation and curettage or endometritis) can cause outflow tract obstruction, leading to secondary amenorrhea.

4. Pregnancy should be ruled out in all women of reproductive age.

III APPROACH TO THE PATIENT

A. Primary amenorrhea. Perform a physical examination to **evaluate secondary sexual development** and assign the patient to one of the three following groups:

1. Normal female secondary sexual characteristics. The presence of normal female secondary sexual characteristics suggests that the patient has normal levels of estrogen, progesterone, and androgens. A **congenital abnormality of the uterus, cervix,** or **vagina** is the most likely cause.

   a. Patient history. Absence of the uterus is usually asymptomatic, whereas an abnormality of the vagina or cervix impairing uterine outflow typically presents with **cyclic crampy pain.**

   b. Pelvic and **bimanual examinations** should be performed to assess for congenital abnormalities, followed by ultrasound of the uterus. An absent or abnormal uterus warrents karyotype analysis. In the presence of a normal uterus, without physical signs of an imperforate hymen or transverse vaginal septum, one should proceed with workup of secondary amenorrhea.

2. Ambiguous external genitalia (male and female characteristics). This finding indicates excess androgen exposure *in utero.*

    a. The most common cause of excess androgen exposure *in utero* is **congenital adrenal hyperplasia.** This diagnosis is confirmed by finding elevated **serum dehydroepiandro-sterone sulfate (DHEAS)** and **17-OH progesterone levels.**

    b. A less likely cause of ambiguous genitalia is **male** or **female hermaphroditism.** Diagnosis is made by **karyotype.**

3. Absent female secondary sexual characteristics. This finding indicates no prior systemic exposure to estrogen. A serum FSH level distinguishes hypothalamic from ovarian pathology.

    a. A **low** or **normal FSH level** (i.e., <20 IU/L) indicates a **hypothalamic** or **pituitary abnormality.**

    b. An **elevated FSH level** (i.e., >20 IU/L) suggests **ovarian failure.** A karyotype analysis should be obtained.

       (1) An **XY karyotype** carries an increased risk of gonadal neoplasm and is treated with gonadectomy and hormone replacement therapy (HRT).

       (2) An **XX karyotype** indicates ovarian insensitivity, premature ovarian failure, or adrenal enzyme deficiency with adrenal hyperplasia.

B. Secondary amenorrhea

HOT KEY

Pregnancy is the most common cause of secondary amenorrhea. A pregnancy test should be performed before undertaking an exhaustive work-up.

---

1. Patient history. Begin by establishing the pattern of the patient's menses, then think about the seven causes of secondary amenorrhea and use them to guide your questions.

    a. Pregnancy. Is the patient sexually active? Does she use contraception, and if so, what form?

    b. Hypothalamic or **pituitary dysfunction.** Is there a history of stress, weight loss, or strenuous exercise?

    c. Hyperprolactinemia. Has the patient noted galactorrhea? What is the patient's medication history?

    d. Thyroid disorder. Does the patient complain of cold intolerance, fatigue, depression, or weight gain? All of these are symptoms of hypothyroidism.

    e. Polycystic ovarian syndrome. Is the amenorrhea chronic? Is there a history of obesity or hirsutism?

    f. Premature ovarian failure. Has the patient experienced "hot flashes" or atrophic vaginitis?

    g. Asherman's syndrome. Does the patient have a history of endometritis, pregnancy, or abortion?

2. **Physical examination**
   a. Galactorrhea, hirsutism, or thyromegaly may be found on physical examination.
   b. The presence of secondary sexual characteristics (indicating estrogen and progesterone production) should be noted.
   c. A pelvic examination should be performed to assess vaginal patency and uterine or ovarian pathology.
3. **Laboratory studies.** An algorithm for evaluating secondary amenorrhea is shown in Figure 45-1.

HOT **KEY** Amenorrhea persisting for more than 6 months following the cessation of oral contraceptive use should not be attributed to the oral contraceptives. A work-up for secondary amenorrhea is appropriate for these patients.

IV TREATMENT DEPENDS ON THE UNDERLYING DISORDER

A. **Primary amenorrhea**
   1. **Congenital abnormalities of the uterus, cervix,** or **vagina.** Some congenital abnormalities can be treated surgically.
   2. **Congenital adrenal hyperplasia** is treated with low-dose dexamethasone to suppress production of androgen precursors.
   3. **Ovarian failure.** Patients with the XY karyotype should have their ovaries removed to reduce the risk of ovarian cancer. All patients with ovarian failure should receive HRT.

B. **Secondary amenorrhea**
   1. **Hypothalamic** or **pituitary dysfunction**
      a. Prolactin-secreting tumors can be treated with bromocriptine to suppress prolactin secretion. Other pituitary tumors and prolactinomas that are unresponsive to medical therapy can be resected, either via a transphenoidal approach or, rarely, craniotomy.
      b. Patients with pituitary failure due to neoplasia, Sheehan's syndrome, or other causes require replacement therapy with steroids (i.e., hydrocortisone, 15 mg every morning and 10 mg every evening), thyroid hormone, and estrogen/progesterone.
   2. **Polycystic ovarian syndrome.** All patients with polycystic ovarian syndrome should be screened to rule out and androgen secreting tumor, which is associated with significantly elevated testosterone or DHEA-S levels. Many benefit from weight loss, which decreases peripheral estrogen formation

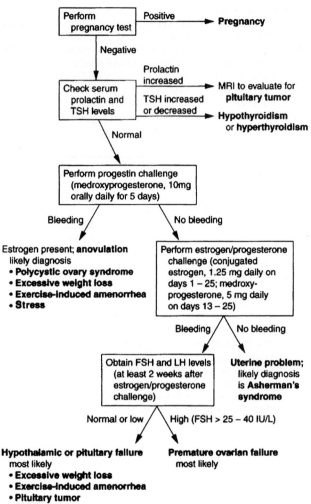

FIGURE 45-1. Approach to the patient with secondary amenorrhea. *FSH* = follicle-stimulating hormone; *LH* = luteinizing hormone; *MRI* = magnetic resonance imaging; *TSH* = thyroid-stimulating hormone.

and insulin resistance. In addition, they should receive one of the following three hormonal therapies:

    a. Oral contraceptives decrease ovarian androgen production and induce withdrawal bleeding to prevent endometrial hyperplasia.

    b. Clomiphene increases FSH production in women who desire fertility.

    c. Terminal progesterone induces withdrawal bleeding.

3. **Premature ovarian failure** is treated with ovariectomy (if the patient has an XY karyotype) and HRT. Women should be screened for osteoporosis and additional risk factors for heart disease. They should be instucted to take calcium supplementation with vitamin D.

4. **Asherman's syndrome** is treated with dilatation and curettage (D&C) or lysis of endometrial adhesions, followed by short-term placement of a pediatric Foley catheter or an intrauterine device (IUD) to maintain the endometrial cavity. Estrogens are given to maintain the endometrial lining.

References

Master-Hunter T, Herman D. Amenorrhea: Evaluation and Treatment. *Am Fam Physician* 2006;73(8):1374–1382.

Practice Guideline of the American Society for Reproductive Medicine: Current Evaluation of Amenorrhea. *Fertility and Sterility* 2004;82 supp 1: s3–9.

46. Abnormal Uterine Bleeding

I INTRODUCTION

A. A **normal menstrual cycle** lasts 21–35 days, of which 2–7 days involve bleeding. The total blood loss during a normal menstrual cycle is 25–80 milliliters. Any menstrual bleeding outside of these parameters is considered abnormal and should be evaluated.

B. Common terms used to describe **abnormal patterns of menstrual bleeding** are defined in Table 46-1. The terminology can be confusing; it is always appropriate to simply describe the abnormality in terms of the cycle length, days of bleeding, or amount of bleeding.

II DIFFERENTIAL DIAGNOSIS.
Abnormal bleeding can be **pregnancy-related** or due to dysfunctional uterine bleeding, which may be **ovulatory** or **anovulatory** (Table 46-2).

A. **Pregnancy-related bleeding** occurs in patients who are pregnant or were recently pregnant.

B. **Ovulatory bleeding** is abnormal bleeding in patients who are ovulating normally. Because ovulation requires a functioning endocrine axis, the hypothalamus, pituitary gland, and ovaries are usually normal in these patients. The endometrium cycles normally, with a proliferative (estrogen-dependent) and a secretory (progesterone-dependent) phase. Ovulatory bleeding is usually attributable to either an **anatomic abnormality** of the uterus, cervix, or vagina or a **bleeding disorder** (see Chapter 73).

C. **Anovulatory bleeding** occurs in patients who are not ovulating normally, which usually indicates an abnormality in one of the organs of the endocrine axis. When ovulation does not occur, estrogen is often present for long periods of time without progesterone, leading to the "unopposed estrogen effect." Unopposed estrogen causes the endo-metrium to continue in the proliferative phase, resulting in periodic shedding of tissue. Bleeding patterns vary, but are often characterized by irregular intervals and irregular amounts.

1. **Hypothalamic-pituitary dysfunction.** Thyroid disease, hyperprolactinemia, excess androgens or cortisol, and stress (emotional, weight loss-related, or exercise–related) can disturb hypothalamic rhythmicity and result in anovulation.

TABLE 46-1. Patterns of Abnormal Uterine Bleeding

Menorrhagia: Prolonged, heavy uterine bleeding occurring at regular intervals

Metrorrhagia: Variable amount of uterine bleeding occurring at frequent, irregular intervals

Menometrorrhagia: Prolonged, heavy uterine bleeding occurring at irregular intervals

Polymenorrhea: Uterine bleeding occurring at regular intervals of less than 21 days

Oligomenorrhea: Uterine bleeding occurring at intervals varying from 35 days to 6 months

Amenorrhea: Absence of uterine bleeding for at least 6 months

Intermenstrual bleeding: Variable amount of uterine bleeding occurring between regular menstrual periods

Dysfunctional uterine bleeding: Abnormal uterine bleeding in which the source is the endometrium; occurs in the absence of anatomic lesions and is most often caused by chronic anovulation

---

2. **Ovarian dysfunction.** Ovarian tumors, polycystic ovary syndrome, or ovarian failure (menopause or premature ovarian failure) may cause anovulatory uterine bleeding.

HOT KEY

Physiologic anovulatory bleeding accompanies normal aging and occurs in perimenarchal and perimenopausal patients. It is common for adolescent girls to experience anovulation and heavy or irregular bleeding for 1–2 years after the onset of menses. Similarly, perimenopausal women have anovulatory cycles that can cause abnormal patterns of bleeding for several years.

III **APPROACH TO THE PATIENT.** Figure 46-1 presents a stepwise approach for evaluating a patient with abnormal uterine bleeding.

A. **Obtain the patient history and perform a general physical examination.**

1. What is the patient's current pattern of menstrual bleeding? Her previous pattern? Has she experienced any post-coital bleeding?

2. Does the patient have any associated symptoms?

3. Has the patient noted any changes in weight or exercise regimen, or experienced excess stress?

TABLE 46-2. Common Causes of Abnormal Uterine Bleeding

Pregnancy-related bleeding
  Ectopic pregnancy
  Threatened or spontaneous abortion
  Retained products of gestation
  Gestational trophoblastic disease
Ovulatory bleeding
  Uterine anomaly
    Uterine carcinoma
    Uterine fibroids
    Uterine polyps
    Adenomyosis
    Foreign body (e.g., intrauterine device [IUD])
    Sarcoma
  Cervical anomaly
    Cervical carcinoma
    Cervical polyps
    Cervicitis
    Condyloma
    Pelvic inflammatory disease (PID)
    Erosion
    Cervical trauma
  Vaginal anomaly
    Vaginal carcinoma
    Vaginal infection (e.g., vaginitis, herpes)
    Vaginal foreign body
    Vaginal trauma
    Adenosis
  Bleeding disorder
Anovulatory Bleeding
  Hypothalmic-pituitary dysfunction
    Physiologic anovulatory bleeding (perimarchal and
      perimenopausal)
    Thyroid disease
    Hyperprolactinemia
    Stress
    Cushing's syndrome (cortisol excess)
    Adrenal or ovarian tumor (androgen excess)
  Ovarian dysfunction
    Ovarian failure
    Ovarian tumor
    Polycystic ovary disease

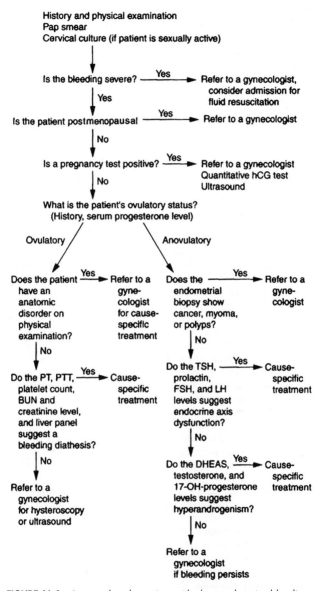

FIGURE 46-1. Approach to the patient with abnormal uterine bleeding. *BUN* = blood urea nitrogen; *DHEAS* = dehydroepiandrosterone sulfate; *FSH* = follicle-stimulating hormone; *LH* = luteinizing hormone; *PT* = prothrombin time; *PTT* = partial thromboplastin time; *TSH* = thyroid-stimulating hormone.

HOT KEY Premenstrual symptoms (e.g., breast tenderness, mood swings, bloating, cramping) accompany ovulation and suggest ovulatory bleeding. Patients with anovulatory cycles often lack premenstrual symptoms.

3. What is the patient's obstetric history, surgical history, past medical history, and medication history? Has she ever had an abnormal pap smear? Does she have a new sexual partner?

HOT KEY Patients who have evidence of severe bleeding on physical examination (e.g., orthostatic vital signs, pallor, brisk bleeding) should be fluid resuscitated, admitted to the hospital, and evaluated emergently by a gynecologist.

B. Attempt to identify an anatomic cause for the bleeding.
   1. Perform a **pelvic examination,** and obtain a **Pap smear.**
   2. Patients who are sexually active should have **cervical cultures** to rule out pelvic inflammatory disease (PID).
C. Narrow the differential diagnosis
   1. **Rule out pregnancy-related bleeding** by performing a **pregnancy test.** All women of reproductive age with abnormal uterine bleeding should have a pregnancy test. If positive, the patient should be referred to a gynecologist. These patients require a quantitative human chorionic gonadotropin (hCG) level and ultrasonographic evaluation to evaluate potential obstetric causes such as miscarriage, ectopic pregnancy and trophoblastic disease.
   2. Rule out iatrogenic causes of bleeding. Anticoagulants, selective serotonin reuptake inhibitors, tamoxifen and hormonal medications such as oral contraceptives or hormone replacemnt therapy may cause changes in bleeding patterns. Patients should be questioned about their use of herbal supplements such as ginko or soy products.
   3. **Determine the patient's ovulatory status.** The **history** is often suggestive of ovulatory status, obviating the need for laboratory testing. However, if the ovulatory status is in question, a **serum progesterone level** can be obtained 1 week before the next expected menses (during the secretory phase). A level greater than 5 ng/ml indicates that ovulation has occurred.
D. Order additional laboratory and imaging tests as appropriate.
   1. **Ovulatory bleeding.** These patients should be evaluated for abnormalities of the vagina, cervix, and uterus, and for bleeding disorders. If a diagnosis is not made after a thorough history, physical examination, and laboratory work-up, referral

to a gynecologist is indicated for imaging of the uterus (hysteroscopy or ultrasound).

2. **Anovulatory bleeding** Postmenopausal women should be referred to a gynecologist for evaluation and offered dilation and curretage.

    a. **Endometrial biopsy.** All patients with anovulation of more than 1 year's duration should be considered for endometrial biopsy because unopposed estrogen is a strong risk factor for the development of endometrial hyperlasia or cancer.

        (1) The biopsy may reveal cancer, polyps, or myomas. Referral to a gynecologist is indicated for these patients.

        (2) Patients with high estrogen levels usually have a thick endometrium, while those with low estrogen levels have a thin endometrium. A thin endometrium suggests an abnormal endocrine axis.

    b. **Evaluate for endocrine axis dysfunction.** If the endometrial biopsy does not reveal cancer, polyps, or myoma, patients with chronic anovulation should be evaluated for endocrinologic abnormalities, which may disrupt the hormonal axis. The following tests should be ordered:

        (1) Thyroid-stimulating hormone (TSH) level, to evaluate for hypo- and hyperthyroidism

        (2) Prolactin level, to evaluate for hyperprolactinemia

        (3) Follicle-stimulating hormone (FSH) and **luteinizing hormone (LH) levels**

            (a) An FSH level greater than 40 IU/L suggests ovarian failure.

            (b) An LH:FSH ratio of more than 2:1 is compatible with polycystic ovary disease.

    c. **Evaluation for hyperandrogenism.** A **dehydro-epiandrosterone sulfate (DHEAS) level, testosterone level,** and **17-OH progesterone level** should be obtained for patients with a negative endocrine axis evaluation or with signs of hyperandrogenism (e.g., hirsutism, virilization).

        (1) Patients with the rapid onset of hyperandrogenism, elevated testosterone levels, or elevated DHEAS levels may have adrenal or ovarian androgen-producing tumors, and gynecology referral is warranted.

        (2) Elevated DHEAS or 17-OH progesterone levels may indicate an adrenal enzyme deficiency.

IV TREATMENT

A. Ovulatory bleeding. Medical management of menorrhagia includes nonsteroidal anti-inflammatory drugs or the progestin-secreting intrauterine device. Surgical treatment entails correction of the anatomic abnormality. Specific bleeding disorders should be addressed by a hematologist.

B. Anovulatory bleeding. Definitive treatment depends on the underlying disorder.

1. **Observation** is appropriate for perimenarchal patients who have mild bleeding that corrects itself within several months.

2. **Oral contraceptive therapy**

   a. **Mild** to **moderate bleeding** can usually be controlled with combination oral contraceptive pills (i.e., each pill contains both estrogen and progesterone). The patient should take 1 tablet daily.

   b. **Moderate** to **severe bleeding** in a perimenarchal patient can be treated with a 21-day package of combination oral contraceptive pills, each containing 30 μg of estrogen. The patient should take one pill three times daily for 7 days, and then stop taking the pills for 7 days. Following withdrawal bleeding (often heavy), she can begin another package of pills, this time taking one tablet daily. After 3–6 months, normal cycling usually resumes and the patient can stop therapy with oral contraceptives if she so desires.

   c. Oral contraceptive pills are an effective method of regulating menstrual cycling in patients with chronic anovulation. Possibly advantageous side effects of therapy with oral contraceptives include contraception and reduced hyperandrogenism.

3. **Progesterone therapy**

   a. Monthly progesterone therapy may be used for women with chronic anovulation who have contraindications to or do not want to take oral contraceptives. Patients should take 10 mg of medroxyprogesterone acetate daily or 200 μg of micronized progesterone for 12 days, during the same time each month. This method does not provide contraception.

   b. Monthly progesterone therapy is appropriate for perimenopausal women who present with anovulatory bleeding. When withdrawal bleeding stops (usually after 3–12 months of therapy), the patient has completed menopause (ovarian failure).

HOT
▶
KEY

An endometrial biopsy (to rule out cancer, polyps, or myoma) should be performed prior to initiating progesterone therapy in a perimenopausal woman.

d. A one-time 12-day course of progesterone may be used for patients without chronic anovulation who have heavy bleeding associated with one anovulatory cycle (once pregnancy has been excluded).

V FOLLOW-UP AND REFERRAL

A. Follow-up. Patients should be seen every 1–2 weeks until a diagnosis is established and bleeding is satisfactorily controlled.

B. Referral to a gynecologist is indicated at several points during the work-up of abnormal uterine bleeding (see Figure 46-1), and whenever uncertainty about a diagnosis or management exists. All postmenopausal women with vaginal bleeding should be referred to a gynecologist.

References

Albers JR, Hull SK, Wesley RM. Abnormal uterine bleeding. *Am Fam Physician* 2004;69(8):1915–1926.

Hatusaka H. The evaluation of abnormal uterine bleeding. *Clin Obstet Gynecol* 2005;48(2):258–273.

47. Pelvic Pain and Dysmenorrhea

....

I INTRODUCTION

A. **Pelvic pain** accounts for as many as one third of office visits to gynecologists, and it is a common problem seen by primary care providers.

B. **Dysmenorrhea** (i.e., painful menstruation) is experienced by as many as 45–95% of women and is severe or disabling in 10%.

II DIFFERENTIAL DIAGNOSIS

A. **Acute pelvic pain.** Patients with acute pelvic pain may present with unilateral or bilateral pain, fever, orthostatic vital signs, an elevated white blood cell (WBC) count, or vaginal bleeding or discharge. Causes of acute pelvic pain can be classified as ovarian, tubal, or extrapelvic (i.e., referred pain).

1. **Ovarian causes** include **ovarian torsion** and **ruptured ovarian cyst.**

2. **Tubal causes** include **ectopic pregnancy** and **pelvic inflammatory disease (PID).**

3. **Extrapelvic causes** include **appendicitis, bowel ischemia, kidney stones,** and **urinary tract infection (UTI).**

HOT **KEY** Many of the causes of acute pelvic pain require emergent intervention to prevent serious complications: ectopic pregnancy can result in massive blood loss, PID can result in sepsis and infertility, and ovarian torsion can result in loss of the ovary.

B. **Subacute or chronic pelvic pain** can be categorized as primary dysmenorrhea, secondary dysmenorrhea, or non-menstrual.

1. **Primary dysmenorrhea** (i.e., **menstrual pain in the absence of underlying organic disease)** is thought to be caused by the production of uterine prostaglandins from endometrial cells during menstruation. The prostaglandins cause dysrhythmic muscle contractions, leading to reduced uterine blood flow and endometrial ischemia.

    a. Patients generally begin to experience pain several months after menarche.

    b. The pain begins with the onset of menstrual flow, lasts 2–3 days, and is usually described as a crampy, lower abdominal pain that radiates to the back or inner thigh. Headache, fatigue, and nausea and diarrhea may accompany the pain.

2. Secondary dysmenorrhea is menstrual pain that has an **organic cause.** Secondary dysmenorrhea should be suspected in women who begin to have menstrual pain after several years of menstruating without pain. Women may report the onset of dyspareunia, intermenstrual bleeding, menorrhagia or postcoital bleeding as well. Causes of secondary dysmenorrhea include the following.

    a. Endometriosis is the presence of functioning endometrial tissue outside of the uterus (e.g., in the peritoneum, bowel wall, bladder, or ovaries). During the menstrual cycle, hormones can influence this extra-uterine tissue, causing it to undergo changes that cause pain.

    b. Adenomyosis is the presence of functioning endometrial tissue in the muscular layers of the uterus. As in endometriosis, hormonal influence may cause growth of this tissue, resulting in pain at the time of menstruation.

    c. Leiomyomata (uterine fibroids) are smooth muscle tumors of the uterus that may cause pain with growth.

    d. Ovarian cysts may cause pain when they grow rapidly or if they undergo intermittent torsion.

    e. Congenital abnormalities can obstruct the normal menstrual flow, leading to fluid accumulation and pressure behind the site of obstruction.

    f. Endometrial polyps are small growths of endometrial tissue that may be associated with pain.

3. Non-menstrual pelvic pain. Non-menstrual causes of pelvic pain produce constant or irregular patterns of pain unrelated to the menstrual cycle.

    a. Gynecologic causes include **pregnancy, PID,** and **intrauterine device (IUD) use.** Although pregnant women often feel uncomfortable, mildly nauseous, or tired, any new pain requires prompt consultation with a gynecologist.

    b. Urologic causes include **UTI, interstitial cystitis** and **kidney stones.**

    c. Gastrointestinal causes include **inflammatory bowel disease, irritable bowel syndrome,** and **constipation.**

    d. Musculoskeletal disorders, such as abdominal wall or low back muscle strain, can be associated with pelvic pain.

    e. Chronic pelvic pain is pain that lasts longer than 6 months with no clear organic pathology.

> **HOT KEY** While it is useful to classify chronic pelvic pain as either cyclic (primary and secondary dysmenorrhea) or non-cyclic (non-menstrual pain), the pattern of pain may vary among individuals with any of the conditions associated with chronic pelvic pain.

III APPROACH TO THE PATIENT

A. Acute pelvic pain

1. **Patient history and physical examination.** A thorough history and physical examination are essential. The approach taken for a patient with acute pelvic pain is similar to that taken for a patient with acute abdominal pain (see Chapter 31 III A–B).

2. **Laboratory studies**
   a. Pregnancy test. If the **urine human chorionic gonadotropin (hCG) pregnancy test** is negative, a **serum hCG level** should be obtained to rule out ectopic pregnancy. (The urine hCG test may remain negative for as long as 6 weeks after conception.)
   b. A **urinalysis, complete blood count (CBC)** with **differential,** and **erythrocyte sedimentation rate (ESR)** are indicated for all patients. The ESR is usually elevated in patients with PID.

3. **Imaging studies. Ultrasound or a computed tomography (CT) scan** of the pelvis is indicated for patients with suspected ectopic pregnancy, appendicitis, or abscess, or when the source of the pain remains unclear.

B. Chronic pelvic pain (Figure 47-1). All patients with chronic pelvic pain should have a thorough **history** and **physical examination,** including a pelvic exam. In addition, all sexually active patients should have a **pregnancy test** and **cervical cultures** for *Neisseria gonorrhoeae* and *Chlamydia trachomatis* (to evaluate for PID). The patient can then be assigned to one of the three diagnostic categories on the basis of this preliminary information.

1. **Primary dysmenorrhea.** If the history, physical examination, cervical cultures, and pregnancy test do not suggest another cause of dysmenorrhea, it is appropriate to initiate therapy for primary dysmenorrhea.

2. **Secondary dysmenorrhea.** Physical examination findings may help define the cause.
   a. **Endometriosis.** Patients may have focal tenderness on examination and nodularity to palpation of the uterosacral

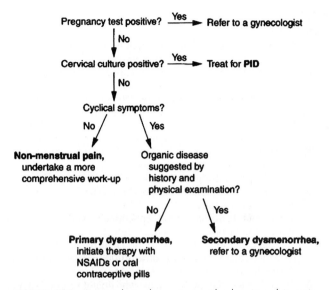

FIGURE 47-1. Approach to the patient with chronic pelvic pain. *NSAIDs* = nonsteroidal anti-inflammatory drugs; *PID* = pelvic inflammatory disease.

ligaments. The diagnosis can only be established with laparoscopy.

   b. Congenital abnormalities may be visualized during speculum examination.

   c. Leiomyomata and **ovarian cysts** can often be palpated during bimanual examination.

3. Non-menstrual pelvic pain

   a. Gastrointestinal disorders. The patient may have a history of constipation (or alternating constipation and diarrhea), nausea, melena, rectal bleeding, or stress-induced symptoms. A more extensive gastrointestinal evaluation is indicated for these patients.

   b. UTI. Patients should have a urinalysis and urine culture to rule out UTI.

   c. PID is suggested by a history of PID, cervical discharge or cervical motion tenderness on examination, or systemic signs of infection.

   d. Musculoskeletal pain. A musculoskeletal source of the pain may be evident on examination (i.e., the lower abdominal or pelvic floor muscles may reveal isolated tenderness).

IV TREATMENT

A. PID may be treated on an outpatient basis if the patient is not pregnant or febrile, has no signs of abscess or peritonitis, and is able to tolerate and comply with oral antibiotic therapy. Antibiotic regimens must cover *C. trachomatis* and *N. gonorrhoeae;* one typical regimen is **ceftriaxone,** 250 mg administered intramuscularly once, followed by **doxycycline,** 100 mg orally twice daily for 14 days plus metronidazole 500 mg orally twice daily for 14 days. Alternative regimens include fluroquinolones (e.g., levofloxacin 500 mg once a day for 14 days with metronidazole for 14 days) or azithromycin (e.g., azithromycin 1 gm po with ceftriaxone 250 mg intramuscularly—particulary for patients who are unlikely to complete 14 days of doxycycline).

B. Primary dysmenorrhea
   1. **Nonsteroidal anti-inflammatory drugs (NSAIDs)** are the initial treatment of choice, and are effective in up to 70% of women. Common regimens are oral **naproxen,** 500 mg taken as needed (up to a maximum dose of 1000 mg daily) or Ponstel 250 mg for the first 2–3 days of menstruation.
   2. **Oral contraceptive pills.** Patients who do not respond to therapy with NSAIDs or who desire contraception can be treated with oral contraceptive pills, which are extremely effective at reducing symptoms.
   3. **Levonorgestrel-releasing intrauterine device.** Along with decreasing the amount of blood loss, this has been shown to significantly reduce dysmenorrhea. However, non-hormonal intrauterine devices may actually INCREASE dysmenorrhea, and women may experience relief with their removal as discussed below.
   4. **Alternative therapies** include heat, thiamine, magnesium and vitamin E supplementation.

C. Secondary dysmenorrhea. Medical treatment (usually with oral contraceptive pills) is often used to manage many of the conditions that can cause secondary dysmenorrhea, but surgical options are available and may be more appropriate for patients desiring pregnancy (some of the conditions can affect fertility). Patients should be referred to a gynecologist for therapy.

D. Non-menstrual pelvic pain. Treatment is cause-specific.
   1. **PID** and **UTI** are treated with appropriate antibiotics.
   2. An **IUD** suspected of causing irritation can be removed.
   3. **Constipation** and **irritable bowel syndrome** may respond to fiber supplementation.
   4. **Chronic pelvic pain,** which is a diagnosis of exclusion, is an incompletely understood syndrome that is best managed with gynecology consultation. Patients may respond to a variety of medical, surgical, and psychosocial treatments.

V FOLLOW-UP AND REFERRAL

A. Pregnant patients with acute pelvic pain and patients with suspected **ovarian torsion** require **immediate gynecologic consultation.**

B. Patients with primary dysmenorrhea should be referred to a gynecologist for laparoscopy when oral contraceptive pills and NSAIDs are not effective at controlling pain. Patients with secondary dysmenorrhea should be referred for gynecologic evaluation whenever the cause is not readily identified and responsive to treatment.

C. Patients with **gastrointestinal symptoms** or **evidence of peritonitis** on physical examination (e.g., rebound, rigidity, guarding) may require imaging (e.g., ultrasound, computed tomography) and **immediate surgical consultation.**

References

ACOG Committee on Practice Bulletins-Gynecolgy: ACOG Practice Bulletin No. 51: Chronic Pelvic Pain. *Obstet Gynecol* 2004;103(3):589–605.

Proctor M, Farquahar C. Diagnosis and management of dysmenorrhea. *BMJ* 2006; 332(7550):1134–1138.

48. Abnormal Vaginal Discharge

I Abnormal vaginal discharge is usually attributable to **vaginitis** (i.e., inflammation of the vaginal wall), which may be due to infection, atrophy, or chemical/foreign body irritants. Less commonly, it may be found in the setting of cervical or vaginal cancer or endometrial disease. Infectious vaginitis is due to one of three causes: **bacterial vaginosis, candidiasis,** or **trichomoniasis.**

B. Normal vaginal secretions are generally clear or white, odorless, and viscous. Progesterone exposure during the luteal phase of the menstural cycle or pregnancy results in a phsyiologic change in vaginal discharge, producing thicker, whiter and more copious amounts. An **abnormal discharge** is usually **yellow, gray,** or **green** and **increased in volume,** and is usually accompanied by **itching, vulvar irritation, dyspareunia, dysuria,** or **vaginal odor.**

II **DIFFERENTIAL DIAGNOSIS.** Abnormal vaginal discharge can be caused by any process that increases or alters secretions from the **vagina, cervix,** or **uterus** (Table 48-1).

A. Vaginitis
1. Infectious vaginitis is the most common cause of abnormal vaginal discharge.
   a. Bacterial vaginosis, the most common cause of vaginitis, results from a **disturbance in the normal vaginal flora.** It is not sexually transmitted. An overgrowth of anaerobes and Gram-negative bacteria (e.g., *Gardnerella vaginalis, Bacteroides* species, *Peptostreptococcus* species, *Mycoplasma hominis*) leads to an increase in the vaginal pH. Patients may be asymptomatic, or they may complain of **itching,** a **"fishy" odor,** or a **whitish discharge.**
   b. *Candida vulvovaginitis,* the second most common cause of infectious vaginitis, is caused by *Candida albicans*, a fungus.
      (1) Patients usually present with a **white, curd-like discharge, vulvar** or **vaginal erythema,** and **itching.**
      (2) Risk factors for symptomatic infection include **pregnancy, diabetes, oral contraceptive use, diabetes, antibiotic** or **corticosteroid use,** and **tight-fitting clothing.**

TABLE 48-1. Differential Diagnosis of Abnormal Vaginal Discharge

Infectious vaginitis
   Bacterial vaginois
   Candida vulvovaginitis
   Trichomonas vaginitis
Chemical irritation/foreign body
Atrophic vaginitis
Cervicitis and pelvic inflammatory disease (PID)
   Neisseria gonorrhoeae
   Chlamydia trachomatis
Herpes simplex virus (HSV) infection
Human papillomavirus (HPV) infection (condyloma acuminatum)
Cervical cancer, vaginal cancer
Endometrial disease (cancer polyps, intrauterine device)

---

    c. ***Trichomonas* vaginitis** is caused by the flagellated protozoan, ***Trichomonas vaginalis***. It is usually sexually transmitted.
      (1) Patients may be asymptomatic, or they may present with a **copious yellow** or **green frothy discharge, vaginal erythema** and **itching, dysuria, dyspareunia,** or a **"strawberry cervix"** (i.e., reddening and petechial hemorrhage of the cervix, a rare finding).

  2. Vaginal Irritation. Increased sexually activity, douches, retained tampons, contraceptive devices, spermicides, and topical medication such as antifungal therapy may all irritate vaginal tissues, which may result in abnormal discharge, with or without associated discomfort.

  3. Atrophic vaginitis is a common cause of discharge in older women. It occurs when lack of estrogen stimulation leads to atrophy and friability of the vagina. Patients usually present with **scant yellow-brown discharge. Dysuria, vaginal itching and dyspareunia** may occur as well.

B. Cervicitis and **pelvic inflammatory disease (PID),** which are caused by *Neisseria gonorrhoeae* or *Chlamydia trachomatis* infection, may be associated with increased cervical secretions, leading to a vaginal discharge. Cervicitis and PID are usually associated with **cervical motion** or **adnexal tenderness** and a **purulent cervical discharge.**

C. Herpes simplex virus (HSV) and **human papillomavirus (HPV) infections** can be associated with vaginal discharge. Both have characteristic lesions that are usually visible during a speculum examination.

D. Cervical cancer, vaginal cancer and **endometrial disease** are rare but important causes of vaginal discharge.

III APPROACH TO THE PATIENT. The goal is to determine whether the discharge is attributable to vaginitis, or to a less common, but potentially more dangerous, condition.

A. Patient history. A thorough history is essential. Areas to focus on include the following:
   1. **Nature of the discharge** (i.e., the amount, color, duration, and odor)
   2. **Associated symptoms** (e.g., itching, dysuria, dyspareunia, abdominal pain, fever)
   3. **Gynecologic history** (i.e., sexual history, menstrual history, prior episodes of discharge, tampon use or douching)
   4. **Medication history**
   5. **Medical history** (i.e., chronic diseases)
   6. **Date of last menstrual period,** as pregnancy will alter what treatments may be offered for many conditions.
B. Physical examination
   1. A **speculum examination** should be performed to examine the cervix for discharge, polyps, or lesions suggestive of herpes, condyloma acuminatum, or cervical dysplasia. Cervicitis is present if a swab inserted into the cervical canal shows a yellow or green exudate.
   2. A **bimanual examination** that reveals adnexal, uterine, or cervical motion tenderness suggests PID as the cause of the discharge.
C. Laboratory studies
   1. A swab of the secretions should be taken from the vagina and placed on two separate microscope slides.
      a. **Potassium hydroxide (KOH) preparation ("whiff" test).** A drop of KOH should be added to one slide. A fishy odor in response to the KOH suggests bacterial vaginosis.
      b. **Wet preparation.** Normal saline should be added to the other slide, and the pH of the discharge should be measured. A pH greater than 4.5 suggests bacterial vaginosis or possible trichomonas infection.
   2. **Microscopic examination.** Both slides should be examined microscopically. A microscopic slide that meets the diagnostic criteria given in Table 48-2 is helpful for ruling in the disease, but a slide that does not reveal a suspected pathogen does not rule out the disease.
   3. **Culture** is much more sensitive than microscopic examination for detecting *Candida* and *Trichomonas* infections.

TABLE 48-2. Diagnostic Criteria for Common Causes of Infectious Vaginitis

Diagnosis	Diagnostic Criteria
Bacterial vaginosis	Amsel criteria* 1. pH > 4.5 2. Clue cells on wet preparation 3. Positive "whiff" test 4. Thin, white, homogenous discharge
Candida vulvovaginitis	Hyphae or budding spores on KOH preparation OR Positive culture
Trichomonas vaginitis	Motile trichomonads on wet preparation OR Positive culture

KOH = potassium hydroxide.
*Three of the four criteria must be met.

HOT KEY Because the three most common causes of infectious vaginitis have similar signs and symptoms, it is important to follow the diagnostic criteria given in Table 48-2 in order to avoid diagnostic error and incorrect treatment.

 IV **TREATMENT**

A. **Infectious vaginitis** is treated with **antibiotics or antifungal therapy.** Several common regimens for each of the three types of infectious vaginitis are given in Table 48-3.

HOT KEY Before initiating treatment, always determine if the patient is pregnant, because some of the medications are contraindicated in pregnancy.

B. **Atrophic vaginitis** does not necessarily require any intervention if the patient is minimally symptomatic. However, it is usually successfully treated with **topical estrogen therapies,** such as creams (2–4 g intravaginally daily for 2 weeks) tablets or rings. **Vaginal lubricants** may also improve symptoms.

TABLE 48-3. Selected Therapeutic Regimens for Infectious Vaginitis

Condition	Drug	Form	Dosage
Bacterial vaginosis*	Metronidazole[†]	Oral	500 mg twice daily for 7 days
			OR
			2 g given as one dose
		0.75% Gel	5 g intravaginally twice daily for 5 days
	Clindamycin	Oral	300 mg twice daily for 7 days
		2% cream sustained release	5 g once
Candida vulvovaginitis[‡]	Clotrimazole	500-mg vaginal tablet	1 tablet once
		200-mg vaginal tablet	1 tablet at bedtime for 3 days
		100-mg vaginal tablet	1 tablet at bedtime for 7 days
	Miconazole	200-mg vaginal tablet	1 tablet at bedtime for 3 days
		100-mg vaginal tablet	1 tablet at bedtime for 7 days
	Butoconazole	2% cream sustained release	5 g intravaginally once
	Terconazole	0.8% cream	5 g intravaginally at bedtime for 3 days
	Fluconazole[§]	Oral	150 mg given as one dose
Trichomonas vaginitis ¶	Metronidazole[†]	Oral	2 g given as one dose
			OR
			500 mg given twice daily for 7 days
	Tinidazole 500 mg	Oral	4 tablets, 1 dose

*Need for treatment in pregnant patients is controversial
[†]Metronidazole is contraindicated in the first trimester of pregnancy and should not be taken with alcohol
[‡]Patients in the first trimester of pregnancy should not undergo treatment for Candida vulvovaginitis.
[§]Fluconazole should not be used during pregnancy
¶Treat the patient and her partner.

C. PID. The treatment of PID is discussed in Chapter 47 IV A.
D. Cervicitis, HSV infection, and **HPV infection.** Treatment is discussed in Chapter 81.

V FOLLOW-UP AND REFERRAL

A. Follow-up. Patients who respond appropriately to therapy do not require scheduled follow-up.
B. Referral
   1. When the diagnosis cannot be established or the abnormal discharge persists despite therapy, referral to a gynecologist is indicated.
   2. Patients with suspected cervical cancer, vaginal cancer or endometrial disease require prompt referral to a gynecologist.

References
ACOG Committee on Practice Bulletins—gynecology: Clinical management guidelines for obstetrician-gynecologists, Number 72: vaginitis. *Obstet Gynecol* 2006; 107(5):1195–1206.
Owen MK, Clenney TL. Management of vaginitis. *Am Fam Physician* 2004;70(11): 2125–2132.

49. Urinary Incontinence

I INTRODUCTION

A. **Urinary incontinence** is **involuntary urine voiding** that presents a **social** or **hygienic problem for the patient** because of the **frequency** with which the incontinence occurs or the **amount of urine** lost with each episode.

B. **Incidence and epidemiology.** The prevalence of urinary incontinence is difficult to assess because many patients are hesitant to discuss the subject with their physicians.

   1. It is estimated that **5%–15% of the general population** in the United States are affected.

   2. Urinary incontinence is **more common with aging:** 15%–30% of elderly people in the community and at least 50% of patients in nursing homes are affected.

HOT KEY

> Always ask elderly patients if they have urinary incontinence.

C. **Physiology of voiding.** Continence is dependent upon a compliant bladder wall and a functional urinary sphincter. The sphincter is comprised of both voluntary skeletal muscle and involuntary smooth muscle.

   1. **Bladder wall.** The **detrusor muscle** forms the bladder wall and consists of three layers of smooth muscle.

      a. **Parasympathetic stimulation** causes the detrusor muscle to contract. **Voiding** is initiated via a reflex arc from the brain stem nucleus, and can be inhibited by higher cortical control.

      b. **Sympathetic (β-adrenergic)** stimulation stretches the bladder dome and relaxes the detrusor muscle.

   2. **Bladder neck** and **proximal urethra. Sympathetic (α-adrenergic)** stimulation causes the bladder neck to contract, maintaining normal continence.

   3. **Pelvic floor muscles.** The skeletal muscle of the pelvic floor is under **voluntary control** via the **pudendal nerve.** Contraction of the pelvic floor muscles prevents emptying of the bladder when the intra-abdominal pressure increases.

▮ DIFFERENTIAL DIAGNOSIS

A. **Acute urinary incontinence**. The causes of acute urinary incontinence can be remembered with the mnemonic, "DAMN DRIPS."

MNEMONIC

Causes of Acute Urinary Incontinence ("DAMN DRIPS")

Delirium
Atrophic urethritis or vaginitis
Medications—e.g., sedative-hypnotics, diuretics, anticholinergics, α-adrenergic agonists or antagonists
Neurologic disorders—e.g., cord compression, cauda equina syndrome
Diabetes mellitus or insipidus
Restricted mobility
Infection—urinary tract infection (UTI)
Psychiatric disorders—e.g., depression
Stool impaction

B. **Chronic urinary incontinence**
   1. **Urge incontinence.** Either **detrusor hyperreflexia** (i.e., involuntary detrusor contraction due to an underlying neurologic disorder) or **instability** (i.e., involuntary detrusor contraction without an underlying neurologic disorder), or urinary sphincter dysfunction may result in a sudden unexpected urge to void that cannot be overcome with voluntary contraction.
   2. **Stress incontinence.** Laxity of the pelvic floor muscles with subsequent weaking of the urinary sphincter can result from **aging, multiparity,** or **surgical** or **neurologic impairment of the bladder neck.** These patients experience incontinence when their intra-abdominal pressure increases and exceeds urethral pressure (during physical exertion, laughting, coughing or sneezing).
   3. **Overflow incontinence.** Bladder outlet obstruction (e.g., as a result of **prostate enlargement)** or decreased detrusor contraction (e.g., as a result of **diabetic neuropathy)** causes the bladder to fill to distention and then overflow.
   4. **Total incontinence.** Rarely, patients are unable to hold any urine at any time. This may be due to nerve damage or surgical disruption of the urinary sphincter, or the formation of a fistula that bypasses the sphincter.

HOT KEY The elderly often have mixed incontinence (i.e., multiple mechanisms contribute).

III APPROACH TO THE PATIENT

A. Patient history

1. **Acute urinary incontinence**. The goal of history–taking is to rule out precipitating causes.

2. **Chronic urinary incontinence.** Attempt to classify the patient's incontinence as urge incontinence, stress incontinence, or overflow incontinence. Some patients may have symptoms of both stress and urge incontinence.

3. **Voiding Diary.** A voiding diary can be very useful to help document specific precipitants, symptoms and circumstances of symptoms.

B. Physical examination. Special attention should be given to the following areas:

1. **Abdominal examination.** Palpate for bladder distention.

2. **Rectal examination.** Look for stool impaction and assess rectal tone, as well as laxity of the pelvic floor.

3. **Pelvic examination.** Look for genital atrophy (evidenced by dryness and loss of pubic hair); bladder, rectal, or uterine prolapse; and pelvic masses.

4. **Neurologic examination**

   a. A motor and sensory examination and gait testing should be performed to assess for underlying neurologic disorders (e.g., stroke, multiple sclerosis).

   b. A mental status evaluation may reveal cognitive problems that could impair the patient's ability to recognize the need to void.

HOT KEY Spinal cord compression (e.g., from metastatic cancer) should always be considered in patients with acute urinary incontinence.

5. **Provocative stress test.** With a full bladder, the patient is asked to cough while in the standing or lithotomy position. Instant urinary incontinence is diagnostic of stress urinary incontinence, while delayed or persistent urinary incontinence suggests detrusor instability (i.e., urge urinary incontinence).

C. Laboratory studies
   1. **Urinalysis.** Urine should be evaluated for white blood cells (WBCs), bacteria, glucose, occult blood, and protein.
   2. **Blood work.** Evaluate the blood urea nitrogen (BUN), creatinine and glucose levels.
D. Post-void residual (PVR) study. A PVR study is usually performed in patients with suspected overflow incontinence [e.g., an elderly man with benign prostatic hyperplasia (BPH)]. A PVR of less than 50 ml is normal, while a PVR greater than 200 ml is considered abnormal. Intermediate values (i.e., a PVR of 50–200 ml) may be abnormal and must be interpreted on an individual basis.
E. Cystometry. Cystometry is used to assess bladder and urethral function during bladder filling. It can be helpful to diagnose detrusor hyperactivity.

IV TREATMENT

A. Nonpharmacologic therapy
   1. **Scheduling regimens** (i.e., behavioral therapy) are primarily used for patients with **urge urinary incontinence.** Patients are advised to void at regular intervals to avoid excessive filling of the bladder.
   2. **Pelvic floor muscle exercises (Kegel exercises)** are primarily used for patients with **stress urinary incontinence.** Patients are taught to contract the periurethral, perianal, and perivaginal muscles simultaneously. A typical regimen is 20 contractions four times daily. Patients should be advised that they should start to see improvement after performing exercises for 4–6 weeks.
   3. **Urinary collection devices.** Patients who remain symptomatic despite other therapies may benefit from urinary collection devices (e.g., condom catheters, special undergarments).
B. Pharmacologic therapy is summarized in Table 49-1.

V FOLLOW-UP AND REFERRAL.

Patients should be referred to a urologist or uro-gynecologist (an option for women) in the following situations:

A. Failure of medical therapy
B. Hematuria, when a cause cannot be identified
C. Cause of incontinence unclear
D. A surgical problem is identified (e.g., a fistula, markedly enlarged prostate, severe laxity of the pelvic floor or prolapse of pelvic organs)
E. Comorbidities related to urinary incontinence (e.g., recurrent UTI, persistent irritative voiding symptoms)

TABLE 49-1. Pharmacological Therapy of Urinary Incontinence

Type of Incontinence	Agent	Dosing Regimen
Urge incontinence	Oxybutynin	2.5–5.0 mg at bedtime, may increase to three times daily
	Oxybutynin, extended release	5–15 mg, once daily
	Imipramine	Start with 10–25 mg at bedtime; increase as needed to 25–150 mg at bedtime
	Tolterodine	1–2 mg, twice daily
	Estrogens (oral, transdermal or topical)	See regimens given for stress incontinence
Stress incontinence	Phenylpropanolamine	25–50 mg, up to 4 times daily
	Estrogens (oral, transdermal, or topical)	Conjugated estrogen, 2 g intravaginally daily for 14 days, then twice weekly
		OR
		Conjugated estrogen, 0.3–1.25 mg orally daily (with a progesterone in women who have not had a hysterectomy)*
	Imipramine	Start with 10–25 mg at bedtime; increase as needed to 25–150 mg at bedtime
Overflow incontinence	Bethanechol	20–100 mg, 4 times daily
	Terazosin	1–10 mg daily[†]
	Prazosin	3–12 mg, divided, 2 or 3 times daily[‡]

*Many other regimens are available.
[†]Increase dose as tolerated.
[‡]Patient should take first dose (1 mg) while still supine.

References

Nygaard IE, Heeit M. Stress urinary incontinence. *Obstet Gynecol* 2004;104(3):607–620.

Wein AJ, Rackley RR. Overactive bladder: a better understanding of pathophysiology, diagnosis and management. *J Urol* 2006;175(3 pt 2):S5–S10.

50. Contraception

....

I INTRODUCTION

A. Many different methods of contraception are available. In order to help patients who seek contraception make the most appropriate choice, primary care physicians must be familiar with the risks and benefits associated with each method. Whenever there is uncertainty about the most appropriate choice, consultation with a gynecologist is recommended.

B. Physicians should assume an active role in counseling and should not rely on patients to introduce the topic of contraception. The value of preventing unwanted pregnancy and sexually transmitted diseases (STDs) cannot be overemphasized.

II CONTRACEPTIVE METHODS.
Table 50-1 lists the common methods of reversible contraception along with the failure rates, advantages, and disadvantages associated with each. The methods of birth control can be remembered using the mnemonic "COITUS."

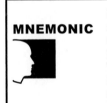

MNEMONIC

Birth Control Methods ("COITUS")
Condoms and other barrier methods
Oral contraceptives and other hormonal methods
Intrauterine device (IUD)
Timing methods
Unprotected (coitus interruptus)
Surgical methods

A. **Barrier methods**
1. **Condoms.** Latex condoms offer significant protection against STDs (including HIV), and should be recommended to all sexually active patients who are not in a monogamous relationship where both partners are known to be free of STDs.
    a. Condoms made from animal intestines do not offer the same protection against STDs.
    b. The female condom has a higher failure rate than the male condom, but does protect the external female genitalia from STDs.

TABLE 50-1. Contraceptive Methods

Method	Mechanism of Action	Failure Rate* with Typical Use	Perfect Use	Disadvantages	Advantages
No method	...	85%	...	...	...
Periodic abstinence	Avoidance of coitus during presumed fertile day	20%	...	...	...
Spermicide alone	Inactivation of sperm 21%		6%	Vaginal irritation	May protect against some STDs
Cervical cap with spermicide	Mechanical barrier, inactivation of sperm	18%	12%	Cervical irritation, may be difficult to fit, Pap smear abnormalities	Protection against STDs
Diaphragm with spermicide	Mechanical barrier, inactivation of sperm	18%	6%	Cervical irritation, increased risk of urinary tract infection	Protection against STDs
Condom					
Male	Mechanical barrier	12%	3%	Allergic reactions	Protection against STDs
Female		21%	5%	Difficult to insert, poor acceptability	Protection against STDs, protection of the external genitalia

(Continued)

TABLE 50-1. Contraceptive Methods (*Continued*)

Method	Mechanism of Action	Failure Rate* with Typical Use	Perfect Use	Disadvantages	Advantages
Oral contraceptives Combined	Suppression of ovulation, changes in cervical mucus and endometrium	3%	0.1%	Thromboembolism and stroke (rare), myocardial infarction in older smokers, nausea, headache, depression	Protection against ovarian and endometrial cancer, PID, fibrocystic breast disease, ovarian cysts, iron-deficiency anemia, and dysmenorrhea
Progestin-only	Changes in cervical mucus and endometrium, possibly suppression of ovulation	3%	0.5%	Irregular, unpredictable bleeding in some	Protection against PID, iron-deficiency anemia, and dysmenorrhea
Intrauterine devices Progesterone T (Progestasert)	Inhibition of sperm migration, fertilization, and ovum transport	2%	1.5%	Increased incidence of ectopic pregnancy	Decrease in menstrual blood loss and dysmenorrhea

Copper T 380A (ParaGard)	Same mechanism of action as progesterone T device	0.8%	0.6%	Uterine perforation (rare), increase in menstrual blood loss	Can be left in place for 10 years
Medroxyprogesterone acetate (Depo-Provera)	Suppression of ovulation, changes in cervical mucus and endometrium	0.3%	0.3%	Menstrual irregularities, headache, weight gain, acne	Effective for 3 months
Levonorgestrel subdermal implants (Norplant)	Similar to progestin-only oral contraceptives	0.09%	0.09%	Menstrual irregularities, headache, weight gain, acne, removal problems	Ease of use, reversibility, effective for 5 years

Modified with permission from the Medical Letter: Choice of contraceptives. Med Lett Drugs Ther 37(941):9, 1995.
PID = pelvic inflammatory disease; STDs = sexually transmitted diseases.
*Percent accidental pregnancy during first year of use. Modified from RA Hatcher, et al: Contraceptive Technology, 16th ed. New York, Irvington, 1994, p113.

   2. Diaphragms and **cervical caps** must be fitted by a trained
      physician. Proper use is associated with a decreased risk of
      STDs, although failure rates are considerably higher than
      with many other methods.
      a. Spermicide must be applied to the cervical side of the bar-
         rier.
      b. The device should be left in place for 6–8 hours after in-
         tercourse.
      c. Women should be refitted for a new diaphragm after child-
         birth or significant changes in weight.
B. Hormonal methods. Combination hormonal contraception (estrogen plus progesterone) is available as pills, a transdermal
   patch or a vaginal ring. Progesterone-only contraception is available as a pill, intramuscular injection, or the levonorgestral intrauterine system.
   1. Oral contraceptive pills (OCPs). Physicians should be famil-
      iar with the many different types of OCPs (Table 50-2). Pa-
      tients respond to these medications differently, and it may be
      necessary to change to a different type of OCP to minimize
      unwanted side effects.
      a. Mechanism of action. OCPs are available in **two main for-
         mulations:** combination (estrogen plus progesterone) or
         progesterone-only.
         (1) Combination pills prevent ovulation by suppressing
            the mid-cycle luteinizing hormone (LH) surge. The
            progesterone component increases the viscosity of
            the cervical mucus and changes the characteristics of
            the endometrium to decrease implantation.
            (a) Combination pills are available in triphasic for-
               mulations, which vary the dose of estrogen, pro-
               gesterone, or both throughout the cycle with the
               goal of decreasing the total hormone dose without
               decreasing efficacy.
            (b) Newer, more potent progestins (e.g., nor-gesti-
               mate, desogestrel) are being used in combination
               pills in lower doses and may be associated with
               fewer side effects.
         (2) Progesterone-only pills are as efficacious as combi-
            nation pills, but they do not prevent ovulation and
            therefore may be associated with higher rates of ec-
            topic pregnancy.
      b. Side effects
         (1) Nausea, breast tenderness, and **fluid retention** are
            often associated with the estrogen component. **In-
            creased appetite, depression, fatigue, acne,** and **hir-
            sutism** may be associated with the progestin compo-
            nent.

TABLE 50-2. Selected Oral Contraceptive Pills

Type	Brand Names	Estrogen Dose*	Progestin Dose	Comments
Combination Pills				
Monophasic formulations	Ortho-Novum 1/35, Norinyl 1 + 35	35 μg	1 mg norethindrone	Now less commonly used due to the development of newer pills containing lower doses of progesterone
	Nordette, Levlen	30 μg	0.15 mg levonorgestrel	
	Lo/Ovral	30 μg	0.3 mg norgestrel	
Triphasic formulations	Triphasil, Tri-Levlen	30 μg	0.5 mg levonorgestrel (days 1–6)	Fewer progesterone-associated side effects† (as compared with monophasic formulations); multiple pill types may make dosing more confusing
		40 μg	0.075 mg levonorgestrel (days 7–11)	
		30 μg	0.125 mg levonorgestrel (days 12–21)	
	Ortho-Novum 7/7/7	35 μg	0.5 mg norethindrone (days 1–7)	
		35 μg	0.75 mg norethindrone (days 8–14)	
		35 μg	1 mg norethindrone (days 15–21)	
Formulations containing the new progestins	Ortho-Cept, Desogen	30 μg	0.15 mg desogestrel	Least androgenic of the combination pills (may cause less acne and hirsutism)
	Ortho-Cyclen	30 μg	0.25 mg norgestimate	
Progesterone-only pills	Micronor, Nor-QD	…	0.35 mg norethindrone	Associated with more breakthrough bleeding, but fewer of the estrogen-dependent side effects‡
	Ovrette	…	0.75 mg norgestrel	

*Estrogen component is ethinyl estradiol.
†Progesterone-associated side effects include increased appetite, depression, fatigue, acne, and hirsutism.
‡Estrogen-associated side effects include nausea, breast tenderness, and fluid retention.

(2) **Breakthrough bleeding** commonly occurs with both combination and progesterone-only pills during the first 3 months of use. The breakthrough bleeding usually becomes much less frequent with combination pills, but may persist with progesterone-only pills. If irregular bleeding persists beyond 3 months, patients should be evaluated for other causes of abnormal bleeding (see Chapter 46).

(3) **Increased blood pressure.** The patient's blood pressure should be monitored for the first few months after the patient begins to take OCPs, and annually thereafter. Combination pills are associated with an increased in blood pressure among women with hypertension, as well as an increased risk of vascular events among women whose hypertension is not well controlled. Women with hypertension who are over 35, who smoke, or whose blood pressure is not well controlled but desire hormonal contraception should be counseled about their risks and offered progestin-only contraceptives.

(4) **Headache.** OCP use may be associated with an increased frequency of headaches in some women. Patients presenting with headache require a thorough evaluation. Patients with persistent headaches may do better with another form of birth control or a switch to progesterone-only pills. Combination pills that contain low doses of estrogen during the first few days of the placebo week (e.g. Mircette) may reduce menstrual migraines.

(5) **Thrombosis** – a small increase in venous thromboembolic disease is seen with OCPs; the risk is increased in women who smoke.

c. **Advantages.** OCPs are associated with a number of important health benefits, in addition to having a low failure rate.

(1) Both combination and progesterone-only pills decrease dysmenorrhea and the amount of uterine bleeding, leading to decreased iron-deficiency anemia among users. In addition, oral contraceptive use lowers the risk of ectopic pregnancy and pelvic inflammatory disease (PID).

(2) Combination OCPs are associated with a decreased risk of ovarian cancer, endometrial cancer, and fibrocystic breast disease.

d. **Risks**

(1) Studies that have examined the risk of **breast cancer** in users of OCPs have yielded contradictory results.

Women at high risk for breast cancer may wish to use another method of contraception.

    (2) OCPs should not be prescribed to women older than 35 years who smoke, because these women are at risk for **myocardial infarction and stroke.** Oral contraceptive pills in the currently used formulations are generally not thought to increase the risk of cardiovascular disease among patients who do not smoke.

  e. Contraindications. Major contraindications to oral contraceptive pill use include:

    (1) A history of thromboembolic disorder, stroke, myocardial infarction, breast cancer, estrogen-dependent tumors, liver disease, or gallbladder disease

    (2) Pregnancy and breast-feeding

2. Transdermal combination patch (Ortho Evra). Ortho Evra delivers combination hormonal therapy and is changed weekly for three weeks, then stopped to allow menstruation. It is not as effective as pills in overweight women. Recent reports have suggested an increased risk of thromboembolic events in women using the patch.

3. Combination hormonal vaginal ring (NuvaRing).

  a. Mechanism of action. Low dose estrogen and progesterone are secreted by a ring placed in the vagina for three weeks. The ring is then removed for a week, during which time menses will occur. The following week a new ring is inserted.

  b. Side effects. The ring is associated with a lower incidence of breakthrough bleeding than OCPs. Unpleasant side effects include foreign body sensation, difficulty with intercourse and expulsion of the ring.

4. Medroxyprogesterone acetate (Depo-Provera) injections are a very effective means of contraception.

  a. Mechanism of action. Medroxyprogesterone acetate suppresses ovulation, thickens the cervical mucus, and alters the endometrial lining to prevent pregnancy.

  b. Administration. Medroxyprogesterone acetate (150 mg subcutaneously) is administered once every 12 weeks.

    (1) Although the injections are effective for 14 weeks, they are generally given every 12 weeks so that the woman has a 2-week "grace period" if she misses her appointment.

    (2) The injection should take place within 5 days of the onset of menses. Women who are more than 2 weeks late for their injections should have pregnancy excluded before reinjection.

  c. Side effects

    (1) Irregular bleeding and **spotting** occurs in almost all women using medroxyprogesterone acetate. After several months of use, the incidence of spotting decreases, and **amenorrhea** is common.

HOT KEY

The amenorrhea associated with medroxyprogesterone acetate use can cause anxiety for patients, who may believe they are pregnant.

(2) **Weight gain** of 2–7 pounds (1–3 kilograms) is common, and **headache, bloating, fatigue, depression,** and **decreased libido** have also been reported.

HOT KEY

Fertility may be delayed for as long as 1 year after stopping medroxyprogesterone acetate injections.

    d. Risks. Medroxyprogesterone acetate injections are not known to increase the risk of breast, ovarian, or endometrial cancer.
  5. Levonorgestrel intrauterine system (Mirena)
    a. Mechanism of action. Mirena ia an intrauterine device that slowly releases levonorgestrel over 5 years, providing excellent contraceptive efficacy.
    b. Side effects. The most common side effect is **irregular bleeding** and **spotting,** which occurs initially in most patients, but eventually many women report decreased bleeding or amenorrhea. An increase in the rates of headaches and acne have been reported due to its hormonal secretion.
    c. Risks. Risks include ectopic pregnancy and expulsion of the device.
C. Non-hormonal Intrauterine devices (IUDs) are one of the most effective contraceptive methods available.
  1. The **copper T 380A device** causes a sterile inflammatory response in the endometrium that is thought to be spermicidal. It is approved for 10 years of use.

HOT KEY

IUDs should not be used in patients who are at risk for bacterial endocarditis because they may cause transient bacteremia.

D. Surgical methods include **vasectomy** and **tubal ligation.** Vasectomy is a less invasive procedure and is associated with fewer complications. Both are very effective methods of **permanent sterilization.** Patients should be advised about the availability of reversible contraception, and should clearly understand the permanency of these procedures.

III FOLLOW-UP AND REFERRAL

A. After initiating any new method of contraception, all patients (including those who have chosen barrier methods) **should have scheduled follow-up,** generally within 2–12 weeks. **Improper use of contraceptives is one of the most common reasons for failure.**

B. Patients who are having **persistent side effects** caused by a hormonal method of contraception may benefit from consultation with a gynecologist.

C. Patients who opt for **Mirena** or a non-hormonal **IUD** must see a physician who is trained in the insertion of these devices.

References

ACOG Committee on Practice Bulletins–Gynecology: Use of hormonal contraception in women with coexisting medical conditions. *Obstetr Gynecol* 2006;107(6):1453, 1467.

Herndon EJ, Zieman M. New Contraceptive Options. *Am Family Physician* 2004; 69(11):853–860.

• •

51. Approach to Joint Aspiration and Joint Injections
....

I Introduction

A. **Joint aspiration (arthrocentesis)** and **injection** can be both diagnostic and therapeutic. Arthrocentesis is the best way to differentiate among infectious, traumatic, inflammatory, degenerative, and metabolic causes of joint disease.

   Intra-articular injection of steroids—once infection has been
excluded—can provide substantial pain relief. Most rheumatol-
ogists limit patients to four joint injections per joint per year,
although there is little evidence that more frequent injections
are harmful.

II Indications and Contraindications for Joint Aspiration

A. **Diagnostic Aspiration**
   1. Acute synovitis
   2. Chronic arthropathy
B. **Therapeutic Aspiration**
   1. Decreases intra-articular pressure
   2. Recurrent aspiration for sepsis
C. **Contraindications**
   1. Injection or aspiration through cellulitis, psoriasis, surface
      blood vessels.
   2. Unstable coagulopathy
   3. Prosthetic joint (without consulting an orthopedic surgeon).

III Technique

A. **Preliminary steps**
   1. **Sterile preparation of the area.** Palpate and mark the area
      with a pen or indentation then clean the overlying skin with

antiseptic. Sterile gloves are not necessary, as long as one uses a no touch technique, but gloves for universal precaution are mandatory.

2. **Anesthesia** is optional. If desired, **ethyl chloride vapo-coolant** can be applied topically, or **1% lidocaine** can be administered subcutaneously.

B. **Joint aspiration**

1. **Assemble your materials.**

   a. **Needles.** A 21-gauge, 1.5-inch needle is sufficient for most aspirations, although aspiration of pus may require a larger (i.e., 18-gauge) needle. A 23 or 25 guage is appropriate for smaller joints.

   b. **Syringes** with a capacity of 2–20 milliliters are preferable. Larger syringes are more cumbersome and are not as effective at removing fluid.

2. **Quickly introduce the needle, aspirating gently until synovial fluid begins to flow.**

   a. If the needle hits cartilage or bone, withdraw the needle partially and reposition it.

   b. Aspirate as much fluid as possible; if necessary, milk fluid toward the needle from another site.

HOT KEY

If a joint injection is planned, do not aspirate to dryness to reduce the risk of needle displacement

---

3. **Send the aspirated joint fluid for cell count, Gram staining, culture,** and **crystal analysis.** If no obvious fluid is obtained, save the material from the needle lumen for culture and crystal analysis.

C. **Therapeutic steroid injection**

1. **Steroid preparations** include **triamcinolone** (the longest acting preparation), **prednisolone,** and **methylprednisolone.**

   a. The dose depends on the size of the joint. For a large joint like the knee or shoulder, 40 mg (1 cc) is used. For a medium joint like the wrist, ankle or elbow, 30 mg is used. Smaller joints like the metacarpophalangeal joint and tendon sheaths need just 10 mg.

   b. A local anesthetic, such as 1–2 ml of 1% lidocaine or 1–2 ml of 0.5% bupivacaine, can be added to the steroid to provide immediate relief of pain until the anti-inflammatory properties of the steroid takes effect.

> **HOT**
> ▶
> Warn patients that the anesthetic will wear off in 2–4 hours resulting in a temporary increase in pain.
> **KEY**

2. **Technique.** Care must be taken to avoid injecting the steroid into tendons or ligaments. Injection should require very little pressure. If resistance is met, withdraw the needle and reposition it until the steroid flows freely into the joint (Table 51-1).

Joint infection as a result of arthrocentesis is extremely rare; nevertheless, worsening pain and swelling after arthrocentesis should raise the concern of an infection.

Many patients complain of a pain flare that lasts for several hours following steroid injection. Such flares are self-limited and may be mitigated by massaging the joint with ice and resting for 12 to 24 hours after injection.

IV ANATOMIC APPROACHES (FIGURE 51-1)

1. **Interphalangeal joints.** Aspirate from the superolateral or superomedial aspect, staying dorsal to the digital vessels and lateral to the extensor tendon (see Figure 51-1A). Use a small needle (22- to 25-gauge) to minimize trauma.
2. **Wrist.** Passively flex the joint 20°–30° to open the joint space on the dorsal aspect of the wrist. Direct the needle into the space distal to the radius, ulnar to the extensor pollicis longus tendon, and radial to the extensor tendon for the index finger (see Figure 51-1B).

TABLE 51-1. Potential Side Effects from Joint Injection or Aspiration	
Side Effect	**Percent Occurrence and Comments**
Flushing	12% (usually from anesthetic)
Post-injection flare	up to 15%
Sepsis	<1:78,000
Subcutaneous atrophy	with peri-artcular injections
Depigmentation	With more superficial injections

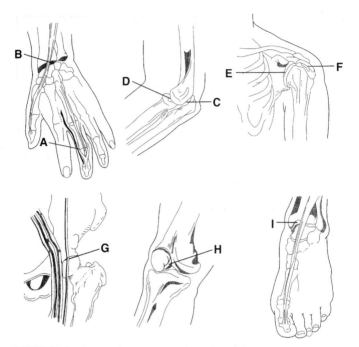

FIGURE 51-1. Approaches to commonly aspirated joints.

3. Elbow

a. Position the arm in 45° flexion. Approach the joint laterally, and enter the joint lateral to the olecranon process and 1 centimeter inferior to the lateral epicondyle (see Figure 51-1C).

b. An alternative approach is to insert the needle just proximal to the head of the radius (see Figure 51-1D).

4. Shoulder

a. To aspirate the **glenohumeral joint,** have the patient sit with her arm relaxed in her lap. Approach the joint anteriorly, holding the needle horizontally. Insert the needle medial to the head of the humerus and below the tip of the coracoid process (see Figure 51-1E).

b. To aspirate the **subacromial bursa,** insert the needle laterally under the acromion, directly into the bursa (see Figure 51-1F).

5. Knee.
Have the patient lie supine with his knee extended but relaxed. Either a medial or a lateral approach may be used. Direct the needle posterior to the patella and anterior to the femoral condyle (see Figure 51-1H).

6. Ankle. Position the patient's foot in slight plantar flexion. Approach the tibiotalar joint slightly medial to the extensor hallucis longus tendon, approximately 1 centimeter above and 1 centimeter lateral to the medial malleolus (see Figure 51-1I).

Reference

Courtney P, Doherty M. Joint aspiration and injection. *Best Practice & Research Clinical Rheumatology* 2005;19(3):345–369.

52. Acute Ankle Pain

I **INTRODUCTION.** Acute ankle pain is one of the most common musculoskeletal complaints. Although most patients presenting with acute ankle pain have a minor injury, as many as one-third of patients experience residual symptoms.

A. Anatomy (Figure 52-1). The ankle is a **hinge joint:** articulations between the distal tibia and fibula form an arch (mortise) that overlies the talus. Stability of the joint is provided by **multiple ligaments.**

B. Mechanisms of injury

   1. Inversion injuries. Inversion of the foot may result in injury of the **lateral ligaments** (i.e., the **anterior talo-fibular, posterior talofibular,** and **calcaneofibular ligaments).**

HOT KEY

Inversion injuries involving the lateral ligaments are the most common ankle injuries.

---

   2. Eversion injuries are much less common than inversion injuries. Because the deltoid ligament (i.e., the ligament that attaches the medial malleolus to the talus) is strong, it is not as prone to rupture as the lateral ligaments. The most common eversion injury is actually a fracture of the lateral malleolus. Therefore, both inversion and eversion injuries usually involve the lateral ankle.

II **DIFFERENTIAL DIAGNOSIS**

A. Ankle sprains. Most ankle injuries are **ligamentous sprains,** usually sustained while playing a sport: basketball, volleyball, and football players are at highest risk. Although sprains are usually related to vigorous activity, any sudden stress on a ligament (such as may occur when stepping off a curb) can result in injury.

   1. The patient may hear a "pop" followed by the sudden onset of acute pain.

   2. Symptoms correlate with the severity of the injury. Usually, the patient is unable to bear weight initially, followed by a

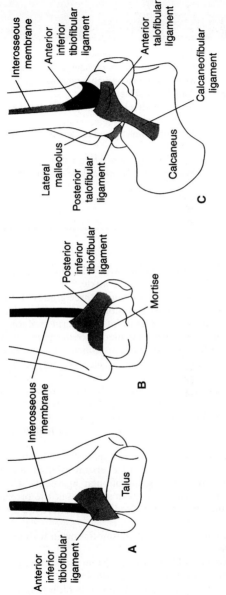

FIGURE 52-1. Distal tibiofibular joint and tibiotalar joint. (A) Anterior view. (B) Posterior view. (C) Lateral view. (Redrawn with permission from Steinberg GC, Baran DT, Akins CM. *Ramamurti's Orthopaedics in Primary Care*, 2e. Baltimore: Williams & Wilkins, 1992.)

TABLE 52-1. Classification of Ankle Sprains	
Grade	**Criteria**
First degree	Stretching of the ligament No instability or impairment of functional ability Mild tenderness and pain on stress
Second degree	Partial tear of the ligament Mild to moderate instability and impaired functional ability Moderate swelling and tenderness on initial examination
Third degree	Complete rupture of the ligament Marked instability of the joint resulting in minimal functional ability Marked swelling, tenderness, and ecchymosis on initial examination

feeling of the ankle "giving way" and the development of marked ecchymosis around the ankle.

   3. Sprains are usually assigned one of three grades (Table 52-1).

B. **Ankle fracture.** The most common fractures (in order of decreasing frequency) are fracture of the lateral malleolus of the fibula, fracture of the medial malleolus of the tibia, bimalleolar fractures, and fractures of the talus. Smoking and a high body mass index are associated with ankles fractures, but low bone mineral density does not appear to contribute. Fractures are considered unstable if 2 or more sites of significant injury are present such as lateral malleolar fracture with deltoid ligament disruption or bimalleolar fractures.

C. **Bone contusion.** Trauma may lead to contusion of the lateral or medial malleolus.

D. **Syndesmosis injuries,** also known as high ankle sprains, may accompany severe inversion or eversion injuries and involve the inferior and transverse tibiofibular ligaments. They most often occur in collision sports. In some cases, the proximal interosseous membrane is involved as well. There are 3 types of injury:

   1. **Type 1** involves signs of syndesmotic sprain with normal radiographs
   2. **Type 2** has a tibiofibular space >6 mm measured 1 mm above the joint seen on stress radiograph.
   3. **Type 3** has frank diastasis on nonstress radiograph.

E. **Peroneal tendon injuries** include **subluxation, tendinitis,** and **rupture.**

F. Achilles tendon injuries include **rupture** and **tendinitis.** Abrupt dorsiflexion of the foot (such as might occur following a jump) is the usual cause of tendon rupture.

III APPROACH TO THE PATIENT

A. Patient history
1. What were the circumstances surrounding the injury?
2. How long ago did the injury occur?
3. Was the patient able to bear weight immediately after the injury occurred?

B. Physical examination
1. Document any ecchymosis or swelling. Swelling anterior or inferior to the malleolus should be differentiated from supramalleolar swelling which may indicate fracture or syndesmotic injury.
2. Assess peripheral sensation and distal pulses.
3. Palpate the pedal and posterior tibial pulses.
4. Palpate the bones, tendons, and ligaments of the ankle and foot. Pay particular attention to the:
    a. Medial and lateral malleoli (especially the posterior edges)
    b. Lateral ligaments
    c. Achilles and peroneal tendons
    d. Navicular and cuboid bones
    e. Base of the fifth metatarsal bone
5. Determine whether the patient is able to bear weight and take four steps.
6. Perform specific tests as necessary (Figure 52-2).
    a. Anterior drawer test (see Figure 52-2A). Position the patient so that she is sitting or lying down with her knee slightly flexed. Make sure the ankle is positioned at a 90° angle to the leg. With one hand on the tibia and the other hand on the back of the heel, try to draw the foot forward. Rupture of the anterior talofibular ligament (i.e., the first lateral ligament injured by an inversion injury) is indicated by instability.
    b. Squeeze test (see Figure 52-2B). Squeeze the tibia and fibula together at midcalf, then assess for pain in the distal ankle. A positive test suggests injury of the **syndesmotic ligaments.**

HOT

▶

A syndesmosis injury should be suspected in patients with chronic pain after an ankle sprain.

KEY

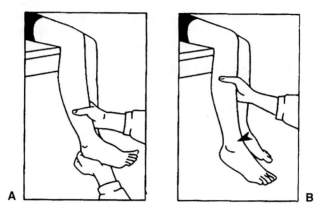

FIGURE 52-2. (A) Anterior drawer test. Instability when the foot is pulled forward suggests rupture of the anterior talofibular ligament. (B) Squeeze test. Pain in the distal ankle (*arrow*) suggests injury of the syndesmotic ligaments.

      c. Thompson test. Position the patient so that she is prone, with her foot extending off the edge of the table, and squeeze the gastrocnemius-soleus complex. Normally, this maneuver results in plantar flexion, but in patients with **Achilles tendon rupture,** the foot will not flex.

      d. Peroneal tendon examination should be performed when there is pain or a "snapping" sensation over the lateral malleolus. Tendon injury is suggested by subluxation when the patient everts her foot against resistance.

C. Imaging studies
   1. Radiography
      a. Indications. Radiographs are obtained for patients who meet the criteria described in the **Ottawa rules.**
         (1) Ankle films should be ordered to rule out an ankle fracture if pain is present near either malleolus and the patient:
            (a) Cannot bear weight immediately after the injury and for four steps during the evaluation, **or**
            (b) Has bone tenderness at the posterior or inferior edge of either malleolus
         (2) Foot films should be ordered to rule out a foot fracture if pain is present at the midfoot and the patient:
            (a) Cannot bear weight immediately after the injury and for four steps during the evaluation, **or**

(b) Has bone tenderness at the navicular bone, the cuboid bone, or the base of the fifth metatarsal bone

---

HOT KEY

Studies that have been done to validate the Ottawa rules have demonstrated that their sensitivity is high (95%–100%) but their specificity is low (15%–40%). Thus, if all three of the criteria are **not** met one can be comfortable ruling out an ankle fracture, but many patients who do meet one of the criteria do not have an ankle fracture.

---

b. Views
  (1) Ankle films
    (a) Anteroposterior, lateral, and **oblique views** are the standard views. The main objective is to rule out fracture, and if one is found to determine whether or not there has been displacement of bone.
    (b) Stress anteroposterior ankle films may be obtained if no fracture is seen but significant swelling and tenderness are present on examination. Widening of the ankle mortise suggests a tear in either the medial deltoid ligament or the lateral collateral ligament (or both).

HOT KEY

Suspect a talar dome fracture in a patient with persistent pain after a sprain. These fractures are characterized radiographically by a small necrotic fragment of bone on the articular surface of the talus.

---

  (2) Foot films. Standard views include **anteroposterior, internally rotated oblique,** and **lateral views.**
  (3) Fibula films should be obtained to evaluate the possibility of a high fibular fracture in patients suspected of having a syndesmosis injury.
2. Magnetic resonance imaging (MRI) is often performed to confirm a suspected peroneal tendon injury. It is recommended for ankle injury with medial echymoses and chronic sprains that are still symptomatic 4 months after injury.

IV TREATMENT

A. Ankle sprains

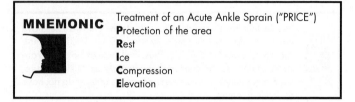

MNEMONIC Treatment of an Acute Ankle Sprain ("PRICE")
Protection of the area
Rest
Ice
Compression
Elevation

1. Ice should be applied for 15–20 minutes every 1–2 hours, and the ankle should be immobilized by wrapping it with an elastic bandage. This treatment should be continued for 24–48 hours.
2. Nonsteroidal anti-inflammatory drugs (NSAIDs) can be used for pain control.
3. Patients with grade II or III sprains should be seen by an orthopedist within 24–48 hours.
4. **Functional rehabilitation** is recommended including early active range of motion, proprioceptive training and peroneal strengthening especially in the injured athlete.
5. Use of crutches for grade I and II sprains is discouraged. A short period of **protective bracing** may be helpful.
6. **Return to activity** usually occurs after 3–5 days for a grade I strain, 1–3 weeks for a grade II sprain, and up to 6 months for a grade III sprain.

B. Ankle fractures

1. Fractures of either malleolus that are small and undisplaced can be treated with a short leg walking cast. The ankle should be immobilized for 8 weeks.
2. Undisplaced fractures of both malleoli, the calcaneus, or the base of the fifth metatarsal bone and single malleolar fractures that show displacement should be immobilized in a short leg sugar-tong splint and the patient should be referred to an orthopedist for treatment.
3. Open fractures, neurovascular compromise or fracture dislocations must be referred to an orthopedic surgeon immediately.

HOT **KEY** Ankle fracture-dislocation is an orthopedic emergency because blood flow may be compromised and avascular necrosis of the navicular bone can occur. Immediate reduction is recommended.

4. Splinting a non-emergent fracture should be done at 90 degrees (in neutral position) to provide support and control pain. Usually a short-leg posterior splint is sufficient.

HOT KEY

If significant swelling or deformity is present, a bulky dressing should be placed prior to splinting to allow for further swelling while maintaining stability.

C. Syndesmosis injuries
 1. **Type 1** is treated similar to a simple sprain.
 2. **Type 2** is treated with a non-weightbearing short-leg cast for 4 weeks followed by weightbearing in an immobilization boot for 4 more weeks.
 3. **Type 3** requires immediate referral to an orthopedic surgeon for possible stabilization.
 4. **Return to activity** for type 1 and 2 is about 8 to 12 weeks.
D. Peroneal tendon subluxation. Patients require orthopedic surgery for reduction and immobilization.
E. Achilles tendon injuries
 1. **Achilles tendinitis** can be treated conservatively with rest, heat, stretching exercises, and nonsteroidal anti-inflammatory drugs (NSAIDs).
 2. **Achilles tendon rupture** warrants referral to an orthopedist for immediate surgical repair.

V FOLLOW-UP AND REFERRAL

A. Most patients with first-degree sprains can be managed in a primary care setting, and usually can resume normal activities after about 4 weeks.
B. Patients with second- or third-degree sprains, fractures, or tendon rupture must be evaluated by an orthopedic surgeon within 48 hours. Any patient with signs of neurovascular compromise should see an orthopedist immediately. Two indications for operative fixation are loss of joint congruency and loss of joint stability.

References
Saluta J, Nunley JA. Managing foot and ankle injuries in athletes. *J Musculoskel Med* 2006;23:195–201.
Bachmann LM, Kolb E, Koller MT, et al. Accuracy of Ottawa ankle rules to exclude fractures of the ankle and mid-foot: systematic review. *BMJ* 2003;326:417.

53. Acute Knee Pain

I **INTRODUCTION.** The anatomy of the knee is shown in Figure 53-1.

II **DIFFERENTIAL DIAGNOSIS (TABLE 53-1)**

A. Fractures. The **patella, tibial plateau,** and **fibular head** can all sustain fractures following trauma.

B. Joint space disorders include **infection, inflammatory arthritis,** and **osteoarthritis (OA).**

C. Ligament injuries (sprains)
   1. The **medial (tibial) collateral ligament, lateral (fibular) collateral ligament, anterior cruciate ligament,** and **posterior cruciate ligament** are all susceptible to sprains.
      a. **Collateral ligament injuries** are usually caused by stress in the medial or lateral direction (e.g., a blow to the lateral aspect of the knee could result in medial collateral ligament rupture).
      b. **Cruciate ligament injuries** are usually caused by hyperextension stress.
   2. **Classification.** Sprains are usually graded as **first- degree** (no laxity), **second-degree** (some laxity), or **third-degree** (complete disruption).

D. Meniscal tears may be traumatic or atraumatic. A history of injury while the knee was flexed and twisting is typical.

E. Patellar tendinitis ("jumper's knee"), often seen in patients who play basketball or participate in track and field, occurs when overuse results in microscopic tears of the patellar tendon.

F. Bursitis usually results from **direct trauma** or **overuse** and can affect the **prepatellar, pes anserinus, superficial intrapatellar,** or **deep intrapatellar bursae.**

G. Patellofemoral syndrome is often seen in runners. The syndrome usually results from malalignment of the femur, patella, and tibia. Patellofemoral syndrome can lead to patellar chondromalacia.

H. Referred pain (i.e., from the ipsilateral hip)

III **APPROACH TO THE PATIENT**

A. Patient history. A careful history gives important clues to the source of the pain. Consider the following questions:
   1. Was there a mechanism of injury?

2. Where is the pain located?
3. Was the onset sudden or insidious
4. Is there an effusion, and if so, how soon did it appear?
5. Do any activities exacerbate the pain (e.g., twisting, squatting, ascending or descending stairs)?
6. Is there a history of prior problems in the knee or other joints?
7. Is there associated stiffness, locking, catching, snapping, grinding, or crepitus?

HOT **KEY** Complaints of the knee "buckling" or "giving out" are common, and are actually not specific as to the location of the injury. These symptoms may simply be indicative of quadriceps muscle weakness.

B. Physical examination
1. **Inspection.** Loss of the infrapatellar indentations signals an effusion. Compare the appearance of the affected knee with the unaffected knee.
2. **Palpation**
   a. Check for joint line and bony tenderness.
   b. Evaluate for effusions by pushing down on the kneecap.
   c. Tenderness outside of the knee joint may suggest bursitis or tendinitis.
3. **Range of motion assessment.** Evaluate the knee's range of motion while feeling for crepitus. True "locking" of the knee (i.e., a sudden inability to completely extend the knee) usually indicates a meniscal tear, a cruciate ligament rupture, an osteochondral fracture, or a loose body.

HOT **KEY** A true locked knee is an emergency! Arthroscopy is necessary for definitive diagnosis.

---

4. **Special maneuvers**
   a. **Evaluation for patellar tendinitis.** With the knee fully extended, evaluate for tenderness at the superior or inferior pole of the patella.
   b. **Valgus** and **varus stress testing** can be used to evaluate the **collateral ligaments.** With the knee slightly flexed (to about 10°) place one hand above and the other below the knee and then "bend" the knee laterally and medially. Laxity suggests a collateral ligament injury.

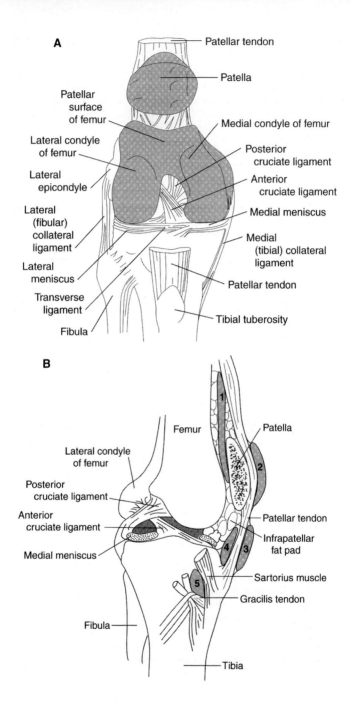

A

Patellar tendon

Patella

Patellar surface of femur

Medial condyle of femur

Lateral condyle of femur

Posterior cruciate ligament

Lateral epicondyle

Anterior cruciate ligament

Lateral (fibular) collateral ligament

Medial meniscus

Medial (tibial) collateral ligament

Lateral meniscus

Patellar tendon

Transverse ligament

Tibial tuberosity

Fibula

B

Femur

Patella

Lateral condyle of femur

Posterior cruciate ligament

Anterior cruciate ligament

Patellar tendon

Medial meniscus

Infrapatellar fat pad

Sartorius muscle

Gracilis tendon

Fibula

Tibia

TABLE 53-1. Clinical Manifestations of Disorders That Can Cause Acute Knee Pain

Disorder	Clinical Manifestations
Fracture	Tenderness, inability to bear weight on limb, effusion (tibial plateau fractures)
DJD	Chronic pain, bland effusion
Infection	Joint erythema, warmth, and effusion
Inflammatory arthritis	Joint erythema, warmth and effusion
Ligament injury	Laxity on stress testing
Meniscal tear	Pain with twisting motion, locking, joint line tenderness, positive McMurray's test, positive Apley test (with compression)
Patellar tendinitis	Tenderness at the superior or inferior pole of the patella
Bursitis	Tenderness, often accompanied by erythema, warmth, and swelling
Patellofemoral syndrome	Anterior knee pain at rest, crepitus, pain while ascending stairs, pain with compression of the patella, positive apprehension test (i.e., patient resists lateral movement of the patella)

DJD = degenerative joint disease.

HOT

Laxity with straight-leg valgus and varus testing suggests multiple ligament tears.

KEY

---

    c. Drawer and **Lachman's tests.** These tests are used to evaluate the **cruciate ligaments.** Have the patient lie supine with his knee flexed at either a 20° angle (Lachman's test)

FIGURE 53-1. Anatomy of the knee. (*A*) Anterior view, emphasizing the collateral ligaments. (*B*) Sagittal view with the medial condyle removed. The bursae are numbered: 1 = suprapatellar; 2 = prepatellar; 3 = superficial infrapatellar; 4 = deep infrapatellar; 5 = pes anserinus. (Part *A* redrawn with permission from Moore KL, Agur AMR. *Essential Clinical Anatomy*, 3rd ed. Baltimore: Lippincott Williams & Wilkins, 2006. Part *B* redrawn with permission from Byank RP, Beatie WE. Exercise-related musculo-skeletal problems. In *Principles of Ambulatory Medicine*, 7th ed. Edited by Barker LR, Fiebach NH, Kern DE, Thomas PA, Ziegelstein RC, Zieve PD. Baltimore: Lippincott Williams & Wilkins, 2006.)

or a 90° angle (drawer test). Place both of your hands just below the knee and pull, as if you were opening a drawer. Anterior movement of the tibia indicates an anterior cruciate ligament disruption.

HOT KEY

Lachman's test is more sensitive than the drawer test for a ligament tear.

    d. McMurray's test. This test can be used to evaluate a **meniscal tear.** With the patient supine, flex and extend her knee, first with the foot internally rotated and then with it externally rotated, while palpating with the opposite hand for popping or locking of the knee.
    e. Apley compression-distraction test. This test can be used to evaluate the knee for **meniscus** and **collateral ligament injuries.**
        (1) Meniscus injury. With the patient prone and the knee flexed at a 90° angle, apply a gradual downward force on the leg and then internally and externally rotate the foot. Pain with compression suggests meniscus injury.
        (2) Collateral ligament injury. Repeat the maneuver while applying upward traction on the leg rather than downward pressure. Pain with this maneuver suggests a collateral ligament injury.
C. Laboratory studies. Diagnostic joint aspiration (see Chapter 51) should be performed in patients with an effusion.

HOT KEY

Aspiration of gross blood suggests a serious injury (usually a fracture or ligament tear).

D. Imaging studies. A plain film of the knee in the setting of acute injury should be ordered if the patient meets any one of the following criteria, known as the **Ottawa rules:**
    1. 55 years or older
    2. tenderness at the head of the fibula
    3. isolated tenderness of the patella
    4. unable to flex the knee to 90°
    5. unable to bear weight on the limb immediately after the injury and at the time of evaluation

IV TREATMENT

A. **General measures. Rest, ice,** and **elevation** often help to relieve swelling, which can delay recovery.

HOT

KEY

In patients with large or bloody effusions, aspirating the effusion may alleviate some of the patient's symptoms.

B. **Specific therapies**
   1. **Fractures.** Patients should be referred to an orthopedist after the fracture has been immobilized.
   2. **Osteoarthritis(OA)** see Chapter 57

HOT

KEY

Because NSAIDs may exacerbate certain medical conditions (e.g., peptic ulcer disease, renal insufficiency, bleeding diatheses), consider a patient's history before prescribing an NSAID.

---

   3. **Ligament injuries.** Treatment depends on the patient's level of activity. Most patients with these types of injuries should see an orthopedic surgeon or sports medicine specialist.
      a. **Anterior cruciate ligament injuries** may be treated conservatively in an inactive person but early surgical repair is recommended in an athletic individual.
      b. **Posterior cruciate ligament injuries** are usually associated with other ligament injuries, and surgery is usually required.
      c. **Medial** and **lateral collateral ligament tears** commonly require only immobilization followed by rehabilitation.
   4. **Meniscal tears** may heal spontaneously if they are peripheral, but **many require surgical repair.** Most patients should be referred to an orthopedist after the knee is immobilized.
   5. **Bursitis**
      a. Bursal **aspiration** for diagnostic purposes and to rule out infection. **Compression dressing** and **knee padding** may be needed after aspiration to help the bursal walls reapproximate.
      b. If the **WBC >1400 cell/mm³**, infection is assumed. Serial aspirations should be done until the fluid is sterile.

c. **Antibiotics** should be used if infection is suspected (e.g., prepatellar bursitis often results from infection). Oral antibiotics are usually sufficient.

d. **Rest, heat,** and **NSAIDs** are usually used to treat bursitis.

e. If the patient can't tolerate **NSAIDs** and infection has been ruled out, a **glucocorticoid injection** may be performed.

HOT

Patients with pes anserinus bursitis should be advised to sleep with a pillow between their legs.
KEY

---

6. **Patellar tendinitis** is difficult to treat. Patients should be advised to reduce their activity level and perform exercises designed to stretch and strengthen the quadriceps and hamstring muscles.

 FOLLOW-UP AND REFERRAL. Patients with persistent undiagnosed knee pain should be referred to an orthopedist or sports medicine specialist for diagnosis and treatment.

Reference
Jackson JL, O'Malley PG, Kroenke K. Evaluation of acute knee pain in primary care. *Ann Intern Med* 2003;139(7):575–588.

54. Shoulder Pain

. . . .

I. INTRODUCTION

A. Incidence. Approximately 1 in 5 adults experiences shoulder pain during his or her lifetime.

B. Anatomy (Figure 54-1). The clinically relevant components of the shoulder joint can be remembered as "4-3-2-1."

MNEMONIC	Anatomy of the Shoulder Joint ("4-3-2-1")
	4 muscles ("SITS") — **s**upraspinatus, **i**nfraspinatus, **t**eres minor, **s**ubscapularis (rotator cuff)
	3 joints — acromioclavicular, sternoclavicular, glenohumeral
	2 tendons — supraspinatus, biceps
	1 bursa — subacromial

II. DIFFERENTIAL DIAGNOSIS

A. Subacromial bursitis and **supraspinatus tendinitis** result in essentially the same clinical illness. Repetitive overhead motion (e.g., serving in tennis or throwing a baseball) is the usual cause.

B. Adhesive capsulitis ("frozen shoulder") usually results from prolonged immobility due to pain from another disorder (e.g., subacromial bursitis).

C. Rotator cuff tears can occur in young adults who subject the joint to extreme overuse (e.g., in baseball pitchers). In older adults, even minor trauma to the shoulder can cause a rotator cuff tear.

D. Osteoarthritis (OA) usually affects the acromioclavicular joint; much more rarely, the glenohumeral joint is affected.

E. Bicipital tendinitis results from overuse (e.g., repeated flexion-extension or pronation-supination of the elbow).

F. Glenohumeral instability is subluxation or dislocation of the glenohumeral joint secondary to prior trauma.

G. Referred pain. Cervical disk disease, an apical lung tumor, pleural disease, myocardial ischemia or infarction, and subdiaphragmatic processes (e.g., gallbladder disease, abscess, free air) should all be considered as possible causes of shoulder pain.

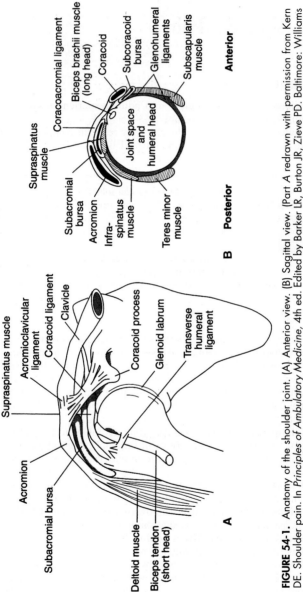

FIGURE 54-1. Anatomy of the shoulder joint. (A) Anterior view. (B) Sagittal view. (Part A redrawn with permission from Kern DE. Shoulder pain. In *Principles of Ambulatory Medicine*, 4th ed. Edited by Barker LR, Burton JR, Zieve PD. Baltimore: Williams & Wilkins, 1995, p 849. Part B modified with permission from Pansky B. *Review of Gross Anatomy*. New York: Macmillan, 1979.)

APPROACH TO THE PATIENT. Approximately 85% of cases of shoulder pain can be diagnosed by history and physical examination alone. Clinical findings for each of the common causes are given in Table 54-1.

> **HOT KEY**
> Most cases of shoulder pain are caused by subacromial bursitis, supraspinatus tendinitis, rotator cuff tear, or adhesive capsulitis.

A. Patient history. Key points include the following.
  1. What is the **patient's age?** Rotator cuff tears are more common in patients older than 50 years.
  2. Was the **onset sudden?**
     a. A **sudden "pop"** while lifting overhead suggests a **rotator cuff tear.**
     b. The **onset of pain** is usually **gradual** in **subacromial bursitis** and **supraspinatus tendinitis.**
  3. Are there any **aggravating factors?**
     a. **Difficulty brushing one's hair** or **nocturnal pain** caused by rolling over onto the shoulder may signify the **impingement syndrome** (i.e., repetitive friction between the acromion and the greater tuberosity of the humerus leads to inflammation of the rotator cuff and bursa). **Subacromial bursitis, supraspinatus tendinitis,** or **small rotator cuff tears** can all cause the impingement syndrome and therefore have similar clinical presentations.
     b. **Pain as a result of curling the arm** (e.g., lifting a pot away from the stove) suggests **bicipital tendinitis.**
     c. **Pain that occurs when the patient reaches behind herself** (e.g., to put on a coat or fasten a bra) may signify **adhesive capsulitis.**
B. Physical examination
  1. **Palpation.** Palpate the acromioclavicular joint, the subacromial bursa, the glenohumeral joint, and the bicipital groove for tenderness, which may be a sign of OA, bursitis, adhesive capsulitis, or bicipital tendinitis, respectively.
  2. **Range of motion assessment**
     a. **Active range of motion**
        (1) Have the patient reach behind his head and touch the opposite shoulder to test abduction and external rotation.
        (2) Ask the patient to reach behind his back with his hand in the "hitchhiker" position and touch the ipsilateral

TABLE 54-1. Clinical Manifestations of the Common Causes of Shoulder Pain

Disorder	History	Physical Examination	Imaging
Subacromial bursitis	Pain with overhead activity (e.g., shampooing hair)	Point tenderness over the subacromial area	None necessary
Supraspinatus tendinitis	Nocturnal pain that interferes with sleep	Painful arc (60°–120°) with active range of motion	
Adhesive capsulitis	Diffuse, dull ache Decreasing function (e.g., difficulty putting on a coat)	Diffuse tenderness Decreased active and passive range of motion	None usually necessary; arthroscopy can detect decreased capsular volume
Rotator cuff tear	Patient may describe hearing or feeling a sudden "pop" Pain with overhead activity; patient may be unable to lift arm without assistance Nocturnal pain	Point tenderness over subacromial area Painful arc (60°–120°) with active range of motion Positive impingement sign Weakness	MRI
Bicipital tendinitis	Anterior shoulder pain, exacerbated by lifting or curling (e.g., lifting a pan off the stove top)	Tenderness over bicipital groove Pain with resisted forearm supination	None necessary

DJD of the acromioclavicular joint	Pain over the acromioclavicular joint	Tenderness over the acromioclavicular joint Pain with crossed-chest adduction test	Plain films may show narrowed joint space and osteophyte formation
Glenohumeral instability	Severe pain after acute event Patient often holds arm close to body with unaffected hand	Neurovascular compromise in some patients	Plain films are diagnostic
Referred pain	Diffuse, progressive pain that overlaps anatomic boundaries Pain can radiate below elbow	Preserved range of motion Other findings depend on the cause	Plain film of shoulder and chest Additional studies guided by clinical suspicion

DJD = degenerative joint disease

shoulder blade to test adduction and internal rotation. Note the highest spinous process reached for future comparisons.

   b. Passive range of motion. If the active range of motion is decreased, test the passive range of motion.

      (1) In **impingement disorders,** the active range of motion is decreased due to pain, but the passive range of motion is preserved.

      (2) In **adhesive capsulitis,** both the active and the passive range of motion are decreased.

3. Weakness may be secondary to a rotator cuff tear, a brachial plexus lesion, or cervical disk disease.

4. Special maneuvers

   a. Impingement sign. Have the patient elevate her arm with the elbow flexed (like a military salute) against resistance. Pain with this motion indicates the **impingement syndrome.**

   b. Drop arm test. Have the patient hold the affected arm in 90° of abduction. Place downward force on the patient's outstretched arm at the wrist and note any pain or weakness. In patients with severe pain, it may be necessary to inject the subacromial bursa with lidocaine prior to performing this test.

      (1) Weakness is indicated by arm drop and suggests a **significant rotator cuff tear.**

      (2) Pain without weakness usually indicates **supraspinatus tendinitis** or **subacromial bursitis.**

   c. Resisted supination test. Have the patient attempt supination while you apply resistance at the wrist. Pain with this test suggests **biceps tendinitis.**

   d. Head compression test. With the patient seated, apply firm downward pressure on the top of her head. Neck pain or radicular symptoms suggest **cervical disk disease.**

5. Neuromuscular examination is important for patients with glenohumeral instability. Evaluate the brachial and medial pulses and the sensory and motor function of the forearm, wrist, and hand.

C. Imaging studies

1. Plain film radiography can assess for fractures, arthritis, calcific tendinitis, destructive bone lesions, and the bony morphology of the acromion.

   a. Usually, an anteroposterior view in internal and external rotation, a lateral view, and a scapular view are obtained.

   b. Cysts on the greater tuberosity may reflect rotator cuff disease.

2. Magnetic Resonance Imaging (MRI) and arthrography

    a. MRI has become the **gold standard** for detecting **rotator cuff tears** replacing arthrography, although arthrography might be helpful in detecting partial thickness tears.

    b. Arthrography can also be used to diagnose **adhesive capsulitis;** reduced contrast capacity of the joint space is suggestive.

3. **MRI** is noninvasive, readily available, and is accurate as arthrography for diagnosing partial and complete **rotator cuff tears.**

4. **Ultrasonography** is rarely used in the assessment of shoulder pain, but can be useful for diagnosing a **large rotator cuff tear.**

IV TREATMENT

A. Impingement syndromes and **bicipital tendinitis.** Therapy is only moderately effective for these patients. Fewer than 50% of patients undergoing multimodal therapy will be asymptomatic after 1 year.

    1. Pharmacologic therapy

      a. Nonsteroidal anti-inflammatory drugs (NSAIDs) should be tried initially. Common regimens include ibuprofen, 400–800 mg orally, three times daily for 2 weeks, or naproxen, 250–500 mg orally twice daily for 2 weeks.

      b. Corticosteroid injections (see Chapter 51 II C) may be used if NSAID therapy fails or is contraindicated. Injections may be slightly more effective than NSAIDs, but in the absence of definitive data on safety and efficacy, they should be administered no more than four times a year.

    2. Exercise

      a. Passive range of motion exercises should be initiated immediately. The patient should be shown how to perform pendulum and other passive range of motion exercises at home. Patient-oriented literature is available to demonstrate and reinforce the importance of practicing these exercises.

      b. Active range of motion exercises. Physical therapy involving a combination of **isometric exercises** (performed with elastic tubing), **shoulder shrugs,** and **wall push-ups** can be **started 2 weeks after initiating NSAID therapy** or administering a corticosteroid injection. These exercises strengthen the rotator cuff muscles.

    3. Monitoring. The patient should return 2–4 weeks after beginning active range of motion exercises so that the physician can assess the patient's progress and the effectiveness of pharmacologic therapy.

B. Rotator cuff tears

1. **Small rotator cuff tears** are managed conservatively, as described in IV A. Small, uncontrolled trials that have examined the safety and efficacy of steroid injections in the treatment of small rotator cuff tears have suggested that steroid therapy is moderately beneficial and not deleterious in these patients.

2. **Moderate** to **large rotator cuff tears** are best managed with **surgery** (arthroscopic or open techniques may be used). Aggressive and supervised **physical therapy** is necessary after surgery; rehabilitation can take 6–9 months.

C. Adhesive capsulitis. The recovery from adhesive capsulitis is slow and requires persistent physical therapy.

1. As in the treatment of impingement syndromes, **NSAIDs** and **exercise** are the mainstays of therapy. The patient should begin immediately with passive range of motion exercises (e.g., pendulum exercises) and advance to active range of motion exercises (e.g., wall push-ups).

2. The role of **corticosteroid injections** in the treatment of adhesive capsulitis is controversial. Studies in a small number of patients showed that intra-articular steroids may improve range of motion without causing demonstrable harm.

3. **Shoulder manipulation** under anesthesia can be considered for patients with recalcitrant disease.

D. Glenohumeral instability. The primary care provider should temporarily immobilize the shoulder with a **splint** and refer the patient to an **orthopedic specialist.**

E. Osteoarthritis

1. **Conservative management** with **physical therapy** and **acetaminophen** or **NSAIDs** should be tried.

2. Mixed injections of **lidocaine** and **short-acting steroids** can also provide relief.

> **HOT KEY**
>
> Conservative therapy is appropriate for all patients with shoulder pain, except for those with moderate to large rotator cuff tears or glenohumeral instability.

V FOLLOW-UP AND REFERRAL

A. Referral to an **orthopedist** is appropriate for patients with moderate to large rotator cuff tears or glenohumeral instability. Patients who fail to obtain significant relief of symptoms after 4 weeks of conservative therapy should also be referred, regardless of the cause of the shoulder pain.

B. A **physical therapist** can integrate the home exercises described in the patient literature with a more formal exercise program. Consultation with a physical therapist also helps to ensure patient compliance.

References

Gomoll AH, Katz JN, Warner JJ, Millett PJ. Rotator cuff disorders: recognition and management among patients with shoulder pain. *Arthritis & Rheumatism* 2004;50(12):3751–3761.

Mitchell C, Adebajo A, Hay E, Carr A. Shoulder pain: diagnosis and management in primary care. *BMJ* 2005;331(7525):1124–1128.

55. Elbow Pain

I **INTRODUCTION.** The elbow allows positioning of the hand in space via flexion-extension and pronation-supination. Pain or dysfunction can originate in any structure of the elbow (i.e., bone, ligaments, tendons, nerves, bursae, joint space), referred from the wrist or shoulder or from a cervical radiculopathy.

II **DIFFERENTIAL DIAGNOSIS.** Elbow disorders can be caused by trauma, overuse, nerve compression, infection, or systemic disease.

A. **Fractures** of the distal humerus, radial head, or olecranon (proximal ulna) are usually caused by direct trauma. Older patients with osteoporosis are much more susceptible to elbow fractures.

B. **Dislocations.** Elbow dislocations are relatively common. Posterior displacement of the radius and ulna accounts for most elbow dislocations and usually results from falling on an extended, abducted arm.

C. **Ligament injuries** are typically seen in athletes, especially those who are required to throw a ball.
  1. The **medial (ulnar) collateral ligament** is affected most often.
  2. The **pain** is **usually medial** and located just **below the epicondyle.** The pain worsens when valgus stress is applied while the elbow is held in the flexed position.

D. **Epicondylitis**
  1. **Lateral epicondylitis (tennis elbow, tendinitis)** most commonly results from **overuse**. The **pain** is **usually lateral** and located just **below the epicondyle.**
  2. **Medial Epicondylitis (golfer's elbow)** pain is well localized also. It is aggravated by lifting with contraction of the **wrist flexors**.

HOT KEY

Overuse injuries usually involve the patient's dominant extremity.

E. **Nerve entrapment.** The **ulnar nerve** is affected more often than the radial or medial nerves. There can be sensory (and occasionally motor) symptoms in the 4th and 5th digit.

1. Pressure over the cubital tunnel (during intoxication or coma or from trauma) or cumulative injury from repeated elbow flexion and extension can result in ulnar neuropathy.
2. Clinical manifestations include medial elbow or forearm pain and hand clumsiness that worsens with activity.

F. **Olecranon bursitis** can result from **trauma** or **infection.** Clinical manifestations include pain and "goose egg" swelling as a result of fluid collection.

G. **Arthritis.** Infectious arthritis, inflammatory arthritis (e.g., rheumatoid arthritis, spondyloarthritis, gout, pseudogout), and osteoarthritis from secondary causes can all affect the elbow joint. Patients complain of effusion and acute elbow pain that increases with movement.

H. Referred Pain. This is usually decribed as a deep ache not related to elbow motion. It can be accompanied by parasthesias, but lacks local signs. It can be aggravated by shoulder or neck movement.

III APPROACH TO THE PATIENT

A. **Patient history.** Answers to the following questions can help to narrow the differential diagnosis.
1. Was the **onset of symptoms** abrupt or gradual? The abrupt onset of pain and a "popping" sound are worrisome for a ligament tear.
2. Where is the **pain located?**
3. **Is there swelling or decreased range of motion?**
4. Are there **associated symptoms** (e.g., numbness, swelling, loss of function)?
5. What is the patient's **exercise** and **work history?** Overuse injuries are common.
6. Is there a **history of trauma?**
7. Is there a **history of arthritis at other joints?**

B. **Physical examination**
1. **Inspection**
   a. **Olecranon bursitis** is suggested by a **tender, localized fluid collection** over the olecranon (i.e., the "funny bone").
   b. **Rheumatoid arthritis**
      (1) **Rheumatoid nodules** may be seen on the extensor surface of the elbow.
      (2) Always examine the hands and feet for **signs of systemic arthritis.**
   c. **Elbow dislocation.** Patients with elbow dislocations usually hold the **limb close to the body at a 45° angle.**

   2. **Palpation**

     a. Tenderness **just below the lateral epicondyle** may suggest **lateral epicondylitis.**

     b. Tenderness **1–2 centimeters below the lateral epicondyle** may suggest **elbow joint arthritis.**

   3. **Range of motion assessment.** The elbow's range of motion, including **flexion-extension** and **pronation-supination,** should be evaluated.

     a. Septic arthritis usually results in severe pain that limits the patient's range of motion.

     b. In patients with lateral epicondylitis, passive–flexion-extension of the elbow is painless, but forced pronation-supination is painful.

   4. **Neurologic examination** is necessary to rule out entrapment syndromes.

     a. **Weakness, atrophy,** or **sensory deficits** imply nerve involvement.

     b. **Tinel's sign.** Tapping over the ulnar nerve in the cubital tunnel between the medial epicondyle and the olecranon may elicit shock-like pain in a patient with nerve compression.

   5. **Distal neurovascular examination** is mandatory for a patient with a dislocated elbow to rule out nerve entrapment (common) and circulatory compromise (rare). The brachial and radial pulses and the sensory and motor function of the fingers and wrist should be evaluated.

   6. If these examinations are normal, examine the neck, shoulder and wrist for a source of **referred pain**.

C. Laboratory studies. When clinical suspicion warrants it, aspiration and analysis of joint or bursal fluid should be carried out as described in Chapter 51. The joint fluid should be sent for a cell count, Gram staining, culture, and crystal analysis to rule out infection or crystal-induced arthritis. A bursal white blood cell count of >1000 mm^3 is suggestive of infection or inflammation.

D. Imaging studies

   1. **Radiography.** In the setting of trauma, plain radiographs of the elbow should be obtained to rule out fracture or dislocation. Anteroposterior views of the elbow in the neutral position and in supination, as well as a lateral view with the elbow held at a 90° angle, are most useful.

   2. **Magnetic resonance imaging (MRI)** of the elbow may be useful if a ligament tear is suspected.

E. Nerve conduction studies are used to confirm a diagnosis of nerve entrapment, especially when a more proximal lesion (e.g., radiculopathy, plexopathy) cannot be excluded on the basis of the physical examination.

TREATMENT

A. **Fractures and dislocations**
   1. **Simple, nondisplaced fractures** of the radius or olecranon can be splinted. The patient should see an orthopedic surgeon within 1 week.
   2. **Displaced fractures, dislocations,** or **fractures associated with nerve palsy** require expedient orthopedic consultation.
B. **Ligament tears** are best treated with **rest.** Operative repair is possible but challenging, and is usually attempted only in competitive athletes or in the setting of a complete tear.
C. **Lateral and medial epicondylitis** is treated with **rest** and **nonsteroidal anti-inflammatory drugs (NSAIDs, followed by physical therapy.**
   1. A **counterforce brace** placed circumferentially on the proximal forearm may improve pain by alleviating strain on the affected tendon, but this is no substitute for rest and NSAIDs.
   2. **Injection of corticosteroids** adjacent to, but not in, the tendon sheath may be used if necessary.
   3. **Operative treatment** is rarely required.
D. **Nerve entrapment** is treated initially with **rest** and **elbow padding** during activity. **Operative decompression** and **transposition of the ulnar nerve** is considered when the pain lasts longer than 6 weeks or evidence of motor de-nervation exists.
E. **Olecranon bursitis**
   1. **Infectious bursitis** is treated with repeated **aspiration** of the bursal fluid and oral **antibiotics** (e.g., cephalexin or dicloxacillin, 250–500 mg orally three times daily for 7–10 days).
   2. **Traumatic bursitis** is treated with **aspiration, immobilization,** and **NSAIDs. Local corticosteroid injections** (see Chapter 51) can also be used once infection has been excluded.
      a. Ibuprofen, 400–800 mg orally three times daily for 5–7 days, is often used.
      b. Maintaining the elbow in flexion opposes the two walls of the bursa and aids healing.
F. **Arthritis** is treated according to its cause.
   1. **Septic arthritis.** Patients require **intravenous antibiotic therapy** and **repeat aspirations** of infected joint fluid. Orthopedic referral and arthroscopic decompression may be required if cell counts, pain, and swelling do not resolve in 2–3 days.
   2. **Inflammatory arthritis.** Symptomatic relief most commonly includes **NSAIDs, acetaminophen,** or intra-articular injections of **corticosteroids.**

Reference
Anderson BC. Office Orthopedics for Primary Care: Diagnosis and Treatment, 2nd ed. Philadelphia: WB Saunders, 1999.

56. Wrist and Hand Pain

APPROACH TO THE PATIENT. All patients with wrist injuries must be carefully evaluated because in many cases, the diagnosis of a serious disorder must be made on the basis of clinical, rather than radiographic, evidence.

A. **Patient history.** Important features of the history include when the trauma occurred, the position of the wrist at the time of injury, and a complete recreational and occupational history.

B. **Physical examination**
   1. Assess vascular perfusion, neurologic function, and muscle tone, bulk, and strength of the affected hand.
   2. In examining the wrist, pay particular attention to focal pain, tenderness, or swelling, and any maneuvers that exacerbate the pain. Muscle atrophy is a sign of chronic disease.

C. **Radiographic evaluation.** Anteroposterior and lateral views should be obtained for all patients with wrist injuries. Special views (e.g., oblique or carpal tunnel views) may be obtained as clinical suspicion warrants.

 HOT KEY The space between each carpal bone should be approximately equal to the other carpal-carpal spaces; enlargement of a space may indicate a ligament injury, while closure of a space may indicate a displaced carpal bone.

WRIST FRACTURES. The bones of the wrist are shown in Figure 56-1.

A. **Types of fractures.** Table 56-1 summarizes the clinical features and treatment of each type of wrist fracture.
   1. **Scaphoid fractures** account for 80% of all carpal injuries.
   2. **Triquetrum fractures** are second in incidence to scaphoid fractures.

 HOT KEY Fractures of the hamulus ("hook") of the hamate are often misdiagnosed as sprains.

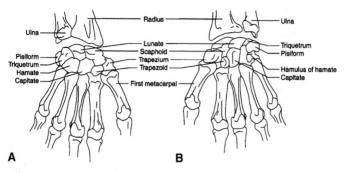

FIGURE 56-1. Bones of the wrist.

B. Treatment
1. **Conservative therapy** entails **rest, immobilization, ice, elevation,** and **nonsteroidal anti-inflammatory drugs (NSAIDs).**
2. **Physical therapy** is an important adjunct to successful rehabilitation.
C. Follow-up and referral. When in doubt, it is always a safe policy to either obtain immediate orthopedic evaluation, or, when this is unavailable, to immobilize the wrist with a splint or short arm cast and have the patient follow up with an orthopedist the following day.

III   LIGAMENT INJURIES. Figure 56-2 shows the ligaments of the wrist and their relation to the scaphoid, lunate, capitate, radius, and ulna. The clinical findings and treatment of ligament injuries of the wrist are summarized in Table 56-2.

A. Scaphoid dislocations usually result from falling on an outstretched and hyperextended wrist.
B. Lunate dislocations occur when the lunate is displaced in a volar direction. **Carpal tunnel syndrome** can be a complication of lunate dislocations.
C. Perilunate (capitate) dislocations are characterized by dorsal displacement of the capitate, while the lunate remains in correct alignment with the radius. Perilunate dislocations are often accompanied by **scaphoid fractures.**
D. Ulnar or radial dislocations result from disruption, degeneration, or tearing of the **triangular fibrocartilage** as a result of chronic mechanical stress or inflammation. The triangular fibrocartilage, a thick band of connective tissue that connects the ulnar-radial articulation to the first carpal row, provides stability during wrist weight-bearing and grasping.

TABLE 56-1. Wrist Fractures					
Bone	Mechanism of Injury	Signs and Symptoms	Radiographic Findings	Complications	Treatment
Scaphoid	Falling on an outstretched and dorsiflexed hand	Tenderness in the anatomical snuffbox	Loss of the scaphoid fat pad stripe	Nonunion and avascular necrosis	Thumb spica cast for 14 days; follow-up with orthopedist in 1–2 weeks
Lunate	Compression; chronic stress	Chronic wrist pain; often patient has no recollection of incipient event	Fragmentation of the lunate with distal collapse	Avascular neurosis of fragment	Conservative therapy; arthroplasty may be necessary for severe fractures
Triquetrum	Falling on an outstretched, dorsiflexed, ulnar-deviated hand	Swelling and tenderness of the dorsal-ulnar wrist	Dorsally displaced fractures on oblique films	Ulnar nerve injury	Short arm cast for 4 weeks; follow-up with an orthopedist in 2 weeks
Trapezium	Direct trauma to the thenar eminence with the hand outstretched and the thumb in adduction	Pain and swelling at the base of the thumb; immobility of the thumb in some cases	Fracture lines seen on routine views	Displacement	Short arm cast for 4 weeks; displaced fractures must be reduced by an orthopedist

Capitate	Falling on an outstretched hand with slight radial deviations or direct trauma to the volar wrist	Pain, tenderness, and swelling in the mid-volar aspect of the wrist	Instability of the "stacked" arrangement of the capitate, lunate, and radius on lateral views (with dislocation)	Avascular necrosis	Short arm cast and immediate follow-up with an orthopedist (fracture usually requires open reduction)
Hamate	Falling on an outstretched hand or direct trauma to the volar wrist	Pain and swelling over the hypothenar eminence; pain increases with gripping or swinging a gripped object	Anteroposterior films may demonstrate loss of the cortical ring	Ulnar neuropathy and flexion tendon rupture	Cast for 4 weeks (only when patient cannot tolerate symptoms) and follow-up with an orthopedist in 2 weeks; surgical excision for fractures of the hamulus ("hook")

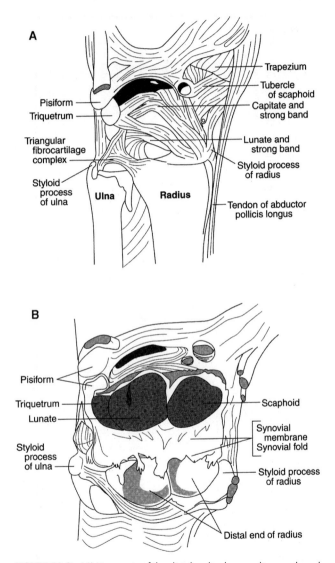

FIGURE 56-2. (A) Ligaments of the distal radioulnar, radiocarpal, and intercarpal joints, anterior view. (B) Dissection of the right radiocarpal joint, opened anteriorly. (Redrawn with permission from Moore KL, Dalley AF. *Clinically Oriented Anatomy,* 5th ed. Baltimore: Lippincott Williams & Wilkins, 2005, p 868.)

TABLE 56-2. Ligamentous Injuries of the Wrist

Dislocation	Signs and Symptoms	Diagnosis	Treatment
Scaphoid	Pain with dorsiflexion and point tenderness at the scaphoid-lunate joint	Anteroposterior films demonstrate a gap between the scaphoid-lunate joint of more than 3 mm	Volar wrist splinting and surgical consultation within 24–72 hours
Lunate or perilunate (capitate)	Minimal swelling and tenderness, chronic wrist pain, patient usually has no recollection of incipient event	Lateral films show disruption of the normal "stacked" alignment of the capitate, lunate, and radius	Volar wrist splinting and surgical consultation within 24–72 hours
Triangular fibrocartilage complex	Pain at the volar-ulnar side of the wrist	Excessive mobility of the wrist on performing the "shuck" test*; wrist arthrography or MRI is definitive	Conservative therapy (i.e., splinting) and follow-up with an orthopedist in 1–2 weeks; physical therapy

MRI = magnetic resonance imaging.
*"Shuck" test: The examiner stabilizes the radial side of the wrist, while moving the ulnar wrist in an anteroposterior direction. Excessive mobility of the wrist implies triangular fibrocartilage disruption, degeneration, or tear.

> **HOT KEY** While some patients with fractures need immediate orthopedic evaluation, all patients with ligament injuries need early referral for surgical therapy. Early recognition and referral is often the difference between successful correction and long-term wrist instability and disability.

IV **Tendon Injuries** of the wrist and hand are summarized in Table 56-3.

A. **DeQuervain's tenosynovitis** is thickening and narrowing of the tendon sheath of the extensor brevis and abductor longus pollicis muscles as a result of repetitive gripping.

B. **Acute calcific tendonitis,** which is caused by hydroxyapatite deposition in the tendons, may mimic DeQuervain's tenosynovitis and is treated similarly.

C. **Intersection syndrome ("squeaker's wrist")** is inflammation surrounding the tendon sheaths as they pass under the first and second compartments of the wrist (peri-tendinitis).

D. **Tendon rupture** rarely occurs in the wrist, except in association with hamulus of the hamate fractures. Fractures of the hamulus can fray the flexor digiti minimi tendon.

E. **Myxoid cyst (synovial cyst, synovial ganglion).** A myxoid cyst is a synovial cyst on the dorsal surface of the wrist or hand. These cysts originate from either a tendon or a joint and usually result from trauma or overuse.

> **HOT KEY** Carpometacarpal osteoarthritis, characterized by dorsal wrist pain that increases with wrist flexion and extension, can present as a tendinitis-like syndrome.

V **Neurovascular Injuries**

A. **Vascular injury** is rare. The usual cause is repetitive trauma at the ulnar aspect of the wrist, leading to the formation of an ulnar artery aneurysm and subsequent thrombosis or spasm of the artery. Baseball catchers, handball players, and waitstaff who repeatedly receive blows to the wrist from swinging kitchen doors are typical patients.

   1. **Clinical findings.** Symptoms are related to arterial insufficiency (e.g., cold digits, mottling, pain, paresthesias). A mass (i.e., the aneurysm) may be palpable.

   2. **Diagnosis.** Arteriography is the diagnostic test of choice.

TABLE 56-3. Tendon Disorders of the Wrist

Disorder	Signs and Symptoms	Diagnosis	Treatment
DeQuervain's tenosynovitis	Pain in the extensor and abductor tendons of the thumb	Pain on Finkelstein's test*	Conservative therapy with splinting, NSAIDs, and avoidance of repetitive gripping motions; refractory cases may require injection of lidocaine and steroids at the radial styloid
Intersection syndrome	Pain and crepitus with gripping and flexion of the wrist	(Pain is more proximal than that seen with DeQuervain's tenosynovitis); considerable dorsal swelling	Conservative therapy
Tendon rupture	Pain and weakness of the involved tendon	History of trauma and weakness on exam	Splinting and orthopedic referral within 24–72 hours
Myxoid cyst	Firm cyst that is usually not tender on the dorsal surface of the wrist; patient may report mild pain over the dorsal ganglion	Jelly-like material on aspiration	Aspiration with a large-bore needle followed by steroid injection; surgical excision usually required to prevent recurrence

NSAIDs = nonsteroidal anti-inflammatory drugs.
*Finkelstein's test: Examiner folds the patient's thumb onto his palm and deviates the wrist in an ulnar direction.

    3. Treatment. Immediate referral to a vascular surgeon is indicated.

B. Carpal tunnel syndrome (median neuropathy) is discussed in Chapter 67.

C. Ulnar nerve entrapment is rare and is usually seen in association with sports or occupational activities that require power gripping with weight-loading on the hypothenar eminence (e.g., power lifting, gripping a baseball bat).

    1. Clinical findings. Paresthesias of the fourth and fifth digits are usually seen. Absence of paresthesias on the dorsal ulnar aspect of the hand is common. Interosseous wasting may be seen in long-standing injury.

    2. Diagnosis. The diagnosis is usually made clinically. Radiographs are needed for patients who have a history of trauma to exclude hamate fracture or dislocation.

    3. Treatment entails wrist padding. Surgical decompression is usually recommended because steroid injections are precluded and splinting is usually ineffective.

Reference

Daniels JM, Zook EG, Lynch JM. Hand and wrist injuries: Part I. Nonemergent evaluation. *Am Fam Phys* 2004;69(8):1941–1948.

57. Osteoarthritis (Degenerative Joint Disease)

I **INTRODUCTION.** Osteoarthritis (OA) was sometimes termed degenerative joint disease (DJD) because it was thought to be a normal result of aging. However, OA is a consequence of multiple factors, including joint integrity, genetics, local inflammation, mechanical forces, cellular and biochemical processes.

A. OA may be either **monoarticular** or **polyarticular.** It has a predilection for joints with maximal load. The most frequently affected joints include the:
   1. **Distal interphalangeal (DIP) joints**
   2. **Proximal interphalangeal (PIP) joints**
   3. **Thumb** [i.e., the carpometacarpal (CMC) joints]
   4. **Knee**
   5. **Hip**
   6. **Spine**

> **HOT KEY**
>
> If a patient has OA in the hand, they are at increased risk of OA elsewhere.

B. OA may be either **primary (idiopathic)** or **secondary** (i.e., occurring in damaged or abnormal joints).**Idiopathic OA** may be **localized** or **generalized** (>3 joints). Although typically non-inflammatory, there is a hereditary destructive variant. **Predisposing factors for OA** include:
   1. Increasing age
   2. Female gender
   3. Obesity (especially at 18 years of age)
   4. Major joint trauma
   5. Repetitive joint stress (except running)
   6. Chronic inflammatory arthritis (calcium pyrophosphate deposition disease [CPPD], Gout, Rheumatoid Arthritis [RA], Spondyloarthritis [SpA])
   7. Congenital and developmental joint defects
   8. Metabolic and endocrine disorders (e.g., hemochromatosis, Wilson's disease, ochronosis, acromegaly, diabetes mellitus, hyperparathyroidism, hypothyroidism, Paget's disease)

9. Type II collagen mutations
10. Nutritional disorders (e.g., Kashin-Beck disease)

HOT **KEY**

Elbow, wrist and ankle involvement are rare in idiopathic OA. If these joints are involved, look for secondary causes of OA.

II   DIFFERENTIAL DIAGNOSIS. Other causes of monoarticular and polyarticular arthritis must be ruled out, (see Chapters 59 and 60) including:

A. **Crystal-induced arthritides** (e.g., gout, CPPD)
B. **Joint infection** (bacterial, spirochetal, or viral)
C. **Inflammatory arthritides** (i.e., RA, SpA)
D. **Joint trauma**
E. **Neoplasia**

HOT **KEY**

In a patient who has "inflammatory OA," suspect crystal-induced arthritis on OA.

III   APPROACH TO THE PATIENT. The patient history and physical examination findings establish the diagnosis.

A. **Patient history.** Patients over the age of 40 may develop gradual onset of joint **pain** exacerbated by activity and relieved by rest. Morning **stiffness** may accompany pain, but typically resolves within 30 minutes of awakening.
B. **Physical examination**
   1. Local findings include **decreased range of motion, crepitus, small effusions, minimal local warmth and tenderness,** and **bony enlargement.**
   2. **Heberden's nodes** and **Bouchard's nodes** are hard, nontender nodules that represent bony outgrowths of the DIP joints and PIP joints, respectively.

HOT **KEY**

Nodal OA is associated with repetitive activity in patients with genetic predisposition and is 10 times more likely in women than in men.

C. **Radiographic studies.** Plain films may demonstrate joint space narrowing, osteophytes, subchondral bone sclerosis, and cysts. Magnetic resonance imaging (MRI) might show bone marrow edema.

D. **Laboratory studies** should be sent (including erythrocyte sedimentation rate and rheumatoid factor) although they are usually unremarkable but may help identify the underlying cause in patients with secondary OA. Synovial fluid analysis typically reveals a white blood cell (WBC) count of less than 2000/mm^3 with a mononuclear predominance (see Table 59-1).

IV TREATMENT. No treatment has been shown to slow the progression of OA. Management strategies focus on controlling pain and minimizing disability.

A. **Pharmacologic therapies**
   1. **Acetaminophen** is the drug of choice. Some studies have found it to be less efficacious than nonsteroidal antiinflammatories (NSAIDs) at controlling pain.
   2. **NSAIDs** should be used with caution; these agents may cause peptic ulcer disease, renal insufficiency, bleeding diatheses, and may be associated with an increase in cardiovascular events.
   3. **Opiates** should be used only in acute exacerbations or when other treatments have failed or are contraindicated.
   4. **Corticosteroid injections** provide temporary relief but may result in articular cartilage breakdown. Injections should generally not be given more than four times per year (per joint), although there is no data to support that more is dangerous.
   5. **Topical Capsaicin and NSAIDs** might be benificial in patients who cannot tolerate oral agents.
   6. **Hyaluronic acid joint injection** has mixed efficacy with no benefit over NSAIDs.
   7. **Glucosamine and Chondroitin sulfate** have mixed efficacy secondary to poor studies. A recent large trial found no benefit except in a subgroup of patients with more severe disease.

B. **Nonpharmacologic therapies**
   1. **Reassurance, education** and **social support** has been associated with a decrease in pain.
   2. **Weight loss** or the use of a **cane, crutches,** or a **walker** can help to reduce the load on the joint. It has been shown that a 10 pound weight loss over 10 years decreases the odds of developing knee OA by 50 percent.
   3. **Orthoses** or **braces** can be used to correct body malalignment. Lateral wedge insoles have proven benefit.

4. **Rest** is recommended only for short periods of time (12 to 24 hours) for acute inflammation and/or pain after which passive joint motion and exercise should resume.

5. **Physical therapy.** Moderate activity is indicated to maintain muscle strength and range of motion. Evidence suggests improvement in clinical outcomes with therapy.

C. **Surgical therapies**

1. **Knee arthroscopy** has not been shown to have benefit.

2. **Joint arthroplasty** is indicated for patients with debilitating disease that is refractory to medical therapy. Uncontrolled pain is the primary indication for surgery.

3. **Spinal laminectomy, fusion,** or **both** is indicated for patients with intractable pain resulting from OA and spinal stenosis.

V FOLLOW-UP AND REFERRAL

A. All patients should be referred to an occupational and physical therapist for assistance in developing an exercise regimen.

B. Patients with debilitating disease should be referred to an orthopedic surgeon or neurosurgeon.

Reference
www.rheumatology.org/publications/guidelines/oa-mgmt.asp

58. Gout

I **INTRODUCTION.** Gout is a disease of disordered purine metabolism that results in elevation of the serum uric acid level and attacks of arthritis. The clinical presentation ranges from occasional attacks of monoarticular arthritis to a debilitating chronic polyarticular arthritis accompanied by erosive bony changes.

A. Pathogenesis. Gout stems from the episodic or constant elevation of the serum uric acid to a level that exceeds 7.0 mg/dl. At this concentration, the serum is saturated with monosodium urate, and the excess is deposited in both articular and extra-articular tissue. Deposition of urate in the tissues leads to inflammation.

HOT **KEY** Pseudogout [calcium pyrophosphate deposition disease (CPPD)] is often difficult to distinguish from gout clinically. Pseudogout tends to be accompanied by chondrocalcinosis that is visible radiographically and patients usually have normal uric acid levels.

B. Epidemiology. Gout characteristically affects men older than 30 years and women after menopause. The mean age of onset in men is 48 years.

II **CLINICAL MANIFESTATIONS OF GOUT**

A. Articular manifestations

1. **Arthritis.** Typically, the involved joint is **swollen, warm, erythematous,** and **extremely tender.** The onset of symptoms is **acute,** usually evolving over 24–48 hours. If untreated, acute attacks usually resolve within days to weeks.

   a. The arthritis is typically **monoarticular,** or **oligo-articular** and **asymmetric.**

      (1) The **first metatarsophalangeal (MTP) joint of the foot** is the most common site for first attacks. Other sites commonly involved include the **instep of the foot,** the **ankle,** and the **knee.**

      (2) If untreated, the disease may result in an asymmetric arthritis with shortened pain-free periods and

involvement of more joints, including those of the upper extremities.

   b. Precipitants include trauma, surgery, exposure to cold, infection, medications (incuding diuretic use and agents that affect uric acid levels), and alcohol consumption.

HOT

75% of patients experience a recurrent attack within 2 years of the initial attack.

KEY

---

   2. Tophaceous gout is characterized by the development of yellowish-white nodular collections of urate crystals in the subcutaneous tissue, bone, cartilage, and joints.
      a. The tophi are usually painless, but lead to erosive destruction of cartilage and bone.
      b. Tophaceous gout usually develops approximately 10 years after the initial attack; however, some patients may present initially with tophi.
B. Renal manifestations
   1. Nephrolithiasis. Radiolucent uric acid kidney stones may precede gouty arthritis. Uric acid stones may serve as a nidus for other types of kidney stones.
   2. Uric acid nephropathy is reversible acute renal failure that is caused by the precipitation of crystals in the renal tubules and collecting ducts. Uric acid nephropathy often occurs when a dramatic increase in uric acid production (e.g., as a result of tumor lysis in patients receiving chemotherapy for leukemia) elevates the urinary uric acid levels.
   3. Urate nephropathy is chronic renal insufficiency secondary to interstitial deposits of uric acid. Urate nephropathy occurs in the setting of severe gout or with comorbid conditions.

III **CAUSES OF GOUT.** Gout results from **hyperuricemia,** which can be caused by decreased urate excretion or increased urate production.

A. Decreased urate excretion is the cause of hyperuricemia in **90% of patients.** Causes include renal disease, alcohol, and drugs (e.g., low-dose salicylates, diuretics). However, in most patients, the cause of decreased urate excretion is unclear.
B. Urate overproduction. Causes include inborn errors of metabolism (e.g., Lesch-Nyhan syndrome), myelo- and lymphoproliferative diseases, hemolysis, alcohol, psoriasis, obesity, and therapy with chemotherapeutic agents.

IV APPROACH TO THE PATIENT

A. Patient history and **physical examination findings** are described in II A 1.

B. Laboratory studies

1. **Serum uric acid level.** Although approximately 95% of patients have a serum uric acid level of more than 7.5 mg/dl when serial measurements are taken during an attack, as many as 25% of patients have normal uric acid levels on a single measurement. Note that hyperuricemia alone is not sufficient for the diagnosis.

2. **Joint fluid analysis.** In a patient with acute arthritis, joint fluid analysis is the most reliable way of diagnosing gout and excluding other diagnoses. During acute attacks, joint aspiration has a sensitivity of approximately 85%.

   a. The fluid sample should be sent for crystal analysis, Gram stain and culture, and a total leukocyte count with differential. (See Table 59-1.)

   b. In patients with gout, the fluid is **predominantly neutrophilic** with at least some **intracellular monosodium urate crystals.** The crystals are **needle-shaped** with **negative birefringence** under polarized microscopy (i.e., they appear yellow when aligned parallel to the plane of polarized light and blue when perpendicular to it).

HOT KEY

Crystals in **p**seudogout appear rhomboid and have **p**ositive birefringence (i.e., the crystals parallel to the light appear blue and those perpendicular to it appear yellow.)

3. **Tophi aspiration.** A wet mount may reveal clusters of urate crystals.

4. **Urinalysis.** A 24-hour urine collection can be used to classify patients as urate overproducers or underexcreters. Overproducers will demonstrate uric acid excretion of more than 800 mg/day on a regular diet, whereas underexcreters will show uric acid excretion of less than 800 mg/day on a regular diet.

C. Radiographic studies. Radiographs are usually normal early in the disease. Later, the bone has "punched out" erosions with sclerotic borders and an overhanging margin. The articular surface tends to be relatively well preserved.

V TREATMENT

A. Asymptomatic hyperuricemia does not warrant therapy because most of these patients never develop gout.

B. Acute gouty arthritis

1. Bed rest and **warm soaks** provide symptomatic treatment.

2. Pharmacologic therapy

a. Nonsteroidal anti-inflammatory drugs (NSAIDs) are the drugs of choice for the treatment of acute gouty arthritis. Use with caution in patients with chronic kidney disease and gastrointestinal risk. The NSAID should be prescribed at the highest approved dose until inflammation has resolved (e.g., indomethacin, 25–50 mg orally every 8 hours). It is most effective when prescribed early.

HOT

▶

KEY

Aspirin is usually avoided because salicylates cause renal uric acid retention at low doses and uricosuria at higher doses.

---

b. Colchicine can be used for patients who cannot tolerate NSAIDs.

(1) To be effective, colchicine must be taken early during an attack.

(2) The dose is 0.6 mg orally every hour until symptoms resolve, gastrointestinal side effects occur, or a total dose of 6 mg has been administered. (Gastrointestinal side effects are dose-limiting in as many as 80% of patients.)

c. Glucocorticoids

(1) Intra-articular corticosteroid injection (e.g., **triamcinolone,** 10–40 mg, depending on the size of the joint) is a alternative to NSAID and colchicine therapy for patients with monoarticular arthritis who are intolerant of the alternatives.

(2) Systemic corticosteroid therapy (e.g., **prednisone** starting at 30 to 50 mg orally for 1 to 2 days and tapered over 7–10 days) is an alternative for patients with polyarticular involvement who are not good candidates for NSAID or colchicine therapy.

C. Intercritical gout (i.e., between acute attacks)

1. Uric acid-lowering therapy is indicated for those with hyperuricemia and recurrent attacks of arthritis, chronic tophaceous gout, or nephropathy. **The goal is to lower the serum uric acid level to less than 6.0 mg/dl.**

a. Lifestyle modifications include **weight loss, decreased alcohol consumption,** and **avoidance of diuretics** and **purine-rich foods** (e.g., meat, sea-food, legumes).

b. Pharmacologic therapy should be started only after all signs of an acute attack have resolved. The choice of drugs may be made empirically or based on the results of a 24-hour urine collection.

  (1) Allopurinol is a xanthine oxidase inhibitor that decreases the production of uric acid.

  (a) Indications. Allopurinol is the drug of choice for patients who meet any of the following conditions:

  (i) Urate overproduction

  (ii) Chronic tophaceous gout

  (iii) Renal disease with a serum creatinine level that exceeds 2.0 mg/dl or a creatinine clearance of less than 80 ml/min

  (iv) History of urinary stones

  (b) Dose. The initial dose is 100 mg daily for 7 days; this dose is then titrated up to 300 mg every day.

  (i) The dose should be limited to 100 mg per day for those with creatinine clearance less than 40 ml/min and 200 mg per day for those with a creatinine clearance of 60–80 ml/min.

  (ii) Concomitant use of 6-mercaptopurine or azathioprine warrants a reduction of the dose of those drugs to 25% of the usual dose.

  (c) Side effects. If a patient who requires allopurinol develops a mild rash, desensitization is a possibility. However, desensitization is not warranted for those with severe reactions, such as exfoliative dermatitis, hepatitis, or interstitial nephritis.

  (2) Febuxostat, a novel nonpurine selective inhibitor of xanthine oxidase that has been found to effectively reduce the levels of serum uric acid. At this time, its FDA approval is pending.

  (3) Rasburicase, a recombinant uricase decreases uric acid levels by degrading uric acid to allantoin. At this time, it is indicated in the setting of chemotherapy for hyperuricemia prophylaxis.

  (4) Uricosuric agents can be used for patients with evidence of decreased uric acid excretion, lack of urinary stones, and relatively normal renal function (i.e., a serum creatinine level of less than 2 mg/dl).

  (a) Probenecid can be given at an initial dose of 250 mg orally twice daily; the dose can be increased as needed up to a maximum dose of 2.0 g per day.

    (b) Sulfinpyrazone can be given at an initial dose of 50 mg orally twice daily; the dose can be increased to a maximum of 300– 400 mg per day in 3–4 divided doses.

  2. **Prophylaxis against recurrent attacks** is indicated for at least 6 months after initiating uric acid-lowering therapy.

    a. Colchicine is the drug of choice. The usual dose is 0.6 mg orally twice daily. In the setting of renal insufficiency, 0.6 mg orally once daily should be used.

    b. NSAIDS may also be used for prophylaxis.

    c. Low dose **prednisone** is an alternative when NSAIDs and colchicine are contraindicated.

References

Becker MA, Schumacher HR Jr, Wortmann RL, et al. Febuxostat compared with allopurinol in patients with hyperuricemia and gout. *N Engl J Med* 2005;353:2450–2461.

Terkeltaub RA. Clinical practice. Gout. *N Engl J Med* 2003; 349:1647.

59. Monoarticular Arthritis

I INTRODUCTION. When a patient presents with joint complaints, the list of possible causes seems enormous. However, the number of possibilities can be lowered considerably by answering the following questions:

A. Is the arthritis monoarticular or polyarticular?
B. Which joints are involved? For example:
    1. Distal interphalangeal (DIP) joint involvement is often attributable to osteoarthritis (OA) or psoriatic arthritis.

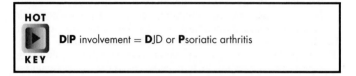

> **HOT KEY**
>
> **DIP** involvement = **D**JD or **P**soriatic arthritis

    2. Wrist involvement is often attributable to rheumatoid arthritis.
    3. First metatarsophalangeal (MTP) joint inflammation can be caused by gout, rheumatoid arthritis (RA) or OA.

II CAUSES OF MONOARTICULAR ARTHRITIS. It is important to diagnose a monoarticular arthritis quickly in order to prevent permanent joint damage and, in some cases, sepsis. The mnemonic "If I Make The Diagnosis, No More Harm" will help you recall the most important causes of monoarticular arthritis.

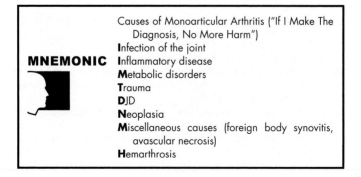

MNEMONIC

Causes of Monoarticular Arthritis ("If I Make The Diagnosis, No More Harm")
Infection of the joint
Inflammatory disease
Metabolic disorders
Trauma
DJD
Neoplasia
Miscellaneous causes (foreign body synovitis, avascular necrosis)
Hemarthrosis

A. **Infection of the joint** must be considered first because it is potentially life-threatening. Commonly implicated organisms include *Streptococcus, Staphylococcus* and *Neisseria gonorrhoeae.* **Less common but important causes include Lyme disease, syphilis, mycobacterial and fungal infection.**

B. **Inflammatory disorders** (e.g., **psoriatic arthritis, RA, reactive arthritis,** and other **systemic lupus erythematosus [SLE]).** Although these diseases usually are oligo or poly-articular (see Chapter 60), they may begin as a monoarticular swelling and thus have to be considered after other causes have been ruled out. Sarcoidosis and hepatitis C associated arthropathy should be considered.

C. **Metabolic disorders** include **gout** and **pseudogout** (calcium pyrophosphate deposition disease, CPPD)]. These disorders are discussed in Chapter 58.

D. **Trauma** to a joint (e.g., torn ligament, bone fracture) can lead to hemarthrosis or internal joint derangement. The patient should always be asked about a history of trauma to the affected joint.

E. **OA** can cause monoarticular or polyarticular arthritis.

F. **Neoplasia** is a rare cause of monoarticular swelling but should be considered. Examples include **osteoid osteoma** and **pigmented villonodular synovitis.**

G. **Miscellaneous causes** include **foreign body synovitis** and **avascular necrosis.**

H. **Hemarthrosis.** Bleeding into a joint, when not related to trauma, is usually associated with **clotting disorders** (e.g., hemophilia) or **anticoagulant therapy.**

III APPROACH TO THE PATIENT

A. **Patient history**
   1. A history of joint complaints that resolve spontaneously might imply a crystal-induced or other noninfectious etiology. Remember, infections are more likely to occur in a damaged joint.
   2. Identifying sexual risk factors is important, especially in young patients.
   3. Does the patient use intravenous drugs?
   4. Does the patient have a prosthetic joint?

B. **Physical examination.** The physical examination is useful for:
   1. Determining which joints are involved. The knee is the most commonly infected joint.
   2. Excluding periarticular processes that may mimic arthritis (e.g., cellulitis, bursitis, tendinitis)
   3. Discerning signs that suggest specific causes (e.g., skin evidence of psoriasis)
   4. Range of motion should be restricted in an infected joint.

C. Other diagnostic modalities
1. **Plain radiographs** of the affected joint are sometimes helpful (e.g., when OA, pseudogout, or fracture is the cause of the joint pain), but generally, radiographs are not useful.
2. **Arthrocentesis** and **joint fluid analysis** is the **mainstay of diagnosis** and should be performed in most patients, especially if infection is a consideration (Table 59-1).

HOT

KEY

Because the synovial fluid white blood cell count (WBC) may be low early in the disease course, always consider infection, regardless of the joint fluid analysis results. Re-aspiration of the joint after 24 hours is indicated if infection is suspected and the initial joint fluid analysis is inconclusive.

---

3. **Synovial biopsy** and **arthroscopy** should be considered if the diagnosis is still unclear.

IV TREATMENT DEPENDS ON THE UNDERLYING DISEASE

A. Joint infection
1. **Arthrocentesis.** Serial aspirations should be obtained for 5–7 days to decrease pain, minimize the risk of joint damage, and minimize the risk of failed antibiotic treatment.
2. **Empiric antibiotic therapy** should be directed against the most common pathogens. Gram stain and culture are used to guide further treatment.
   a. If the Gram stain is negative, **ceftriaxone** (plus gentamycin if pseudomonus is suspected).
   b. If the Gram stain reveals Gram-positive cocci, **cefazolin (plus vancomycin for nursing home patients).**
3. **Surgical intervention** is required for nonresolving infections to ensure adequate drainage of the infected joint or if the patient refuses serial taps.

B. Gout. The treatment of gout is discussed in Chapter 58 V.
C. Inflammatory disorders
1. **RA.** The treatment of RA is discussed in Chapter 60 IV A.
2. **Spondyloarthritis (SpA).** The treatment of SpA is discussed in Chapter 60 IV C.
D. OA. The treatment of OA is discussed in Chapter 57 III.

V FOLLOW-UP AND REFERRAL

A. Referral to a **rheumatologist** is indicated when the diagnosis remains in question despite initial testing.

TABLE 59-1. Joint Fluid Analysis*

	Normal	Noninflammatory	Inflammatory	Septic
WBCs/mm^3	<200	200–10,000	10,000–100,000	>100,000
%PMN	<25%	<25%	50%–90%	50%–100%
Possible causes	...	DJD, trauma, aseptic necrosis	Collagen-vascular diseases, crystal-induced disease, TB, mycotic infections	Pyogenic bacterial infections

DJD = degenerative joint disease; PMNs = polymorphonuclear neutrophils; TB = tuberculosis; WBCs = white blood cells.
*Results in different diseases may be variable.

B. Referral to an **orthopedic surgeon** is indicated for patients with infection that is not responsive to needle aspiration and therapy with appropriate antibiotics.

References

Garcia-De La Torre I. Advances in the management of septic arthritis. *Rheum Dis Clin North Am* 2003;29:61–75.

Kumar S. Managing acute monoarthritis in primary care practice. *J Musculoskel Med* 2004;21:465–472.

60. Oligoarticular and Polyarticular Arthritis

I **INTRODUCTION.** In order to organize the many causes of polyarticular arthritis, classify them as belonging to one of four main categories: classic seropositive, classic seronegative, atypical seronegative or miscellaneous (Table 60-1).

A. Autoimmune—classic seropositive. These disorders are characterized by **symmetric swelling** and the presence of **autoantibodies.**

B. Autoimmune—classic seronegative. Usually HLA B27 associated oligo or polyarticular arthritis involving peripheral joints, entheses and/or the axial joints. They are characterized by the **early onset of disease** (usually before the age of 40 years), and the **absence of autoantibodies** (hence the term "seronegative").

C. Atypical Seronegative. The absence of **autoantibodies** in the presence of a classic disease. (i.e. seronegative rheumatoid arthritis (RA) meeting classification criteria in the absence of **rheumatoid factor**).

D. Miscellaneous causes. Many other illnesses present with polyarthritis. These can easily be remembered in the following manner: one gonorrheal, two spirochetal, three viral, four infiltrative, and five "other."

II **CAUSES OF POLYARTICULAR ARTHRITIS**

A. Autoimmune—classic seropositive
   1. **RA** is a chronic systemic inflammatory disease primarily involving the synovial membranes of multiple joints.
      a. Epidemiology. The disease affects women twice as often as men, and the usual age at the time of onset is 20–40 years.
      b. Clinical manifestations. In order to diagnose RA, four of seven diagnostic criteria must be present (i.e., You must **AMASS** 4 of 7 to **RX** a patient with RA):

TABLE 60-1. Common Causes of Polyarticular Arthritis

Autoimmune—classic seropositive
Rheumatoid arthritis
Systemic lupus erythematosus (SLE)
Systemic sclerosis
Polymyositis
Overlap syndrome

Autoimmune—classic seronegative
Ankylosing spondylitis
Psoriatic arthritis
Reactive arthritis
Arthritis related to enteric disorders (e.g., inflammatory bowel disease, Whipple's disease, enteric infection)

Miscellaneous
1. Gonorrheal—disseminated gonococcal infection
2. Spirochetal—Lyme disease, secondary syphilis
3. Viral—HIV, hepatitis B, parvovirus
4. Infiltrative-sarcoidosis, amyloidosis, hemochromatosis, tophaceous gout
5. Other—degenerative joint disease (DJD), Still's disease, inflammatory bowel disease, rheumatic fever, vasculitis

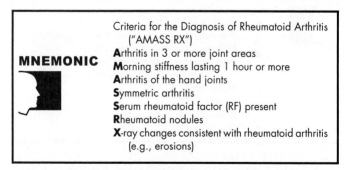

MNEMONIC

Criteria for the Diagnosis of Rheumatoid Arthritis ("AMASS RX")
Arthritis in 3 or more joint areas
Morning stiffness lasting 1 hour or more
Arthritis of the hand joints
Symmetric arthritis
Serum rheumatoid factor (RF) present
Rheumatoid nodules
X-ray changes consistent with rheumatoid arthritis (e.g., erosions)

(1) **Major symptoms** include malaise, fever, morning stiffness, and progressive symmetric swelling of the small joints. The onset of symptoms is insidious.

(2) **Extra-articular findings** may include subcutaneous nodules, serositis, lymphadenopathy, and rarely splenomegaly.

(3) **Radiographic findings** classically include periarticular osteopenia, joint erosions, and, occasionally, subluxation of the joints and upper cervical spine.

(4) Laboratory findings. Eighty-five percent of patients are **RF-positive. Anti-cyclic citrullinated peptide (CCP) Antibodies** are more specific for RA and are associated with erosive disease.

2. **Systemic lupus erythematosus (SLE)** is a multisystemic autoimmune disorder.

   a. **Epidemiology.** Eighty-five percent of all patients are women 20–40 years of age.

   b. **Clinical manifestations.** The criteria for diagnosis are helpful to remember because they include the major clinical manifestations of the disease. The presence of 4 of the 11 criteria makes the diagnosis. In our medical school, in order to pass, we needed to know the 11 criteria for SLE; therefore, we were all in "P-MOAD"—7 Ps and M O A D. The first two Ps are positive lab tests; the next five Ps are arranged from head to toe. Let's go through it:

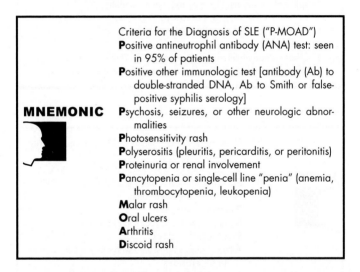

MNEMONIC	Criteria for the Diagnosis of SLE ("P-MOAD")
	Positive antineutrophil antibody (ANA) test: seen in 95% of patients
	Positive other immunologic test [antibody (Ab) to double-stranded DNA, Ab to Smith or false-positive syphilis serology]
	Psychosis, seizures, or other neurologic abnormalities
	Photosensitivity rash
	Polyserositis (pleuritis, pericarditis, or peritonitis)
	Proteinuria or renal involvement
	Pancytopenia or single-cell line "penia" (anemia, thrombocytopenia, leukopenia)
	Malar rash
	Oral ulcers
	Arthritis
	Discoid rash

3. **Systemic sclerosis (scleroderma)** is characterized by fibrosis of the skin and internal organs leading to dysphagia, pulmonary fibrosis, and cardiac and renal disease.

   a. **Clinical manifestations**

   (1) **Symptoms.** Raynaud's disease (seen in 90% of patients) and arthralgias are usually early symptoms.

   (2) **Laboratory findings.** Antibodies that are—specific for scleroderma include anti-topoisomerase (Scl-70), anti-nucleolar antibody, and anti-centromere antibody.

    b. There are **two forms** of systemic sclerosis.

        (1) Diffuse systemic sclerosis affects 20% of patients.

        (2) Limited systemic sclerosis (CREST syndrome). CREST syndrome is the syndrome of **c**alcinosis, **R**aynaud's phenomenon, **e**sophageal motility dysfunction, **s**clerodactyly, and **t**elangiectasia. Those with CREST syndrome have a decreased risk of renal involvement, a higher risk of pulmonary hypertension, increased incidence of anti-centromere antibodies, and a better prognosis.

B. Autoimmune—classic seronegative

The spondyloarthritides (SpAs) are a group of diseases that are HLA B27 associated. There are differentiated forms delineated here and undifferentiated forms. Undifferentiated SpA is the symptoms of inflammatory back pain and or acute anterior uveitis and or enthesitis without radiographic findings of sacroiliitis on plain films.

    1. Ankylosing spondylitis (AS) is the prototype SpA. It is characterized by the gradual onset of inflammatory back pain usually in those younger than 40 years, progressive limitation of anterior flexion of the lumbar spine, and radiographic evidence of sacroiliitis. HLA-B27 is present in approximately 90% of patients who have AS. The disease affects men two to three times as often as women.

    2. Psoriatic arthritis, occurring in as many as 20% of patients with psoriasis, is characterized by a destructive arthritis, often of the distal interphalangeal (DIP) joints, dactylitis, nail pitting, and onycholysis.

    3. Reactive arthritis is classically characterized by the clinical triad of **conjunctivitis, urethritis,** and **arthritis**— the patient cannot "see, pee, or bend at the knees." There is often a preceding diarrheal illness or sexually tramsmitted infection and most cases resolve spontaneously.

    4. Inflammatory bowel disease is associated with polyarthritis. Ten to twenty percent of patients with Crohn's disease or ulcerative colitis develop arthritis. Articular symptoms tend to flare concomitantly with the activity of the bowel disease. All patients in the category of SpA have the potential to develop inflammatory back pain and sacroiliitis and therefore AS. The probability increases when HLA B27 is positive.

C. Miscellaneous causes

    1. Gonorrheal infection. Disseminated gonococcal infection (caused by *Neisseria gonorrhoeae*) may result in migratory polyarthralgias of the large joints, tenosynovitis, fever, and/or a pustular rash.

    2. Spirochetal infection

    a. Lyme disease (caused by *Borrelia burgdorferi*) is charac-
terized by flu-like symptoms, erythema migrans, neurologic problems (e.g., facial nerve palsy, meningitis), cardiac
disease, and/or a chronic or recurrent large joint arthritis.

    b. Secondary syphilis can involve almost any part of the body,
including the joints.

3. Viral infection. The three common viral causes of polyarticular arthritis include **HIV, hepatitis virus (B and C),** and **parvovirus.**

4. Infiltrative disorders include **sarcoidosis, amyloidosis, hemochromatosis,** and **tophaceous gout;** biopsy of the joint or other
affected organs is usually necessary to make the diagnosis.

5. Other disorders

    a. Osteoarthritis (OA) may be the most common cause of
polyarticular arthritis and is discussed in detail in Chapter 57.

    b. Still's disease is a form of juvenile idiopathic arthritis that
also affects adults. It is characterized by spiking fevers,
arthritis, and an evanescent, salmon-colored rash.

    c. Rheumatic fever is a delayed sequela of pharyngitis caused
by a group A streptococcus, although rarely seen now.
Classic clinical manifestations include a migratory polyarthritis, fever, carditis, chorea, and subcutaneous nodules.

    d. Vasculitis is discussed in Chapter 87.

III **APPROACH TO THE PATIENT.** Because polyarticular arthritis
has many causes, clinical, laboratory, and radiographic features are used to establish a diagnosis.

A. Patient history

    1. A history of symmetric large- and small-joint arthritis with
morning stiffness suggests autoimmune arthritis.

    2. Asymmetric, additive, or migratory arthralgias are suggestive
of an infectious or crystal-induced arthritis.

    3. A history of exposure to ticks or sexually transmitted disease,
or the presence of a rash or fever increases the likelihood of
infectious arthritis.

B. Physical examination. The physical examination is useful for:

    1. Determining which joints are involved

    2. Evaluating extra-articular manifestations of disease (e.g.,
oral ulcers, alopecia, and rash may suggest SLE; calcinosis,
sclerodactyly, and telangiectasias may suggest CREST syndrome)

C. Laboratory studies
1. Serologic studies
   a. RF, ANA, Antibody to double-stranded DNA, and extractable nuclear antibodies [i.e., Smith, Ro, La, anti-centromere, anti-histone, or anti-ribonuclear protein (anti-RNB)] are appropriate when a symmetric polyarthritis is present and clinical findings suggest RA or SLE.

   b. Anti-topoisomerase (Scl-70), anti-nucleolar, and anti-centromere antibody tests are indicated if scleroderma or CREST is the suspected diagnosis.

   c. Antibodies to *Borrelia burgdorferi* and the Venereal Disease Research Laboratory (VDRL) test can be used to evaluate for Lyme disease and syphilis, respectively.

HOT KEY

Patients with SLE may have false-positive VDRL test results.

2. Genetic testing for HLA-B27.
Eighty to ninety percent of patients with AS are HLA-B27 positive. However, genetic testing is not generally helpful because 10% of people of western European descent without AS test positive.

 IV TREATMENT depends on the underlying disease.

A. Autoimmune—classic seropositive
1. Rheumatoid arthritis
   a. Nonsteroidal anti-inflammatory drugs (NSAIDs) are a mainstay of treatment.

   b. Disease modifying anti-rheumatic drugs (DMARDs) are indicated for active synovitis or erosive disease (e.g., prednisone, hydroxychloroquine, sulfasalazine, methotrexate, azathioprine, leflunomide, Rituxumab, CTLA 4-Ig, and tumor necrosis factor [TNF] alpha blockers) alter autoimmunity, thereby slowing disease progression. These agents should be given only after consultation with a rheumatologist.

2. SLE.
Like rheumatoid arthritis, SLE is treated with NSAIDs and immunosuppressive agents (e.g., hydroxychloroquine, azathioprine, mycophenolate mofetil, cyclophosphamide).

Immunosuppressive agents should only be prescribed in consultation with a rheumatologist.

3. **Systemic sclerosis.** Because the disease is refractory to most immunosuppressive therapies, treatment is aimed at relieving symptoms.

    a. D-Penicillamine, glucocorticoids, or colchicine have been used to treat severe cases.

    b. Treatment should be tailored to the patient. Consultation with a rheumatologist is recommended.

B. Autoimmune—classic seronegative

  1. Ankylosing spondylitis

    a. Physical therapy is indicated to preserve the patient's range of motion.

    b. NSAIDs (e.g., indomethacin) are used for pain relief, but are not traditionally thought of as disease modifying.

    c. Sulfasalazine may be beneficial when there is peripheral joint involvement, but has no efficacy for axial disease. Initially, 500 mg of sulfasalazine may be given daily. The dose can be increased in 500-mg increments each week until the patient's symptoms improve or a maximum dose of 3 g (divided into two or three doses daily) is reached. A complete blood count should be checked after initiating therapy and frequently thereafter, as sulfasalazine has been associated with cytopenias.

    d. TNF and α blockers are extremely efficacious in treating AS. This class of drugs is reserved for patients with moderate to severe disease activity. Patients are required to have a negative tuberculin skin test prior to starting therapy or be treated with isoniazid for 6 to 9 months. There is an increased risk of tuberculosis reactivation with these agents.

  2. Psoriatic arthritis is treated with NSAIDs, methotrexate, azathioprine, sulfasalazine and/or TNF α blockers.

C. Miscellaneous causes. The treatment strategy usually entails addressing the underlying cause (e.g., antibiotics for infectious arthritis, phlebotomy for hemochromatosis, glucocorticoids for sarcoidosis, allopurinol for tophaceous gout). The treatment of DJD is discussed in Chapter 57.

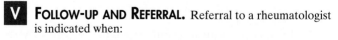

V **FOLLOW-UP AND REFERRAL.** Referral to a rheumatologist is indicated when:

A. The diagnosis remains in question despite initial testing

B. Immunosuppression is required to control joint symptoms refractory to NSAIDs

C. There is any evidence of ongoing joint damage

Reference

Richie AM, Francis ML. Diagnostic approach to polyarticular joint pain. *Amer Fam Phy* 2003;68(6):1151–1160.

61. Low Back Pain

I **INTRODUCTION.** As many as 90% of adults experience low back pain at some time.

A. Low back pain is second only to upper respiratory tract infection as the most common reason to visit an internist.

B. The cost of back pain in terms of work hours lost exceeds that of ischemic heart disease.

II **CLINICAL MANIFESTATIONS**

A. Five percent of patients with back pain have inflammatory back pain (IBP). Commonly, this occurs before the age of 40 and is characterized by an insidious onset, lasting longer than 3 months. It is associated with morning stiffness and improves with exercise. IBP responds dramatically to non-steroidal anti-inflamatory drugs (NSAIDs).

B. Fewer than 5% of patients with low back pain have **sciatica** (i.e., pain that radiates into the buttock and down one leg to below the knee). This symptom complex is seen with nerve root compression, a form of radiculopathy (i.e., nerve root disease). The distribution is dermatomal.

C. Fewer than 1% of patients have **cauda equina syndrome,** an acute radiculopathy characterized by bowel and bladder disturbances (usually urinary retention), saddle anesthesia, and bilateral neurologic deficits.

HOT KEY Cauda equina syndrome is a surgical emergency! Patients with signs or symptoms of cauda equina compression require emergent magnetic resonance imaging (MRI) or computed tomography (CT) scanning and surgical evaluation.

III **DIFFERENTIAL DIAGNOSIS**

A. Back pain as a result of disorders of the vertebrae and disks. Disorders of the vertebrae and disks account for most cases of low back pain. The pain is usually related to one of the following processes.

1. Spondylosis is degenerative changes of the disks and facet joints.

2. **Spondylolisthesis** is forward displacement of a lumbar vertebra onto the one below it.

3. **Disk herniation** usually occurs posterolaterally and can result in nerve root compression. Ninety-five percent of disk herniations occur at disk L4-L5 (affecting the L5 root) or disk L5-S1 (affecting the S1 root). Massive midline herniation can cause cauda equina compression.

4. **Spinal stenosis.** Degenerative changes of the facet joints and the ligamentum flavum cause narrowing of the spinal canal, resulting in compression of the spinal cord. The classic symptom of spinal stenosis is **neurogenic claudication (pseudoclaudication),** which is characterized by poorly localized buttock and leg pain that is exacerbated by walking. Walking downhill is worse than walking uphill because flexion typically alleviates the compression caused by the spinal stenosis.

HOT

▶ In patients with spinal stenosis, walking **down** causes pain levels to go **up.**

KEY

B. **Back pain as a result of systemic disease**

1. **Malignancy. Metastatic disease** from breast, lung, or prostate cancer is the most common form of malignancy-related back pain. **Primary tumors, multiple myeloma,** and **lymphoma** should also be considered. Patients with a malignancy often experience unrelenting nocturnal pain.

2. **Infection.** Local infections, such as **osteomyelitis, diskitis,** and **epidural abscess,** can cause low back pain.

3. The **Spondyloarthritides,** including **ankylosing spondylitis, inflammatory bowel disease, reactive arthritis and psoriatic arthritis** can cause IBP.

4. **Vertebral compression fractures** as a result of **osteoporosis** can cause low back pain in elderly patients and those who take steroids for long periods.

C. **Referred visceral pain.** Low back pain can be a symptom of:

1. **Aortic aneurysm**

2. **Urologic disorders** (e.g., calculi, pyelonephritis, prostatitis)

3. **Gastrointestinal disorders** (e.g., colorectal or peptic ulcer disease, pancreatitis)

4. **Gynecologic disorders** [e.g., endometriosis, pelvic inflammatory disease (PID)]

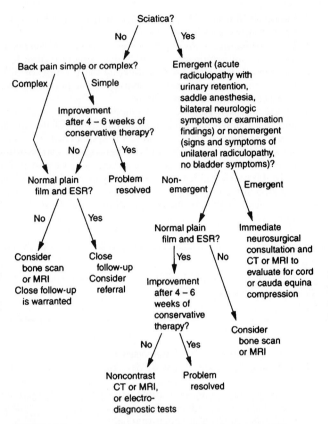

FIGURE 61-1. Approach to the patient with low back pain. *CT* = computed tomography; *ESR* = erythrocyte sedimentation rate; *MRI* = magnetic resonance imaging. (Modified with permission from Wipf JE, Deyo RA: Low back pain. In Branch WT (ed): *Office of Practice of Medicine,* 3rd ed. Philadelphia, WB Saunders, 1994, p 654.)

IV APPROACH TO THE PATIENT (FIGURE 61-1)

A. Patient history. Care should be taken to evaluate the patient's risk factors for a **systemic cause** (e.g., malignancy, infection) of low back pain. Risk factors include:
1. Age greater than 50 years
2. History of cancer or intravenous drug abuse
3. Signs or symptoms of systemic disease (e.g., fever, weight loss, lymphadenopathy)

B. Physical examination

1. **Spinal examination.** Inspect the spine for deformity, palpate for point tenderness, and assess the patient's range of motion.

2. **Neurologic examination.** A directed neurologic examination can be used to screen for radiculopathy.

   a. **Straight-leg raising test.** With the patient supine, lift the patient's leg with the knee extended. If radicular pain occurs when the leg is elevated 30°–60° off the table, the test is positive.

      (1) This test is sensitive for identifying **nerve root irritation,** but not very specific.

      (2) A positive crossed straight-leg raising test (i.e., sciatica is reproduced in the affected leg by lifting the opposite leg) is much more specific for **herniated disk,** but is not very sensitive.

   b. **Screening motor examination.** More than 95% of disk herniations occur at the L4-L5 disk (affecting the L5 root) or the L5-S1 disk (affecting the S1 root) and the remaining 2%–5% occur at the L2-L3 disk or the L3-L4 disk (affecting the L3 and L4 roots, respectively). A screening motor examination should be performed in all patients.

      (1) Have the patient rise from the chair and do a heel walk and a toe walk. Check extensor hallucis longus function (by testing the big toe strength) and evaluate the ankle jerk and knee jerk.

      (2) Table 61-1 reviews the neurologic findings associated with impingement of these roots.

HOT KEY

If the patient has bilateral symptoms or bowel or bladder retention or incontinence, the physical examination should also include a careful perineal sensory examination and evaluation of rectal tone and the sacral reflexes to evaluate for possible cauda equina syndrome.

---

3. **General examination.** If the history has raised the possibility of back pain as a result of a **systemic disorder** or **referred visceral pain,** a more general examination should be performed. For example:

   a. **Abdominal examination** (to rule out aneurysm in an elderly patient with known vascular disease)

   b. **Joint examination** (if the history suggests a spondyloarthritis)

   c. **Lymph node examination** and a more thorough **evaluation for masses** (if malignancy is suspected)

TABLE 61-1. Neurologic Findings In Disk Herniation

Affected Nerve Root	Motor Findings	Sensory Findings*	Reflexes
L3, L4	Difficulty rising from chair (loss of knee extensor function) or performing heel walk	Anterior knee and medial calf	Decreased or absent knee jerk reflex
L5	Difficulty performing heel walk; decreased strength in foot and big toe dorsiflexion	Medial forefoot (first web space)	Reflexes intact
S1	Difficulty performing toe walk; foot eversion and plantar flexion	Lateral foot	Decreased or absent ankle jerk reflex

*Decreased sensation or paresthesias.

C. Laboratory studies. Most patients do not require routine laboratory tests. An **erythrocyte sedimentation rate (ESR)** and **C-reactive protein (CRP)** may be helpful if there is high suspicion for infection, inflammatory disease, or malignancy.

D. Imaging studies

1. **Plain films.** Degenerative changes are ubiquitous in patients older than 40 years and lumbar films yield 20 times the radiation of a chest radiograph; therefore, radiographs are indicated only for the following patients:

   a. Those with risk factors for a systemic cause of low back pain (see IV A)

   b. Those who have sustained significant trauma

   c. Those in whom the history suggests spondyloarthritis.

   d. Those who take steroids or have advanced osteoporosis

   e. Those with significant neuromotor deficits

   f. Selected patients who have failed to respond to conservative therapy

2. **Bone scan.** If plain films increase the suspicion for cancer or infection, a bone scan is indicated. Bone scans are normal in patients with multiple myeloma.

3. **MRI** and **CT with myelogram** must be selectively ordered because these studies are associated with a high incidence of **false-positive results.**
   a. An MRI or CT with myelogram should be performed immediately in patients with suspected malignancy or infection, or any evidence of cauda equina syndrome.
   b. These tests are appropriate for the pre-operative assessment of patients who require surgery for persistent or progressive radiculopathy.

E. **Classification.** Most cases of low back pain cannot be assigned a precise pathoanatomic diagnosis. Nevertheless, it is important to classify the patient's low back pain as either simple or complex on the basis of the clinical findings because this distinction affects the recommended work-up (see Figure 61-1).
   1. **Simple low back pain.** Two-thirds of patients have simple low back pain (i.e., no risk factors for or signs of underlying pathology and a normal neurologic examination).
   2. **Complex low back pain.** Patients either have an abnormal neurologic examination, or they have risk factors for a systemic cause of low back pain.

V TREATMENT

A. **Conservative therapies.** For most patients, even those with radiculopathy, symptoms improve with conservative therapy within 4–6 weeks.
   1. **Bed rest.** Bed rest is generally not beneficial for patients with suspected disk herniations. A gradual return to normal activity should take place within 1–2 weeks.
   2. **Pharmacologic therapy**
      a. **Analgesics**
         (1) **NSAIDs** are effective (e.g., ibuprofen, 800 mg orally as needed, up to 3 times daily). Caution should be used in patients with gastrointestinal risk or renal disease. **Acetaminophen** or **aspirin** may also be tried.
         (2) **Opioids** should be used sparingly. They have no clear benefit over NSAIDs in most patients, are associated with central nervous system (CNS) side effects, and may lead to dependency.
      b. **Muscle relaxants.** In selected patients, a muscle relaxant (e.g., cyclobenzaprine, 10 mg twice daily) may be useful, but use should be limited to 1–2 weeks.
      c. **Steroid injections** are controversial.
      d. **Tricyclic antidepressants** may have efficacy for reducing pain.

3. **Education.** Patients should be educated about the cause of back pain and reassured about the expected course and recovery.
4. **Other approaches**
   a. **Physical therapy.** Patients with prolonged symptoms may benefit from an exercise program.
   b. **Chiropractic manipulation** may be helpful for patients with simple mechanical low back pain, but should be avoided in patients with radiculopathy.
   c. **Yoga** may be beneficial in patients with back pain.
   d. **Traction** is probably not useful.
B. **Surgery** is better for relieving radicular symptoms than for relieving back pain. Relief of symptoms is more rapid with surgery, but long-term outcomes of both surgery and conservative therapy often are similar. Indications for surgery in patients with herniated disks include:
   1. **Cauda equina syndrome**
   2. **Severe** or **progressive neurologic deficit**
   3. **Persistent neuromotor deficit** after 4–6 weeks of conservative therapy
   4. **Persistent sciatica, sensory deficit,** or **reflex loss** in a patient with a **positive straight-leg raising test, consistent clinical findings,** and **favorable psychosocial circumstances** (e.g., realistic expectations and no evidence of depression, substance abuse, or excessive somatization)

References
Carragee EJ. Persistent low back pain. *N Engl J Med* 2005;352:1891–1898.
Deyo RA, Weinstein JN. Primary care: low back pain. *N Engl J Med* 2001;344:363–370.
Speed C. Low back pain. *Br Med J* 2004;328(7448):1119–1121.

PART IX

NEUROLOGY

• •

62. Headache

I **INTRODUCTION.** Headaches affect more than 90% of the population and are one of the most common reasons for office and emergency room visits. Although most headaches are symptoms of benign conditions, it is crucial to identify the small percentage of headaches that signal life-threatening disease.

II **DIFFERENTIAL DIAGNOSIS.** The mnemonic below conveniently divides the differential into "common" and "less common" causes of headache.

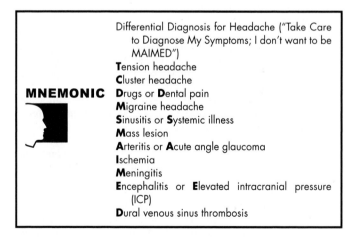

	Differential Diagnosis for Headache ("Take Care to Diagnose My Symptoms; I don't want to be MAIMED")
MNEMONIC	**T**ension headache
	Cluster headache
	Drugs or **D**ental pain
	Migraine headache
	Sinusitis or **S**ystemic illness
	Mass lesion
	Arteritis or **A**cute angle glaucoma
	Ischemia
	Meningitis
	Encephalitis or **E**levated intracranial pressure (ICP)
	Dural venous sinus thrombosis

A. Common causes
  1. Tension headache. Patients often describe a "band-like" sensation of tightening around the head. The pain is likely muscular in origin, and it may be precipitated by stress. Tension

headaches are generally differentiated from migraines by the absence of both associated symptoms (e.g., nausea, vomiting, photophobia) and family history.

2. **Cluster headaches** occur almost exclusively in middle-aged men. These headaches are usually unilateral, centered around the orbit, and described as sharp, stabbing, and severe, often with unilateral autonomic symptoms (stuffy nose, tearing of the eye). The headache often occurs at the same time each day and generally lasts 5–60 minutes. The headaches last for several months, resolve spontaneously, and then recur (hence the name "cluster").

3. **Drugs.** Nitroglycerin, histamine-2 (H_2) blockers, nonsteroidal anti-inflammatory drugs (NSAIDs), nifedipine, atenolol, digoxin, theophylline, and many other medications can all cause headache.

4. **Dental pain.** Patients with abscesses, caries, or infections of the gingiva may complain of a headache or facial pain.

5. **Migraine headaches** show a strong familial pattern. The pain is usually described as unilateral, pulsating, and exacerbated by physical activity. Patients commonly have photophobia, phonophobia, nausea, and vomiting. An aura (i.e., premonitory symptoms such as visual abnormalities, vertigo, or taste sensations) may be present (migraines are classified as occurring with or without aura).

6. **Sinusitis** characteristically causes a frontal or retro-orbital headache that is exacerbated by leaning forward (see Chapter 10). This diagnosis must be made with caution as many patients with migraine or tension headache may have evidence of asymptomatic sinus disease if CT scanning is performed, leading to unnecessary treatment.

7. **Systemic conditions.** Many systemic illnesses can cause headaches (e.g., **common cold, malignant hypertension, fever, carbon monoxide poisoning**).

B. **Less common causes**

1. **Mass lesions.** The presentation varies, but new symptoms, progressive symptoms, or neurologic abnormalities are suggestive features.

   a. **Tumors** often produce subacute, progressive, unilateral pain. The classic symptoms of morning headache, vomiting, and increased pain with the Valsalva maneuver are seen only in a minority of patients in whom intracranial pressure is elevated.

   b. **Abscesses** are usually associated with fever and abnormal neurologic symptoms and signs.

   c. **Subdural hematoma.** Although a history of trauma in the previous weeks is suggestive, the patient may not recall the incident (this is especially true with elderly patients).

   d. **Intraparenchymal** or **subarachnoid hemorrhage** usually results from the rupture of a small blood vessel or berry aneurysm respectively. The time from the onset of headache until maximal pain is usually only seconds in contrast with migraine and tension headache in which a slow build-up to maximal pain occurs over minutes to hours.

2. **Arteritis and other connective tissue diseases**
   a. **Temporal arteritis** should be considered in patients older than 50 years who present with a new headache with visual abnormalities or jaw claudication.
   b. **Other connective tissue diseases** [e.g., systemic lupus erythematosus (SLE), polyarteritis nodosa, Wegener's granulomatosis] can be associated with arteritis (e.g., cerebral vasculitis) and headache.

3. **Acute angle glaucoma** should be considered in an older patient who presents with a new, frontal headache.

4. **Ischemia.** Stroke and transient ischemic attacks (TIAs) should be considered in patients with risk factors for these conditions.

5. **Meningitis.** Patients may initially present with a headache. Fever, mental status changes, and meningeal signs (e.g., neck pain with neck flexion or hip flexion) may also be present.

6. **Encephalitis** almost always is associated with mental status changes or focal neurologic abnormalities.

7. **Elevated ICP** (as a result of **pseudotumor cerebri** or a **mass lesion)** may cause headache. Papilledema or abnormal neurologic signs are suggestive.

8. **Dural venous sinus thrombosis** is usually associated with a predisposing condition (e.g., pregnancy, malignancy, other hypercoagulable disorders) and is a common cause of stroke in the young.

III **APPROACH TO THE PATIENT.** A thorough history and physical examination can establish the diagnosis in most patients. The goal is to avoid missing any potentially life-threatening cause of headache.

A. **Patient history.** A detailed history of all symptoms associated with the current and past headaches is required. The presence of any of the following symptoms raises "NEW FEARS" and suggests a need for more intensive evaluation.

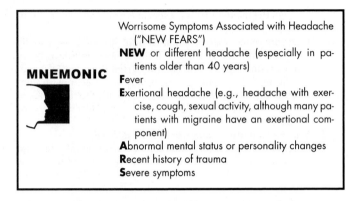

MNEMONIC

Worrisome Symptoms Associated with Headache ("NEW FEARS")

NEW or different headache (especially in patients older than 40 years)

Fever

Exertional headache (e.g., headache with exercise, cough, sexual activity, although many patients with migraine have an exertional component)

Abnormal mental status or personality changes

Recent history of trauma

Severe symptoms

B. Physical examination. A full physical examination is required.
  1. **Papilledema** suggests increased ICP.
  2. **Increased intraocular pressure** is associated with glaucoma.
  3. **Meningismus** (i.e., pain with passive forward neck flexion) suggests meningeal irritation, which can be caused by meningitis or subarachnoid hemorrhage.
  4. A **petechial rash** that is noted first on the lower extremities may be seen with meningococcal meningitis.

HOT KEY Dangerous causes for headache may or may not demonstrate neurological abnormalities; however, if the patient has a headache and a neurological abnormality, a dangerous cause should be presumed.

C. Laboratory studies. Patients who have no worrisome history or physical examination findings generally do not require laboratory testing.
  1. A **complete blood count (CBC), serum chemistries,** and an **erythrocyte sedimentation rate (ESR)** should be obtained for patients with an unclear diagnosis or with worrisome features. The ESR is almost always elevated in patients with temporal arteritis, although it may be elevated in many other inflammatory disorders.
  2. **Cerebrospinal fluid (CSF) analysis** is indicated for patients with suspected meningitis or subarachnoid hemorrhage.

HOT KEY A lumbar puncture should not be performed in patients with focal neurologic signs until a head computed tomography (CT) scan has been performed to rule out increased ICP from a mass lesion.

D. Imaging studies. Head CT or magnetic resonance imaging (MRI) are indicated when clinical and laboratory evaluation do not yield a diagnosis or when intracranial pathology is suspected.

HOT KEY In patients with suspected subarachnoid hemorrhage, a negative CT scan does not rule out the disorder, and lumbar puncture should be performed looking for xanthochromia.

IV TREATMENT

A. Tension headaches can usually be managed with mild analgesics (e.g., acetaminophen, 650 mg every 4–6 hours or ibuprofen, 400–800 mg every 6 hours). Exercise, avoidance of stress, and relaxation techniques may be useful.

B. Cluster headaches
   1. **Acute therapy.** An acute attack can often be arrested by administering **inhaled oxygen** (6 L/min for 10 minutes). **NSAIDs, ergotamine,** and **sumatriptan,** as used for the treatment of migraine headaches (see IV C 1), are also effective.
   2. **Chronic therapy.** A course of **steroids** (e.g., prednisone, 60 mg daily tapered over 2 weeks) may terminate cluster headaches in some patients. Lithium and verapamil are other agents with some efficacy in reducing the number of cluster attacks.

C. Migraine headaches
   1. **Abortive therapy** (Table 62-1) is required during the episode.
   2. **Prophylactic therapy** (Table 62-2) may be considered for patients with frequent attacks (i.e., attacks occurring more than twice a month) or attacks that interfere with the patient's lifestyle. **Beta Blockers** (e.g., atenolol), **tricyclic antidepressants** (e.g., amitriptyline), anticonvulsants (e.g. valproic acid) and **calcium channel blockers** (e.g., verapamil) can be used in the prophylactic treatment of migraine.

D. Sinusitis. Treatment of the sinusitis should resolve the headache (see Chapter 11 VI).

TABLE 62-1. Selected Abortive Treatments for Migraine Headache

Severity of Migraine	Medications	Dose	Cautions
Mild to moderate	Naproxen	500–750 mg orally every 12 hours	May cause gastrointestinal ulceration or bleeding
	Aspirin	650 mg orally every 4–6 hours	Avoid in pregnant women, patients younger than 18 years, and patients with gastrointestinal bleeding or bleeding disorders
	Acetaminophen	500–1000 m orally every 6 hours	Maximum dose is 1.5 g/day in patients with liver disease, best to avoid use of this drug in these patients
Moderate to severe	Sumatriptan and other triptan medications	50–100 mg orally, repeat after 1 hour; maximum dose is 200 mg/day	Contraindicated in patients with CAD Prinzmetal's angina, hypertension, or pregnancy Should not be given concomitantly with ergotamine May cause flushing, neck pain, or chest tightness; first dose should be medically supervised
	Ergotamine	2 mg orally or sublingually, then 1 mg every 30 minutes up to a maximum dose of 6 mg/24 hours	Contraindicated in patients with coronary artery disease (CAD), peripheral vascular disease, or pregnancy Should not be used in combination with sumatriptan

Severe and unrespon-sive	Dihydroergotamine	1 mg intramuscularly; can be repeated twice at 1-hour intervals	Side effects and contraindications are similar to those of ergotamine Should not be given if ergotamine has been used in the past 4 days
	Metoclopramide	10 mg intravenously every 4 hours as needed	May cause dystonia, hypotension, nausea, and vomiting
	Prochlorperazine	10 mg intravenously over 2 minutes	May cause tardive dyskinesia, hypotension, nausea, and vomiting
	Meperidine	25-mg increments intravenously every hour as needed; maximum dose is 1–1.8 mg/kg	May be habituating; use infrequently for severe attacks

TABLE 62-2. Selected Prophylactic Therapy for Migraine Headache		
Medication	**Dose**	**Side Effects**
Atenolol*	50–100 mg orally daily	Depression, fatigue, hypotension
Amitriptyline	10–150 mg orally at bedtime	Xerostomia, urinary retention, drowsiness, cardiac arrythmias
Verapamil	80–360 mg orally daily	Constipation, hypotension, bradycardia

*Use with caution in patients with reactive airway disease.

E. Mass lesions. Patients must be referred to a neurosurgeon or neurologist for evaluation immediately.

F. Temporal arteritis. If the diagnosis is suspected on clinical grounds, patients should be started on prednisone (1 mg/kg/day) and then scheduled for urgent temporal artery biopsy in order to make a definitive diagnosis. Untreated temporal arteritis may lead to permanent blindness.

G. Ischemia. The treatment of cerebrovascular disease is discussed in Chapter 64 V.

H. Meningitis

1. Antibiotics. Any patient with suspected meningitis should receive intravenous antibiotics without delay, even before a lumbar puncture or CT scan is performed. A reasonable initial choice is **ceftriaxone** (2 g every 12 hours) **plus vancomycin** (1 g every 8 hours depending on renal function).

2. Steroids. If bacterial meningitis is suspected, also administer steroids to patients prior to confirming the diagnosis with a lumbar puncture. **Dexamethasone** (10 mg every 6 hours) is often used.

I. Encephalitis. Patients with suspected encephalitis should be started on empiric therapy for herpes simplex virus (HSV) [e.g., **acyclovir,** 10–15 mg/kg intravenously over 1 hour every 8 hours]. A neurologist and/or an infectious disease specialist should be consulted.

J. Pseudotumor cerebri or **hydrocephalus.** These patients require consultation with a neurologist.

V FOLLOW-UP AND REFERRAL

A. Patients with life-threatening causes of headache must be referred to a neurologist, a neurosurgeon, or both. Neurology referral may also be useful for patients with severe migraine headaches or headaches that do not respond to conservative therapy.

B. Patients with non-life-threatening causes of headache should be seen for a repeat examination within 1 month and then as needed, unless symptoms recur.

References

Sandrini G, Friberg L, Janig W, et al: Neurophysiological tests and neuroimaging procedures in non-acute headache: guidelines and recommendations. *Eur J Neurol* 2004;11:217.

Silberstein SD: Practice parameter: evidence-based guidelines for migraine headache (an evidence-based review): report of the Quality Standards Subcommittee of the American Academy of Neurology. *Neurology* 2000;55:754–762.

63. Vertigo

I INTRODUCTION

A. Dizziness is a non-specific term used to describe a variety of subjective sensations. The key first step in evaluation of dizziness is to determine what type of sensation the patient is describing. Faintness and vertigo are the two most common sensations described as dizziness.

B. Faintness is usually described as a sense of **light-headedness** and is usually caused by an insufficient supply of oxygen, blood, or glucose to the brain. Faintness often occurs with hyperventilation or hypoglycemia, or just before a syncopal event.

C. Vertigo, the topic of this chapter, is the illusion of **movement (usually spinning or rocking)** of the patient or the surrounding environment.

    1. Classification. The important distinction to make is between **central (originating in the brain)** and **peripheral (originating in the inner ear)** vertigo.

II CLINICAL MANIFESTATIONS OF VERTIGO. Both central and peripheral vertigo can be associated with nausea, vomiting, gait unsteadiness, and ataxia, and both are exacerbated by head movement. However, several features distinguish central vertigo from peripheral vertigo.

A. Central vertigo

    1. Brain stem, cerebellar, or **cerebral hemispheric signs,** such as asymmetric limb ataxia, focal weakness or numbness, paresthesias, dysarthria, dysphagia, and diplopia, always point to central vertigo, although their absence does not rule out a central etiology.

    2. Nystagmus may be present and can take any form (i.e., horizontal, vertical, or multidirectional). However, nystagmus that is purely in the vertical plane always signifies central vertigo.

    3. Tinnitus or **hearing loss** are **usually not** associated with central vertigo.

B. Peripheral vertigo

    1. There are **no brain stem, cerebellar,** or **cerebral hemispheric signs.**

    2. Nystagmus, which is **invariably present,** occurs unidirectionally, is horizontal and rotatory, and has its fast component toward the side of the normal ear.

3. **Tinnitus** or **hearing loss** are often associated with peripheral vertigo.

III DIFFERENTIAL DIAGNOSIS

A. **Central vertigo.** The most common causes of central vertigo can be remembered with the mnemonic, "SPIN."

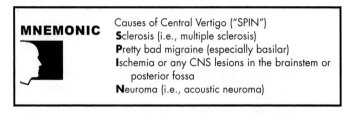

MNEMONIC

Causes of Central Vertigo ("SPIN")
Sclerosis (i.e., multiple sclerosis)
Pretty bad migraine (especially basilar)
Ischemia or any CNS lesions in the brainstem or posterior fossa
Neuroma (i.e., acoustic neuroma)

1. **Multiple sclerosis (MS)** should be considered in young patients with suggestive neurologic symptoms or signs as the lesions in MS often involve the brainstem or posterior fossa.
2. **Migraine** may present with vertiginous spells, although this is somewhat rare and should be a diagnosis of exclusion.
3. **Ischemia.** Ischemia or infarction of the vertebral or basilar arteries can cause ataxia, diplopia, dysarthria, blurred vision, vertigo, dysphagia, and weakness.
4. **Acoustic neuroma.** This common tumor of the cerebellopontine angle usually arises from the vestibular division of the eighth cranial nerve.

B. **Peripheral vertigo** is usually a result of processes that involve the **labyrinth** (inner ear) or **eighth cranial nerve.** The most common causes of peripheral vertigo can be remembered with the mnemonic, "AMPLITUDE."

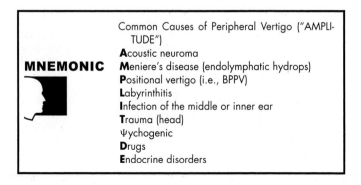

MNEMONIC

Common Causes of Peripheral Vertigo ("AMPLI-TUDE")
Acoustic neuroma
Meniere's disease (endolymphatic hydrops)
Positional vertigo (i.e., BPPV)
Labyrinthitis
Infection of the middle or inner ear
Trauma (head)
Ψychogenic
Drugs
Endocrine disorders

1. **Acoustic neuroma** can cause central vertigo as well as peripheral vertigo.
2. **Meniere's disease** is caused by distention of the endolymphatic compartment within the inner ear. Characteristics include sensorineural hearing loss, aural pressure, and episodic vertigo.
3. **Benign paroxysmal positional vertigo (BPPV)** causes brief episodes of vertigo, which usually last less than 1 minute to 30 minutes and are brought on by head movement.
4. **Labyrinthitis** can occur following a viral upper respiratory tract infection and is characterized by acute, severe vertigo; nausea and vomiting; and hearing loss and tinnitus. Symptoms may last for days to weeks.
5. **Infections other than viral labrynthitis** of the middle or inner ear is a rare cause of vertigo but should be considered in those with evidence of infection (e.g., fever, chills).
6. **Trauma.** Recent head trauma can cause a labyrinthine concussion, producing vertigo that may last for months.
7. **Psychogenic causes** should be considered in patients with a normal neurologic examination who do not have nystagmus, and should be a diagnosis of exclusion.
8. **Drugs.** Aminoglycosides are the most common culprits but many occasionally ototoxic drugs exist.
9. **Endocrine disorders,** such as hypothyroidism and diabetes mellitus, can be associated with vertigo.

IV APPROACH TO THE PATIENT

A. **Patient history.** The cause of the vertigo can be discerned from the history alone in more than 70% of patients.
B. **Physical examination** should focus on the ears, eyes, and nervous system.
   1. Note the presence or absence of ear infection, nystagmus, or neurologic deficits.
   2. The **Nylen-Bárány maneuver** is important in the assessment of BPPV. Have the seated patient turn her head to one side while quickly lying down, so that her head hangs over the edge of the table. Repeat with the other side of the head down after 5 minutes rest. If vertigo is reproduced (along with nystagmus), BPPV is the likely diagnosis.
C. **Laboratory studies** are usually not necessary.
   1. A **thyroid-stimulating hormone (TSH) level** should be ordered if thyroid disease is suspected.
   2. A **serum glucose level** should be ordered if diabetes mellitus is suspected.
D. **Other studies**

1. **Audiometric testing** is useful to evaluate for Meniere's disease or acoustic neuroma in patients with hearing loss or tinnitus.
2. **Brain magnetic resonance imaging (MRI)** is usually indicated if central causes are suspected.
3. **Caloric stimulation, electronystagmography,** and **brain stem auditory evoked potential studies** may be used to distinguish peripheral from central vertigo, or to reach a diagnosis in patients with persistent vertigo.

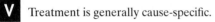 Treatment is generally cause-specific.

A. Central vertigo
1. **Multiple sclerosis.** Therapy with high-dose steroids, immunosuppressants, β-interferon, or copolymer 1 may be useful.
2. **Acoustic neuroma.** These tumors can often be removed surgically.
3. **Stroke or TIA**
   a. **Pharmacologic therapy**
      (1) **Antiplatelets** such as aspirin, clopidogrel, or a combination of aspirin and extended-release dipyridimole may be indicated.
   b. **Risk Factor Modification.** Hypertension, hypercholesterolemia, smoking, and diabetes need to be controlled to prevent further events.
4. **Migraine.** For patients with both migraine headaches and vertigo, β **blockers** or **verapamil** may be helpful.

B. Peripheral vertigo
1. **General symptomatic therapy**
   a. **Pharmacologic therapy.** Medications may prevent CNS adaptation to peripheral vertigo and should not be used for long periods.
      (1) **Diazepam** (2.5–5 mg intravenously once) may terminate the attack and may be appropriate for patients with severe vertigo.
      (2) **Meclizine** (25 mg orally four times daily), **dimenhydrinate** (25–50 mg orally four times daily), or **chlordiazepoxide** (5–25 mg orally three times daily) may benefit those with less severe vertigo.
      (3) **Scopolamine patches** (0.5 mg/day transdermally) are useful for those with recurrent vertigo.
   b. **Exercise.** A mild exercise program can help the adaptation process and improve symptoms.
2. **Meniere's disease.** Treatment is aimed at lowering the endolymphatic pressure.

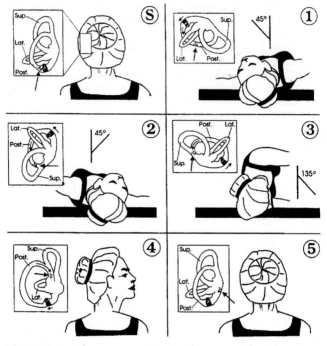

FIGURE 63-1. Epley maneuver. Positioning sequence for left posterior semicircular canal as viewed by operator (behind patient). (Box) Exposed view of labyrinth, showing migration of particles (large arrow). (S) Start—patient seated (oscillator applied). (1) Place head over end of table, 45 degrees to left. (2) Keeping head tilted downward, rotate to 45 degrees right. (3) Rotate head and body until facing downward 135 degrees from supine. (4) Keeping head turned right, bring patient to sitting position. (5) Turn head forward, chin down 20 degrees. Pause at each position until induced nystagmus approaches termination, or for T (latency + duration) seconds if no nystagmus. Keep repeating entire series (1–5) until no nystagmus in any position. From Harwood-Nuss A, Wolfson AB, et al. The Clinical Practice of Emergency Medicine, 3rd Ed. Philadelphia: Lippincott Williams & Wilkins, 2001.

    a. Conservative methods include a **low-salt diet** and **diuretics** (e.g., hydrochlorothiazide, 25–100 mg daily).

    b. Surgical therapy to decompress the endolymphatic sac may be considered for those who remain severely symptomatic despite medications.

3. BPPV. The Epley manuever can be performed to terminate a bout of attacks and by the patient at home when attacks recur (Figure 63-1).

4. Vestibular Neuritis. A recent study suggests benefit from high-dose methylprednisolone for this condition.

VI FOLLOW-UP AND REFERRAL

A. Follow-up. Patients with severe symptoms should be seen frequently (e.g., once or twice a week) until their symptoms subside.

B. Referral

1. When the initial work-up suggests central vertigo, the patient should be referred to a neurologist and for imaging.
2. If brain imaging suggests an acoustic neuroma, consultation with a neurosurgeon is appropriate.

References

Parnes LS, Agrawal SK, Atlas J. Diagnosis and management of benign paroxysmal positional vertigo (BPPV). *CMAJ* 2003;169(7):681–693.

Strupp M, Zingler VC, Arbusow V, et al. Methylprednisolone, valacyclovir, or the combination for vestibular neuritis. *N Engl J Med* 2004;351(4):354–361.

64. Transient Ischemic Attacks

I INTRODUCTION

A. Transient ischemic attacks (TIAs) are **focal losses of neurologic function** that **reverse completely** and are **caused by vascular disease.** Although the formal definition involves a deficit resolving within 24 hours, spells longer than a few minutes usually have evidence of a stroke (infarcted tissue) on imaging.

B. Approximately 50,000 people experience TIAs each year in the United States, and **nearly 11 percent will have an ischemic stroke within 90 days of the event, half of which occur in the first 48 hours.**

C. Role of the primary care physician. The primary care physician must:

1. Identify patients at risk for TIAs and initiate appropriate preventive measures
2. Identify patients with new or recurrent symptoms suggestive of TIAs and arrange for appropriate diagnostic studies and referrals. Consider TIA as "unstable angina" of the brain.
3. Counsel patients regarding the risks and benefits of the various treatment options
4. Assist in preoperative risk assessment of patients being considered for surgical intervention

II CAUSES OF TRANSIENT ISCHEMIC ATTACKS (TIAs)

A. Extracranial atherosclerotic causes responsible for more than 50% of all TIAs and include emboli from **carotid artery disease, vertebrobasilar disease, and aortic arch disease.** Carotid artery disease is the more common of the three.

B. Intracranial causes of TIA include:

1. **Atherosclerosis** of the **cerebral blood vessels**
2. **Inflammation** of the **cerebral blood vessels** [e.g., as a result of systemic lupus erythematosus (SLE), syphilis, or giant cell arteritis]
3. **Hypercoagulable** and **hyperviscosity syndromes** (e.g., antiphospholipid antibody syndrome, polycythemia vera, malignancy)

C. Cardiogenic emboli as a result of arrhythmias, valvular disease, myocardial infarction, or endocarditis can lead to TIAs.

D. Paradoxical emboli [i.e., embolization through a patent foramen ovale or atrial septal defect (ASD)] can result from venous thrombosis, leading to TIAs.

III **CLINICAL MANIFESTATIONS OF TRANSIENT ISCHEMIC AT-TACKS.** The onset of symptoms is **sudden** and without warning, and the **median duration** of the attack is approximately **10 minutes.**

Symptoms of transient, weakness, numbness, aphasia, dysarthria, ataxia, some types of vertigo, or change in vision in one eye are suggestive of TIA.

HOT

TIAs are rarely associated with syncope.

KEY

IV **DIFFERENTIAL DIAGNOSIS.** The following entities must be differentiated from TIAs.

A. Focal seizures are often accompanied by abnormal movements (e.g., clonic movements of a limb). These movements typically start distally in a limb and spread or "march" proximally, occasionally progressing to generalized tonic-clonic seizures.

B. Classic migraines (i.e., migraines with aura) can usually be distinguished from TIAs by the premonition (often visual) of the episode and by associated symptoms (e.g., headache, autonomic arousal with nausea), although some patients will have a focal neurologic deficit such as hemiplegia as the sole manifestation of their aura preceding their headache.

HOT

Headache accompanied by a neurologic abnormality signals a serious CNS disorder until proven otherwise.

KEY

C. Hypo- or hyperglycemic episodes occasionally masquerade as a TIA in patients with diabetes (with hypoglycemia a more common culprit than hyperglycemia).

V **APPROACH TO THE PATIENT.** Evaluation is aimed at excluding other diagnoses and, when TIA is suspected, at identifying the source of the ischemia.

A. Patient history

   1. Delineating the **nature** and the **onset of the symptoms** is important, both for ruling out other conditions and for assessing the urgency of the work-up. Like patients with coronary ischemia and unstable angina, patients with TIA should be strongly considered for admission to expedite workup.

2. Be sure to query the patient about potentially modifiable risk factors for TIA (e.g., cigarette smoking, vascular risk factors).

B. Physical examination. Key features include the following:

HOT KEY Marked hypertension in ischemic stroke and TIA is reactive and serves to perfuse hypoxic areas of the brain. In general, permissive hypertension should be practiced rather than lowering the blood pressure aggressively.

---

1. **Blood pressure assessment.** Hypertension is a risk factor for TIAs.
2. **Cardiovascular examination**
   a. Listen for an **irregular heart rate** and **murmurs** (which may indicate atrial fibrillation, valvular disease or ASD), and evaluate for the **peripheral stigmata of endocarditis** (e.g., Janeway lesions, Osler's nodes, Roth's spots).
   b. Note that generally, the presence or absence of a **carotid bruit** is a poor predictor of the extent of carotid artery disease.
3. **Neurologic examination.** By the time a patient with a suspected TIA receives medical attention, the neurologic examination is usually normal, so abnormal findings should prompt an expedient and thorough work-up. Abnormal findings may include:
   a. **Signs of upper motor neuron lesions,** such as hyperreflexia, increased tone, or an extensor plantar response
   b. **Sensory changes,** such as decreased sensation to light touch, pin prick, or two-point discrimination
   c. **Brain stem findings,** such as cranial nerve deficits
   d. **Language disturbances,** such as aphasia
   e. **Visual field defects**

C. Laboratory studies
1. **General studies**
   a. A **complete blood count (CBC) with platelets** should be obtained to rule out hyperviscosity (from polycythemia) or hypercoagulability (from thrombocytosis).
   b. A **blood glucose level** is particularly important to obtain in patients with known diabetes who are taking insulin or oral hypoglycemic agents.
   c. The **prothrombin time (PT)** and **partial thromboplastin time (PTT)** should be obtained to screen for rare hypercoagulable states (e.g., lupus anticoagulant). It is also

important to have baseline measurements of these parameters for patients who are being considered for anticoagulation therapy.

   d. A **lipid profile** should be obtained to assess for hypercholesterolemia, a modifiable risk factor.

2. **Other studies** may be appropriate to screen for certain conditions if the history or physical examination findings are suggestive.

   a. A **rapid plasmin reagin (RPR)** or **Venereal Disease Research Laboratory (VDRL) test** can be used to screen for
   syphilis.

   b. An **antinuclear antibody test (ANA)** can be used to screen
   for collagen vascular diseases.

   c. A **toxicology screen** should be obtained if cocaine use is a
   possibility.

D. Imaging studies

  1. **General studies**

   a. An **electrocardiogram (EKG)** is important for detecting
   atrial fibrillation, and for looking for evidence of prior
   myocardial infarction. Most patients will need inpatient
   telemetry or outpatient Holter monitoring to screen for
   paroxysmal atrial fibrillation.

   b. **Head computed tomography (CT)** or **magnetic resonance
   imaging (MRI)** should be performed in all patients suspected of having TIAs in order to exclude hemorrhagic
   stroke or mass lesion with hemorrhage.

   c. **Evaluation of the carotid arteries** with CT angiography,
   MR angiography, ultrasound, or catheter angiography can
   accurately identify patients with high-grade stenoses who
   might benefit from surgical carotid endarterectomy or
   stenting.

   d. **Transthoracic echocardiography (TTE)** or **transesophageal echocardiography (TEE)** may be used to detect valvular vegetations, atrial or ventricular thrombi, aortic arch
   atheroma, and patent foramen ovale.

VI **TREATMENT** Focuses on **Stroke Prevention**

A. Risk factor modification

  1. **Control of hypertension.** Both systolic and diastolic hyper-
     tension are independent risk factors for the development of
     stroke.

   a. Antihypertensive therapy is discussed in Chapter 16 IV.

   b. The long-term goal of therapy is to control the patient's
   blood pressure; however, in the setting of an acute unre-
   solved TIA, antihypertensive therapy should be delayed
   until a major stroke has been ruled out. Lowering the

blood pressure during an acute stroke could result in cerebral hypoperfusion.

2. **Cigarette smoking cessation** reduces the risk of stroke.

3. **Control of hyperlipidemia.** Hyperlipidemia is likely to be a risk factor for the development of stroke. The current recommendation is to use the patient's risk factors for coronary artery disease (CAD) as the basis for deciding whether or not to begin therapy aimed at lowering the cholesterol level. (See Chapter 16).

4. **Control of hyperglycemia**. Diabetes is a risk factor for development of stroke in TIA patients and tight glucose control should be initiated if present.

B. Medical therapy

1. **Aspirin** has been shown to decrease the risk of stroke in patients with TIAs.

   a. **Indications.** Aspirin therapy should be initiated in every patient with a TIA who does not require anticoagulation therapy and was not previously on any antiplatelet medications (see V B 3), barring any contraindications to aspirin.

   b. The recommended **starting dose** is usually 81 to 325 mg daily.

2. **Clopidogrel** and a combination of aspirin and extended-release dipyridamole are two other options for antiplatelet medications to prevent stroke in patients who have a TIA while already taking aspirin.

3. **Heparin** or **warfarin** is used rarely for **anticoagulation therapy.**

   a. **Indications**

      (1) **Anticoagulation therapy** is indicated for patients who have atrial fibrillation and who have no contraindications to anticoagulation therapy.

      (2) Other possible indications for anticoagulation include a known thrombus in the left ventricle, a severely depressed ejection fraction (<25–35 percent), and possible large PFOs with associated atrial septal aneurysms.

   b. **Contraindications** to anticoagulation therapy may include:

      (1) Bleeding disorders or a recent history of gastrointestinal bleeding

      (2) A high risk for falling

C. Surgical management. The decision to perform surgery in a patient with TIAs is based on the distribution of the patient's symptoms, the severity of the vascular stenosis, and the patient's surgical risk.

1. **Carotid endarterectomy.** The risk of death or disabling stroke for patients who undergo carotid endarterectomy is approximately 5% in experienced centers. Therefore, certain subsets of patients with TIAs have worse outcomes with surgery than

with medical management. Stenting has emerged as an alternative to endarterectomy, but trials comparing the two are still underway

  a. Patients with **stenoses of 70%–99%** generally fare better when treated by carotid endarterectomy if life expectancy is at least 5 years.

VII FOLLOW-UP AND REFERRAL

A. Neurologic consult

  1. In a patient with a **new TIA,** a neurologist should assist in tailoring the diagnostic work-up and assessing the urgency with which the work-up should be completed, as well as in recommending appropriate therapy.

B. Surgical consult. Consultation with a surgeon is appropriate for patients eligible for carotid endarterectomy.

References

Albers GW, Amarenco P, Easton JD, et al. Antithombotic and thrombolytic therapy for ischemic stroke: the Seventh ACCP Conference on Antithrombotic and Thrombolytis Therapy. *Chest* 2004;126(3 Suppl):483S–512S.

Johnston SC. Clinical practice. Transient ischemic attack. *N Engl J Med* 2002;347(21): 1687–1692.

65. Dementia

I **INTRODUCTION.** Dementia is a syndrome of multiple acquired cognitive deficits that are not attributable to a transient confusional state.

A. Patients exhibit a **decline in cognitive abilities,** resulting in **functional impairment.**

B. Intellectual deterioration occurs in at least two of the following areas: **memory, language, executive function, visuospatial ability,** or **behavioral abnormalities.**

II **CLINICAL MANIFESTATIONS OF DEMENTIA.** Patients with dementing disorders most commonly present with **changes in cognition, function, personality,** or **behavior.** A family member may voice concern, or clinical suspicion may be raised if the patient:

A. Complains of memory loss

B. Reports getting lost, causing an automobile accident, or burning a pot on the stove

C. Fails to keep an appointment

D. Answers questions with increasing vagueness or inaccuracy

E. Has difficulty managing finances, procuring adequate meals, or taking medication as directed

F. Has new depressive or psychotic symptoms

G. Has a disorder commonly associated with dementia (e.g., cerebrovascular disease, parkinsonism, alcoholism)

III **DIFFERENTIAL DIAGNOSIS**

A. **Delirium** is a change in mental status characterized by a disturbance of consciousness, impairment of cognition, and fluctuating signs and symptoms, and can be attributed to an underlying medical condition or drug intoxication. Causes of delirium ("reversible dementia") include:

    1. **Drugs,** such as anticholinergics, opiates, benzodiazepines, antihistamines, and cocaine

    2. **Emotional disorders,** such as mania

    3. **Metabolic or endocrine disorders,** such as hypo- or hyperglycemia, hypercalcemia, uremia, hepatic encephalopathy, hypoxia, and hypercarbia

    4. **Ear or eye dysfunction**

5. **Nutritional deficiencies,** such as vitamin B_{12}, folate, or thiamine
6. **Neurologic disorders,** such as normal pressure hydrocephalus
7. **Trauma** (e.g., leading to a subdural hematoma)
8. **Tumor**
9. **Ischemia** as a result of cerebrovascular disease
10. **Infections,** such as syphilis, meningitis, and systemic infections
11. **Alcohol**

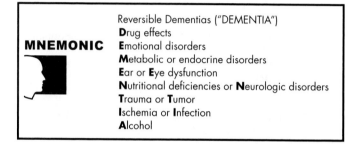

MNEMONIC

Reversible Dementias ("DEMENTIA")
Drug effects
Emotional disorders
Metabolic or endocrine disorders
Ear or **E**ye dysfunction
Nutritional deficiencies or **N**eurologic disorders
Trauma or **T**umor
Ischemia or **I**nfection
Alcohol

B. **Dementia**
1. **Alzheimer's disease.** Patients are **usually older than 60 years,** and the **dementia** is of **insidious onset** and **gradual progression. Memory** is often involved early and prominently.
   a. Although the definitive diagnosis is based on neuropathologic findings, the diagnosis can be presumed on the basis of clinical findings in 90% of patients.
   b. Other neurologic, psychiatric, or systemic diseases that could explain the patient's signs and symptoms must be ruled out.
2. **Vascular dementia** may be associated with a significant stroke, or more commonly it may result from multiple small strokes. Most patients have neurologic signs on physical examination and findings of extensive small vessel disease on neuroimaging.
3. **Dementia with Lewy bodies** is a syndrome in which the patient exhibits at least one of the following:
   a. Parkinsonism developing concurrently with cognitive loss
   b. Visual hallucinations early in the dementia
   c. A changing level of attention and alertness
4. **Frontotemporal dementia** is a series of syndromes in which personality and behavior are affected much earlier than memory.

> **HOT KEY**
>
> Patients with dementia of the Lewy body type exhibit hypersensitivity to neuroleptic agents and this type of dementia is most commonly mistaken for delirium.

IV APPROACH TO THE PATIENT

A. Rule out delirium.

1. A thorough **history** and **physical examination** should be performed, searching for causes of "reversible dementia."
2. **Laboratory studies** to rule out delirium
   a. **General studies.** The following studies should be obtained:
      (1) Complete blood count (CBC)
      (2) Electrolyte panel (including glucose and calcium levels)
      (3) Blood urea nitrogen (BUN) and creatinine levels
      (4) Liver panel
      (5) Thyroid-stimulating hormone (TSH) level
      (6) Vitamin B_{12} and folate levels
      (7) Syphilis serologies
      (8) HIV serology
      (9) Prothrombin time (PT) and partial thromboplastin time (PTT)
      (10) Arterial blood gases (ABGs), possibly including carboxyhemoglobin level
      (11) Toxicology screen
      (12) Urinalysis
   b. **Other studies** may be appropriate, such as:
      (1) Electrocardiography
      (2) Chest radiography
      (3) Lumbar puncture (with an opening pressure)
      (4) Head computed tomography (CT) or magnetic resonance imaging (MRI)
3. **Empiric interventions.** Several agents can be given empirically in an attempt to reverse an acute episode of delirium:
   a. **Thiamine administration.** Malnutrition and alcoholism predispose to thiamine deficiency, which can lead to behavioral changes. Patients should receive thiamine, 100 mg intravenously daily.
   b. **Dextrose administration.** One ampule of **50% dextrose** can be administered intravenously to empirically treat hypoglycemia, if a fingerstick test for glucose is not readily available.

HOT KEY

Alcoholic patients should receive thiamine (100 mg intravenously) prior to dextrose administration to prevent the development of Wernicke-Korsakoff syndrome.

    c. Naloxone hydrochloride administration. Naloxone hydrochloride should be administered if an opiate overdose is suspected. The initial dose is 0.01 mg/kg; higher doses or repeated doses may be required if the patient has respiratory depression or has ingested certain types of synthetic opioids.

B. If delirium is absent, diagnose the particular type of dementia.

    1. Patient history. Questions should be asked of the informant, as well as of the patient.

        a. Characterization of the dementing disorder

            (1) Was the onset sudden or gradual, and how has the disorder progressed?

            (2) What is the nature of the patient's deficits (e.g., memory loss, diminished language skills or other cognitive deficits, personality changes)?

            (3) Does the patient have psychiatric symptoms (e.g., depression, agitation, paranoia, delusions, hallucinations)?

        b. Past medical history

            (1) Does the patient have a history of **cardiac, psychiatric, neurologic,** or **oncologic** disease?

            (2) What is the patient's **alcohol consumption?**

            (3) Is the patient at **risk for HIV?**

            (4) Has the patient experienced **head trauma** recently?

        c. Family history. What is the patient's family–history?

        d. Medication history. Is the patient taking any prescription or over-the-counter drugs?

        e. Social situation. What is the patient's **home environment** like? A disordered living space or the collapse of previously acceptable hygiene and grooming habits is suggestive of dementia and may indicate a need for a caretaker.

    2. Physical examination. The goals of the physical examination are to evaluate the extent of the dementia and to assess any comorbid conditions that may increase the patient's disability. Special attention should be paid to the following areas:

        a. General examination, paying particular attention to signs of thyroid disease (see Chapter 76 III B and Chapter 77 III B)

        b. Cardiovascular examination

    c. Functional examination, including assessment of hearing, vision, and risk of falling

    d. Neurologic examination, including focality, gait, vibration and position sense, and extrapyramidal signs

    e. Mental status examination, including a brief quantitative screen, such as the **Mini Mental State Examination** (Table 65-1), and assessment of the patient's level of consciousness and affect

3. Laboratory and imaging studies

    a. General studies. All patients should receive screening for hypothyroidism (TSH) and B_{12} deficiency.

    b. Specific studies may be warranted, as **dictated by the history and physical examination findings.**

      (1) Neuroimaging studies are appropriate to rule out reversible structural causes of dementia such as hydrocephalus and chronic subdural hematoma.

        (a) CT is the least expensive modality.

        (b) MRI is particularly helpful in HIV-positive patients and patients suspected of having a posterior fossa lesion.

        (c) Positron emission tomography (PET) and **single photon emission computed tomography (SPECT).** These modalities determine disease-specific regional blood flow and glucose metabolism and can distinguish Alzheimer's Disease from Frontotemporal Dementia.

      (2) Neuropsychological studies are especially useful to differentiate the types of dementia and to follow the patient's progress over time.

      (3) An **erythrocyte sedimentation rate (ESR)** can help evaluate malignancy or an inflammatory disorder (e.g., vasculitis) as the cause of the patient's dementia when suspected.

      (4) An **electroencephalogram (EEG)** is rarely indicated, but may help diagnose Creutzfeldt-Jakob disease.

      (5) A **lumbar puncture** can be used to rule out infection (including neurosyphilis), malignancy, and vasculitis.

      (6) A **brain biopsy** is rarely needed, but may be indicated if imaging studies suggest a tumor, vasculitis, or progressive multifocal leukodystrophy (PML).

V   **TREATMENT** of dementia is directed at optimizing the patient's quality of life and functional status.

A. General strategies

    1. Optimize the patient's ability to remain independent. Measures should be taken to maximize the patient's ability to hear, see, and move independently.

TABLE 65-1. Mini Mental State Examination

Maximum Score	Score	
(5)	___	**Orientation** Ask the patient for the date. Then ask specifically for the parts omitted (e.g., "Can you also tell me what season it is?) Award 1 point for each correct answer. ___ ___ ___ ___ ___ year season date day month
(5)	___	Ask the patient in turn, "Can you tell me the name of this: floor? Hospital? Town? County? State?" Award 1 point for each correct answer. ___ ___ ___ ___ ___ state county town hospital floor
(3)	___	**Registration** Ask the patient if you may test his memory. Then say the names of 3 unrelated objects, clearly and slowly, allowing about 1 second between each. After you have named all 3 objects, ask the patient to repeat them. This first repetition determines his score (0-3), but keep repeating the objects until the patient can repeat all 3, up to 6 trials. Award 1 point for each correct answer and record the number of trials. If the patient does not eventually learn 3 objects, recall cannot be meaningfully tested (see below). ___ ___ ___ ___ trial #
(5)	___	**Attention and Calculation** Ask the patient to begin with 100 and count backwards by increments of 7. Stop after 5 subtractions. Award 1 point for each correct answer. ___ ___ ___ ___ ___ ___ 100 93 86 79 72 65 If the patient cannot or will not perform this task, ask him to spell the "world" backwards. Award 1 point for each letter named in correct order. ___ ___ ___ ___ ___ d l r o w

(Continued)

TABLE 65-1. Mini Mental State Examination (*Continued*)

Maximum Score	Score	
(3)	___	**Recall** Ask the patient if he can repeat 3 objects you previously asked him to remember. Award 1 point for each.
(2)	___	**Language** Show the patient a watch and ask him what it is. Repeat for a pencil. Award 1 point for each correct answer
(1)	___	Ask the patient to repeat the sentence after you: "No ifs, ands or buts." Award 1 point for the correct answer.
(3)	___	Give the patient a blank sheet of paper and ask him to follow a 3 stage command: "Take this paper in your right hand. Fold it in half, and place it on the floor." Award 1 point for each part correctly executed.
(1)	___	Ask the patient to read the following statement and do what it says. Award 1 point if the patient performs the action correctly. **CLOSE YOUR EYES.**
(1)	___	Ask the patient to write a sentence for you. Do not dictate a sentence. The sentence must contain a subject and a verb, but grammar and punctuation are not necessary. Award 1 point if the patient performs the action correctly.
(1)	___	Ask the patient to copy the following design. Each figure must have 5 sides and 2 of the angles must intersect. Award 1 point if the patient performs the action correctly.

Total score: ___

Assess the patient's level of consciousness along a continuum:

alert	drowsy	stuporous	comatose

Patient: _____   **Unit:** _____

Examiner: _____   **Date:** _____

Modified with permission from Folsteinn MF, Folsteim SE, McHugh PR. "Mini-mental state." A practical method for grading the cognitive state of patients for the clinician. *J Psychiatr Res* 1975;12(3):189–198.

2. **Avoid exacerbating agents.** The use of centrally acting drugs, including over-the-counter preparations, should be minimized.

3. **Educate the patient and his family.** Caregivers should be educated about behavioral management (see V B), environmental manipulation, safety issues, and the importance of respite. Regardless of the cause of the dementia, patients and their families should be referred to the Alzheimer's Association [http://www.alz.org; (800) 272-3900], a national organization with local chapters that can provide support, education, and referrals (e.g., for daycare programs).

4. **Consider the future.** It is important for the provider to accurately assess the patient's ability to manage finances, drive, cook, get help in an emergency, and ambulate independently in the community, and make recommendations as appropriate.

   a. Discuss and document the patient's wishes for the future use of hospitals, feeding tubes, and nursing homes.

   b. Encourage the patient to establish a Durable Power of Attorney for Health Care.

   c. If the patient is likely to wander, consider a Medic Alert bracelet.

B. **Management of behavioral disturbances** is largely nonpharmacologic. Medications should be used only if the patient has clear psychotic symptoms or is endangering herself or others.

   1. **Nonpharmacologic management.** Providing an outlet (e.g., a safe place to pace or wander, regular activity) is often more effective than medication in managing behavioral disturbances.

      a. **Identify precipitants.** Logging the frequency, timing, and severity of behavioral disturbances can help caregivers identify precipitants. Common precipitants include:

         (1) Delirium

         (2) Depression

         (3) Physical stress (e.g., pain caused by urinary retention or fecal impaction)

         (4) Touch (which the patient may perceive as intrusive)

         (5) Inadequate attention

         (6) Sundowning (i.e., a decline in mental function in the evening)

      b. **Teach caregivers how to interact with the patient.** Caregiver expectations may need to be lowered.

         (1) A **nondemanding, calm, slow approach** to the patient is best.

         (2) **"Talking the patient through"** (i.e., providing reassurance and explanations of actions and events; orienting the patient to reality) is an important aspect of caring for patients with dementia.

(3) Patients respond best to **instructions** that are given **using short, concrete phrases,** with the **emphasis on nouns** rather than adjectives.

c. Minimize the patient's stress.

    (1) Simplify the patient's living environment.

        (a) Play quiet or soothing music.

        (b) Ensure a direct path to the bathroom, kitchen, and bedroom.

        (c) Provide easy mechanics (e.g., door handles instead of doorknobs) and good lighting.

    (2) Structure the patient's day. Setting schedules for sleeping, eating, engaging in activities, and exercising can minimize stress. Overstimulation, as well as understimulation, should be avoided.

2. Pharmacologic management. (Table 65-2)

  a. Antipsychotic agents may be appropriate if the patient exhibits agitation as a result of psychotic ideation. An agent should be selected on the basis of its side effect profile. There is increasing evidence that the newer atypical drugs (e.g., risperidone, olanzapine) may have a small increased mortality associated with their use in this population; therefore, the risk/benefits of these agents must be weighed carefully.

  b. Antidepressant agents. In many patients with possible dementia, depression may coexist.

    (1) Selective serotonin reuptake inhibitors (SSRIs), such as **sertraline, fluoxetine,** and **paroxetine,** have a relatively safe side effect profile and are good choices for treating depression in elderly patients. (Often, a reduced dose is required.)

  c. Antianxiety agents

    (1) Benzodiazepines are indicated for the short-term relief of anxiety, fear, or tension, but are avoided when possible due to their tendency to produce side effects in this population. An agent with a short half-life (e.g., **lorazepam**) should be selected.

C. Pharmacologic treatment of Alzheimer's disease. Several agents are marketed for the treatment of Alzheimer's disease. The patient's cognitive abilities, behavior, and functional status should be assessed every 1–3 months after initiating therapy.

  1. Cholinesterase inhibitors such as donepezil (5 mg daily for 2–6 weeks, then 10 mg daily if tolerated) are probably the most efficacious agents for the treatment of Alzheimer's disease. Therapy with this class of drugs may also help moderate behavioral disturbances.

  2. NMDA receptor antagonists such as memantine (10 mg bid after escalation) have recently been approved as add-on

TABLE 65-2. Pharmacological Management of Behavioral Disturbances in Patients with Dementia

Drug	Dosage	Side Effects
Antipsychotic agents		
Haloperidol	0.5 mg twice daily (one dose given at bedtime), to maximum dose of 1–3 mg/day	High potency side effects (e.g., dystonia, akinesia, dyskinesia)
Risperidone*	0.25 mg twice daily, to a maximum dose of 0.5–4 mg/day	Orthostatic hypotension, parkinsonism
Olanzapine*	2.5–15 mg daily	Stomach pain, nausea, dizziness, xerostomia, constipation
Antidepressant agents		
Trazodone	Initial dose is 25 mg at bedtime, but if necessary, two doses may be given daily, up to a maximum dose of 150 mg/day	Daytime sedation,† priapism (rare)
Sertraline	Initial dose is 25 mg/day; increase dose every 1–2 weeks to a maximum dose of 50–150 mg/day	Gastrointestinal and central nervous system (CNS) effects
Paroxetine	Initial dose is 5 mg/day; increase dose every 1–2 weeks to a maximum dose of 20–40 mg/day	Gastrointestinal and CNS effects
Mood Stabilizers		
Gabapentin	Initial dose 100 mg at bedtime; depending on sedation and effect, the dosage can be increased in 300-mg increments every 2–5 days to a maximum dose of 1200 mg three times daily	Drowsiness, dizziness, nausea

(Continued)

TABLE 65-2. Pharmacological Management of Behavioral
Disturbances in Patients with Dementia (*Continued*)

Drug	Dosage	Side Effects
Valproic acid	Initial dose is 125 mg twice daily; maximum dose is 3000 mg/day	Hepatoxicity, bone marrow suppression, pancreatitis, thrombocytopenia (follow drug levels)
Carbamazepine	200 mg twice daily	Bone marrow suppression (follow drug levels)
Antianxiety agents		
Lorazepam	0.5 mg as needed every 6–8 hours, up to a maximum dose of 6 mg/day	Falls, sedation, paradoxical agitation

*Recent data suggest a small significant increased risk of death in dementia
patients treated with atypical antipsychotics.
†If the patient experiences daytime sedation, increase the bedtime dose and
decrease the morning dose.

therapy for patients with moderate to severe Alzheimer's
disease.

VI FOLLOW-UP AND REFERRAL

A. **Follow-up.** Patients should be seen every 3–6 months to ensure
   optimal management of comorbidities, to monitor patient (and
   caregiver) well-being, and to evaluate the efficacy of pharmacologic therapy.
B. **Referral.** Most patients with dementia can be managed by primary care physicians. However, if the presentation is atypical
   or the diagnosis or management of the disease is difficult, patients can be referred to a neurologist, geriatrician, or geriatric
   psychiatrist.

References
Caselli RJ. Current issues in the diagnosis and management of dementia. *Semin Neurol*
    2003;23(3):231–240.
Schneider LS, Dagerman KS, Insel P. Risk of death with atypical antipsychotic drug
    treatment for dementia: meta-analysis of randomized palcebo-controlled trials.
    JAMA 2005;294:1934–1943.

66. Polyneuropathy

I **INTRODUCTION.** There are three general types of **periph-eral neuropathies:** polyneuropathy, mononeuropathy, and mononeuritis multiplex (multiple mononeuropathies). Of these three, polyneuropathy is the most common and poses the greatest difficulty in differential diagnosis; therefore, it is the focus of this chapter.

A. **Polyneuropathy** is characterized by **symmetrical abnormalities** of **sensation, motor strength,** or **both.**

B. **Mononeuropathy** is characterized by a **focal abnormality** of a single nerve (e.g., carpal tunnel syndrome) and usually results from local nerve compression or stretch.

C. **Mononeuritis Multiplex** is characterized by multiple mononeu-ropathies and often has a vasculitic or infectious etiology. Many causes are treatable and urgent referral to a neurologist is es-sential.

II **CLINICAL MANIFESTATIONS OF POLYNEUROPATHY**

A. **Sensory abnormalities** in the feet are usually the first symptom of most polyneuropathies.

1. **Hypesthesia** (decreased sensation), **anesthesia** (absent sen-sation), **paresthesia** ("pins and needles" sensation without any stimuli), **dysesthesia** (burning sensation with or without stimuli), and **hyperpathia** (exaggerated pain perception) may all be noted. Initially, subjective complaints may not be ac-companied by objective findings.

2. Later, a **pansensory loss in the feet** may occur and progress centrally. Finger involvement often occurs once the knees are affected; eventually, the classic **"stocking-glove" pattern** may be seen.

HOT KEY If a patient has numbness in the legs that extends proximal to the knees and no sensory loss is experienced in the hands, consider a diagnosis other than a polyneuropathy such as a spinal cord problem.

B. **Motor abnormalities** may also occur. Weakness in toe flexors is commonly the first sign. A **diminished ankle reflex** is often seen early in the course of the disease, and a **diminished knee reflex** and **foot drop** may be seen as the disease progresses.

 III **CAUSES OF POLYNEUROPATHY.** The differential diagnosis is long and extensive, many causes can be remembered using the mnemonic, "DANG THERAPIST."

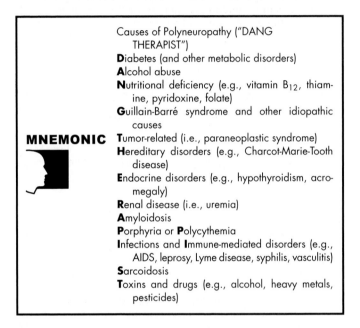

MNEMONIC

Causes of Polyneuropathy ("DANG THERAPIST")

Diabetes (and other metabolic disorders)
Alcohol abuse
Nutritional deficiency (e.g., vitamin B_{12}, thiamine, pyridoxine, folate)
Guillain-Barré syndrome and other idiopathic causes
Tumor-related (i.e., paraneoplastic syndrome)
Hereditary disorders (e.g., Charcot-Marie-Tooth disease)
Endocrine disorders (e.g., hypothyroidism, acromegaly)
Renal disease (i.e., uremia)
Amyloidosis
Porphyria or **P**olycythemia
Infections and **I**mmune-mediated disorders (e.g., AIDS, leprosy, Lyme disease, syphilis, vasculitis)
Sarcoidosis
Toxins and drugs (e.g., alcohol, heavy metals, pesticides)

IV **APPROACH TO THE PATIENT.** Many of the disorders that can cause polyneuropathies are potentially life-threatening if not appropriately diagnosed and treated. Because the differential is extensive and the cause of the polyneuropathy may not be obvious, evaluation of the patient needs to be tailored to the situation. If the diagnosis is not initially apparent, a four-step process may be used to cover most of the possibilities.

A. Take a thorough patient history.
   1. Be sure to ask about **recent events** that may provide a clue to the diagnosis. Specifically, inquire about recent **viral illnesses** (which may suggest Guillain-Barré syndrome), the presence of **similar symptoms in family members or co-workers** (which may suggest a toxic exposure), and **systemic symptoms** (e.g.,

weight loss, which may raise suspicion for an occult malignancy or a chronic infection).

2. Obtain a **medication history.** Some drugs that may be responsible for a polyneuropathy include **phenytoin, isoniazid, hydralazine, dapsone, amiodarone, metronidazole, nitrofurantoin, vincristine, colchicine, antiretroviral medications,** and high doses of **pyridoxine.**

3. Inquire about **toxic exposures.** The most common toxins include **heavy metals** (e.g., arsenic, thallium, lead, mercury), **industrial agents,** and **pesticides** (e.g., organophosphates).

> **HOT KEY** ▶ Remember, common things are common. If diabetes or uremia is present or the patient is a longtime alcoholic, you may not need to look any further.

B. **Assess the time course.** Only a few disorders commonly result in an **acute polyneuropathy** (i.e., one that occurs over a few days).
   1. **Acute axonal polyneuropathies** are are usually caused by **porphyria, intoxications** (e.g., arsenic), or an axonal form of Guillain-Barré.
   2. **Acute demyelinating polyneuropathies. Guillain-Barré syndrome** is the most common type of acute demyelinating polyneuropathy. Classically, all reflexes are lost and CSF examination shows few cells and an elevated protein ("albuminocytologic dissociation"). Nerves to respiratory muscles may become involved. Hospitalization and urgent treatment is warranted.

C. **Perform appropriate laboratory studies** if the diagnosis is not evident. Review the list of possible causes and obtain the laboratory tests that will help you shorten the list. Tests that may be requested include:
   1. Complete blood count (CBC)
   2. Erythrocyte sedimentation rate (ESR)
   3. Renal panel with electrolytes
   4. Fasting glucose and glycosylated hemoglobin levels
   5. Vitamin B_{12} level
   6. Thyroid function tests
   7. Liver panel
   8. Venereal Disease Research Laboratory (VDRL) test
   9. Serum and urine protein electrophoresis
   10. HIV test

D. **Consider occult disorders.** The simple laboratory tests outlined in IV C may not rule out some of the more occult processes (e.g., tumor, vasculitis, sarcoidosis), but they may provide evidence for or against a possible diagnosis (e.g., a normal ESR makes vasculitis less likely). The following tests may be useful in certain clinical settings:

1. **Antinuclear antibody (ANA)** and **serum cryoglobulin assessments** may be used in the evaluation of a suspected vasculitis.
2. **Imaging studies**
   a. **Chest radiographs** may show evidence of sarcoidosis or an occult tumor.
   b. A **computed tomography (CT) scan** may be obtained if an intra-abdominal malignancy is suspected.
3. **Urinary heavy metal** and **porphobilinogen levels** can be used to evaluate the possibility of toxic metal exposures and acute intermittent porphyria, respectively.
4. **Lyme titers** are only useful in the appropriate clinical setting because they lack specificity.
5. **Cerebrospinal fluid (CSF) evaluation**
   a. Findings include high protein levels and a normal cell count ("albuminocytologic dissociation"). in patients with Guillain-Barré syndrome or chronic inflammatory demyelinating polyneuropathy (CIDP).
   b. In patients with AIDS and cytomegalovirus (CMV) polyradiculopathy, findings include pleocytosis and high protein levels.
6. **Electrodiagnostic studies (EMG and nerve conduction studies)** may be performed (if they have not been already) to help categorize whether there is primarily axonal degeneration or demyelination.
7. **Sural nerve biopsy.** The ankle is the easiest place to obtain a cutaneous nerve biopsy.
   a. Nerve biopsy is of low yield in patients with typical polyneuropathies, but should be considered for patients with suspected **mononeuritis multiplex** or in those patients without a clear etiology for their neuropathy.
   b. Because **heredofamilial disorders** often present at an early age and have a characteristic histopathology, a sural nerve biopsy should also be considered for **children.**

V TREATMENT

A. **Relief of neuropathic pain** is usually not easily accomplished. Regimens for the treatment of neuropathic pain are discussed in Chapter 3 IV D 1 and Table 3-4.
B. **Definitive therapies.** Treatment is generally aimed at the underlying disorder (e.g., treating the infection, removing the toxic exposure, replacing the nutritional deficiency). Other specific therapies are as follows:

1. **Diabetic polyneuropathy** is usually progressive. Optimal glucose control has been shown to reduce the development and progression of neuropathy.
2. **Neuropathy associated with renal disease.** Control of uremia with dialysis may slow the progression of the neuropathy.
3. **Guillain-Barré syndrome.** Approximately 85% of patients recover completely or have only mild residual defects. The mortality rate is approximately 3%–4%.
   a. Most patients require hospitalization for observation and **supportive care** (e.g., intubation for respiratory failure, DVT prophylaxis, cardiac monitoring for arrhythmias).
   b. **Plasmapheresis** or IVIG administration is beneficial and should be given urgently (especially within the first 2 weeks of illness).
   c. **Steroids** are not usually effective.
4. **CIDP** may be treated with **steroids, immunosuppressants, IVIG,** or **plasmapheresis.**
5. **Isoniazid overdose** can be treated with **intravenous pyridoxine** (1 gram for each gram of isoniazid ingested).
6. **Acute intermittent porphyria**
   a. **Acute treatment.** Intravenous **glucose** and **hematin** may be needed for acute attacks.
   b. **Chronic treatment** entails **avoiding precipitating factors** (e.g., sulfa drugs) and adhering to a **high-carbohydrate diet.**

VI FOLLOW-UP AND REFERRAL

A. **Referral**
   1. Patients with rapidly progressive disorders (e.g., Guillain-Barré syndrome) require admission to a hospital and urgent consultation with a neurologist.
   2. Referral to a neurologist is also indicated if a specific diagnosis cannot be established after a thorough history, physical examination and laboratory evaluation.
B. **Follow-up.** Patients with an established diagnosis (e.g., vitamin B_{12} deficiency) and stable symptoms may be seen every 1–2 months to evaluate the response to therapy.

References

Grogan PM, Katz JS. Toxic neuropathies. *Neurol Clin* 2005;23(2):377–396.

Sinnreich M, Taylor BV, Dyck PJ. Diabetic neuropathies: classification, clinical features, and pathophysiological basis. *Neurologist* 2005;11(2):63–79.

vanDoorn PA. Treatment of Guillain-Barre syndrome and CIDP. *J Peripher Nerv Syst* 2005;10(2):113–127.

67. Carpal Tunnel Syndrome

I INTRODUCTION

A. Carpal tunnel syndrome—the most common **entrapment neuropathy**—is caused by compression of the **median nerve,** which arises from the C6-T1 nerve roots and innervates the flexor muscles of the wrist and fingers. Carpal tunnel syndrome occurs when the median nerve is compressed within the carpal tunnel at the wrist.

B. Carpal tunnel syndrome affects 0.1% of the population in the United States. Middle-aged women and those with a history of repetitive use of the hands are most often affected.

II CLINICAL MANIFESTATIONS OF CARPAL TUNNEL SYNDROME

A. Pain, paresthesias, or **both** in the distribution of the median nerve (i.e., the thumb, index finger, and middle finger) is the initial complaint. **Aching pain** may radiate into the other fingers of the hand.

  1. The pain is classically **worse at night** and **exacerbated by hand movement.**

  2. **Tinel's sign** and **Phalen's sign** may be positive (each has an approximate sensitivity of 50% and an approximate specificity of 80%).

    a. **Tinel's sign** is positive when percussion (or **t**ouching) the volar area of the wrist produces tingling or pain in the distribution of the median nerve.

    b. **Phalen's sign** is considered positive if pain or paresthesia occur when the patient flexes both wrists to 90° with the dorsal areas of the hands in apposition for 1 minute (reverse **p**raying position).

B. **Sensory loss** and **weakness** or **atrophy of the affected hand muscles** (especially the abductor pollicis brevis) may be present late in the course of the illness.

III CAUSES OF CARPAL TUNNEL SYNDROME.

Carpal tunnel syndrome is most often **idiopathic;** however, it can also occur secondary to several disorders. An easy way to remember the causes of secondary carpal tunnel syndrome is with the mnemonic, "WRIST PAIN."

MNEMONIC

Secondary Causes of Carpal Tunnel Syndrome ("WRIST PAIN")

Work-related
Rheumatoid arthritis
Infiltrative disorders (e.g., amyloidosis)
Sarcoidosis
Thyroid dysfunction (i.e., hypothyroidism) and other endocrine disorders (e.g., diabetes mellitus)
Pregnancy
Acromegaly
Inflammatory tenosynovitis (caused by Reiter's syndrome, gout, soft tissue infection, disseminated gonococcal infection)
Neoplasm (primarily leukemia)

IV   DIFFERENTIAL DIAGNOSIS. Conditions that may be confused with carpal tunnel syndrome include:

A. C6 or C7 cervical radiculopathy
B. Brachial plexus neuropathy (caused by thoracic outlet syndrome)
C. Median nerve compression in the forearm or arm
D. Mononeuritis multiplex
E. Cervical cord abnormalities, such as syringomyelia or demyelinating disease
F. Angina pectoris, if the pain is left-sided

V   APPROACH TO THE PATIENT

A. **Establish the diagnosis.** The diagnosis is usually made on the basis of the **history** and **physical examination.** If the diagnosis is unclear, **nerve conduction studies** can be helpful; however, false-negative results may occur in early, mild cases.
B. **Determine the underlying cause.** Once carpal tunnel syndrome is diagnosed, secondary causes should be considered. Laboratory and imaging studies should only be ordered if the patient has signs or symptoms suggesting an underlying disease. The following studies may provide useful information, depending on the clinical situation:
    1. Erythrocyte sedimentation rate (ESR)
    2. Rheumatoid factor
    3. Complete blood count (CBC)
    4. Fasting blood glucose level

5. Thyroid-stimulating hormone (TSH) level
6. Uric acid level
7. Hemoglobin A_{1c} level
8. Urine pregnancy test
9. Protein electrophoresis
10. Chest radiograph

HOT

Some physicians choose to screen for hypothyroidism and diabetes mellitus in all patients with carpal tunnel syndrome

KEY

VI TREATMENT

A. Conservative measures may be tried first.
  1. **Hand rest.** Resting the hand and modifying repetitive motion activities (e.g., by lowering the keyboard, adjusting the chair height or position, and increasing hand rest time during the workday) may alleviate symptoms.
  2. **Splinting.** A wrist splint should be worn, especially at night.
  3. **Anti-inflammatory medications** (e.g., ibuprofen, 400–600 mg three times daily as needed) can provide symptomatic relief.
B. Surgical decompression. Most patients improve after surgery; however, the prognosis is worse for those with thenar atrophy. There is increasing evidence that early surgical decompression decreases morbidity; therefore, conservative measures should only be tried for a short period of time before surgical referral.

VII FOLLOW-UP AND REFERRAL

A. Follow-up. Patients who are being managed conservatively should see the physician frequently (e.g., monthly), so that the physician can assess the patient's symptoms and the progression of weakness or atrophy. Surgery should be recommended before thenar atrophy occurs.
B. Referral. Consultation with a neurologist is recommended if the diagnosis is unclear.

References

Gerritsen AA, de Vet HC, Scholten RJ, et al. Splinting versus surgery in the treatment of carpal tunnel syndrome: a randomized controlled trial. *JAMA* 2002;288(10):1245–1251.

Viera AJ. Management of carpal tunnel syndrome. *Am Fam Physician* 2003;68(2):265–272.

68. Facial Nerve Palsy

I INTRODUCTION

A. The **facial nerve (cranial nerve VII)** innervates the facial muscles including the muscles of the eyelids. In addition, the facial nerve is involved in dampening sound (via the stapedius muscle) and in taste sensation.

B. It is important to distinguish upper motor neuron weakness, a central nervous system (CNS) disorder, from lower motor neuron facial palsy. The following characteristic usually distinguishes upper motor neuron disease from facial palsy:

1. Voluntary movements of the upper face are preserved in upper motor neuron lesions because the upper forehead muscles are innervated bilaterally. In lower motor neuron lesions, both the upper and lower half of the face are weak.

II DIFFERENTIAL DIAGNOSIS

A. Bell's palsy (idiopathic facial palsy), the most common cause of facial paresis, is a **unilateral lower motor neuron palsy** that occurs fairly abruptly and is thought to be caused by inflammation involving the facial nerve, often as a result of Herpes Simplex infection.

1. **Epidemiology.** Bell's palsy affects men and women equally, with a peak incidence at age 30 years.

2. **Clinical manifestations**
   a. **Symptoms.** The cardinal symptom is **facial paresis.** Other symptoms are not universal, but include **pain around the ear, increased or decreased tearing, subjective facial numbness, hyperacusis,** and **altered taste.**
   b. **Signs** include a **less prominent nasolabial fold** and **weakness of the eyebrow, eyelid,** and **mouth muscles** on the affected side.

HOT **KEY** Features that predict a less than complete recovery for patients with Bell's palsy include age greater than 40 years, hyperacusis, and severe initial pain or paralysis. However, well over 90 percent of all patients will make a full recovery by 3 months.

B. Infection. Many infections can lead to facial nerve palsy; the following are the most common:

1. **Ramsay Hunt syndrome (herpes zoster virus infection).** Facial paresis results from involvement of the geniculate ganglion by a herpes zoster virus infection; usually, vesicles can be seen in the auricle or external auditory canal. This condition is important to identify as antiviral treatment is necessary.
2. **Lyme disease**. A small proportion of patients with Lyme disease develop facial palsies within months of the tick bite.

HOT

Suspect Lyme disease or other less common etiologies in patients with bilateral facial nerve palsy.

KEY

C. **Trauma.** Fracture of the facial bones occasionally affects the facial nerve.
D. **Neoplasia.** Cancer of the ear or parotid gland can lead to facial nerve palsy. Carcinomatous meningitis can also lead to multiple cranial neuropathies.
E. **Demyelinating disorders**
    1. **Guillain-Barré syndrome.** Although weakness usually begins in the legs before involving the upper trunk and face, the **Miller-Fisher variant** of Guillain-Barré syndrome may begin in the face. Bilateral facial weakness is usually the rule.
F. **Heerfordt's syndrome** is parotid enlargement, fever, anterior uveitis, and facial palsy in patients with sarcoidosis.

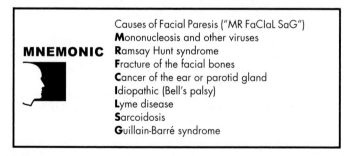

MNEMONIC

Causes of Facial Paresis ("MR FaClaL SaG")
Mononucleosis and other viruses
Ramsay Hunt syndrome
Fracture of the facial bones
Cancer of the ear or parotid gland
Idiopathic (Bell's palsy)
Lyme disease
Sarcoidosis
Guillain-Barré syndrome

III TREATMENT

A. **Bell's palsy (idiopathic facial palsy).** As many as 90% of patients recover fully within 12 weeks; 90%–98% are ultimately satisfied with their recovery.
    1. **Reassurance** is important; many patients believe that they have had a stroke.

2. **Artificial tears** (2 drops four times daily) and the application of a **lubricating ointment** to the affected eye at night are essential if the patient cannot close her eye to prevent corneal abrasions. Patients complaining of eye discomfort should be evaluated for corneal pathology.

3. **Oral corticosteroids** should be considered for patients with severe initial facial pain or paralysis who present within 48 hours of the onset of symptoms. One common regimen is oral prednisone, 60 mg daily for 5 days to start. The dose is then tapered by 10 mg each day over the next week.

4. **Oral antivirals** should be considered for patients who present within 48 hours of the onset of symptoms. One common regimen is oral acyclovir, 800 mg five times a day for 7 days.

5. **Surgery.** Some have considered facial nerve decompression urgently for patients presenting with complete paralysis. There is currently not enough evidence to recommend this treatment.

B. **Secondary facial palsy.** Therapy focuses on supportive care and is aimed at the underlying disorder.

IV FOLLOW-UP AND REFERRAL. Referral to an otolaryngologist or neurologist should be considered if a space-occupying lesion is suspected or the diagnosis is unclear.

References

Gilden DH. Clinical practice: Bell's palsy. *N Engl J Med* 2004;351(13):1323–1331.

Grogan PM, Gronseth GS. Practice parameter: Steroids, acyclovir, and surgery for Bell's palsy (an evidence-based review): report of the Quality Standards Subcommittee of the American Academy of Neurology. *Neurology* 2001;56(7):830–836.

PART X

HEMATOLOGY AND ONCOLOGY

69. Anemia

I **INTRODUCTION.** Anemia is **a manifestation of disease,** not a disease in and of itself.

A. Definition. Anemia is defined as **a decrease in the volume of red blood cells (RBCs) as reflected by the hematocrit (HCT).**
   1. In **men,** a HCT of less than 40% is considered anemic.
   2. In **women,** a HCT of less than 37% is considered anemic.

B. Clinical manifestations of anemia. Patients with anemia may be asymptomatic, or they may complain of **fatigue, dyspnea on exertion,** or **exertional angina.** Signs and symptoms of the underlying disorder may also be present.

C. Classification. Anemia is classified as **microcytic, normocytic,** or **macrocytic** as defined by the **mean corpuscular volume (MCV).**
   1. The **normal MCV** is **80–100 μm^3.**
   2. If more than one disorder is present, the MCV is an average of the different populations of RBCs.

II **MICROCYTIC ANEMIA (MCV <80 μm^3)**

A. Causes of microcytic anemia
   1. **Iron deficiency** is the most common cause of microcytic anemia. It is important to diagnose because it may indicate an underlying gastrointestinal malignancy.
   2. **Thalassemias** are hereditary disorders characterized by a reduction in the synthesis of α or β globin chains.
   3. **Anemia of chronic disease (ACD)** is associated with inflammatory diseases (e.g., rheumatoid arthritis, serious infection, carcinoma).
   4. **Sideroblastic anemias** are a heterogenous group of disorders with altered production of the heme component of hemoglobin (specifically, the generation of the protoporphyrin ring). It is often microcytic, but can be a cause of normocytic or macrocytic anemia. Causes of sideroblastic anemia include:
      a. Inherited disorders

TABLE 69-1. Serum Ferritin Values and Corresponding Likelihood Ratios

Serum Ferritin (μg/L)	Likelihood Ratio
>100	0.2
25–100	Not helpful
15–24	10
<15	50

Based on data from: Guyatt GH, Oxman AD, Ali M, et al: Laboratory diagnosis of iron-deficiency anemia: an overview. J Gen Inter Med 7(2):145–153, 1992.

   b. Drugs and **toxins** (e.g., **L**ead, **I**soniazid, **E**thanol—**LIE**)
   c. Malignancy (e.g., leukemia, lymphoma, myelofibrosis, multiple myeloma, solid tumor)
   d. Collagen vascular disease (e.g., rheumatoid arthritis)
B. Approach to the patient. It is important to differentiate iron deficiency from the other causes of microcytic anemia.
   1. Iron deficiency versus thalassemia
      a. Iron deficiency may be distinguished from thalassemia using the **Mentzer index [MCV divided by RBC count].** A Mentzer index of **less than 13 suggests thalassemia;** one greater than 13 suggests iron deficiency.
      b. An abnormal **hemoglobin electrophoresis** is useful in diagnosing a thalassemia.
   2. Iron deficiency versus ACD
      a. Laboratory studies
         (1) Serum ferritin. This is the most useful test among the iron studies. Likelihood ratios have been established for various ferritin levels. (See Table 69-1) By estimating your pretest probably for iron deficiency and using these likelihood ratios, one can then estimate the posttest probability for iron deficiency (see Chapter 1 III C 3).
            (a) A serum ferritin less than 15 μg/L practically guarantees that the patient has iron deficiency.
            (b) Similarly, a value greater than 100 μg/L essentially rules out the diagnosis.
         (2) Serum transferrin is occasionally helpful because it is usually elevated in iron deficiency and decreased in ACD.
         (3) Soluble transferrin receptor levels may be helpful in mixed cases of anemia of chronic disease and iron

TABLE 69-2. Serum Levels That Differentiate Anemia of Chronic Disease from Iron-Deficiency Anemia*

Variable	Anemia of Chronic Disease	Iron-Deficiency Anemia	Both Conditions[†]
Iron	Reduced	Reduced	Reduced
Transferrin	Reduced to normal	Increased	Reduced
Transferrin saturation	Reduced	Reduced	Reduced
Ferritin	Normal to increased	Reduced	Reduced to normal
Soluble transferrin receptor	Normal	Increased	Normal to increased
Ratio of soluble transferrin receptor to log ferritin	Low (<1)	High (>2)	High (>2)
Cytokine levels	Increased	Normal	Increased

*Relative changes are given in relation to the respective normal values.
[†]Patients with both conditions include those with anemia of chronic disease and true iron deficiency.
(Reprinted with permission from Weiss G, Goodnough L. Anemia of chronic disease. N Engl J Med 352(10):1011–1023, 2005.

deficiency with a normal ferritin. The receptor levels remain unchanged in cases of ACD alone but are increased in the setting of iron deficiency. (See Table 69-2)
   b. **Bone marrow biopsy** remains the gold standard for diagnosing iron deficiency, and is the usual method of diagnosing sideroblastic anemia.

III MACROCYTIC ANEMIA (MCV) >100 μm^3)

A. **Megaloblastic anemia** is caused by defects in DNA synthesis. Causes of megaloblastic anemia include:
   1. **Vitamin B_{12} (cobalamin) deficiency**
      a. **Causes** of vitamin B_{12} deficiency include **pernicious anemia, gastrectomy, blind loop syndrome, pancreatic**

insufficiency, ileal resection or bypass, and **Crohn's disease** of the distal ileum. Dietary deficiency of vitamin B_{12} is rarely a cause because the body's vitamin B_{12} stores can last for 3–5 years. Strict vegans may become deficient.

   b. Clinical manifestations of vitamin B_{12} deficiency may include gastrointestinal disturbances (e.g., anorexia, diarrhea, glossitis) and a neurologic syndrome consisting of paresthesias, imbalance, and occasionally, dementia.

HOT KEY Approximately 10% of patients with vitamin B_{12} deficiency will not be anemic; therefore, vitamin B_{12} levels should be checked in patients with suspected vitamin B_{12} deficiency regardless of the hematocrit.

  2. Folate deficiency
    a. Causes. Folate deficiency is almost always the result of **inadequate dietary intake.** Body stores of folate last only 3–5 months after intake ceases. **Several drugs interfere with folic acid metabolism (e.g. phenytoin and trimethoprim).** Other rare causes of folate deficiency include **tropical sprue, chronic hemolytic anemia, pregnancy and hemodialysis.**
    b. Clinical manifestations. Gastrointestinal complaints may occur but there are no neurologic sequelae.
  3. Drugs (e.g., **methotrexate, azathioprine, zidovudine**) can be associated with megaloblastic anemia.

HOT KEY Practically all patients taking zidovudine (for the treatment of HIV) have an elevated MCV; therefore, this finding can aid in gauging compliance with the medication.

HOT KEY The finding of hypersegmented polymorphonuclear neutrophils (PMNs) on the peripheral blood smear strongly suggests megaloblastic anemia.

B. Chronic liver disease causes a macrocytosis as a result of ineffective erythropoiesis and acute blood loss.

C. **Reticulocytosis.** Reticulocytes are larger than normal RBCs. Patients with reticulocytosis can have MCV readings that are increased but usually less than than 110 μm^3.

D. **Alcoholism** produces erythrocyte membrane abnormalities, leading to macrocytic anemia.

E. **Hypothyroidism** causes macrocytic anemia via an unclear mechanism.

HOT KEY

Macrocytosis + neurologic symptoms = vitamin B$_{12}$ deficiency, alcoholism, or hypothyroidism.

F. **Myelodysplasia.** There are five myelodysplastic syndromes that are characterized by ineffective hematopoiesis:
   1. **Refractory anemia**
   2. **Refractory anemia with ringed sideroblasts**
   3. **Refractory anemia with excess blasts**
   4. **Refractory anemia with excess blasts in transformation**
   5. **Chronic myelomonocytic leukemia**

IV **NORMOCYTIC ANEMIA.** An **absolute reticulocyte count** is one of the first tests ordered in patients with normocytic anemia. The absolute reticulocyte count allows the anemia to be classified as **proliferative** or **hypoproliferative** (Figure 69-1).

A. **Proliferative normocytic anemia** is characterized by erythrocyte loss or destruction.
   1. **Hemolysis.** Laboratory clues include **elevated lactate dehydrogenase (LDH), decreased haptoglobin** and increased **total and indirect bilirubin levels.** If concerned for hemolysis, the **peripheral smear** must be examined. Based on the morphology of the erythrocytes (e.g., schistocytes, sickle cells or spherocytes) the cause of the hemolytic anemia may be determined.
      a. **Microangiopathic hemolytic anemia (MAHA)** is characterized by intravascular shearing of RBCs, resulting in schistocyte formation. A few of the important causes of MAHA are listed here.
         (1) **Disseminated intravascular coagulation (DIC).** In acute DIC, the major concern is bleeding, whereas in chronic DIC, thrombosis is more of a problem.

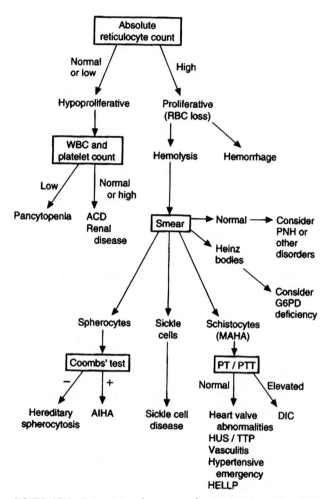

FIGURE 69-1. Determining the cause of normocytic anemia. *ACD* = anemia of chronic disease; *AIHA* = autoimmune hemolytic anemia; *DIC* = disseminated intravascular coagulation; *G6PD* = glucose-6-phosphate dehydrogenase; *HELLP* = hemolysis, elevated liver enzymes, and low platelet count syndrome; *HTN* = hypertension; *HUS/TTP* = hemolytic-uremic syndrome/thrombotic thrombocytopenic purpura; *MAHA* = microangiopathic hemolytic anemia; *PNH* = paroxysmal nocturnal hemoglobinuria; *PT* = prothrombin time; *PTT* = partial thromboplastin time; *RBC* = red blood cell; *WBC* = white blood cell. (Modified with permission from Saint S, Frances C. *Saint-Frances Guide to Inpatient Medicine.* Baltimore: Lippincott Williams & Wilkins, 2004, p 335.)

MNEMONIC Causes of DIC ("MOIST")
Malignancy
Obstetric complications
Infection
Shock
Trauma

    (2) Hemolytic-uremic syndrome/thrombotic thrombocy-topenic purpura (HUS/TTP). The triad of HUS is hemolysis, uremia, and thrombocytopenia. TTP is hemolytic-uremic syndrome accompanied by fever and neurologic changes. In general, if uremia is the prominent disorder, the disease is referred to as HUS. If the central nervous system (CNS) manifestations are more significant, then TTP is the appropriate term.

HOT
▶
KEY
An LDH level less than 1000 U/L makes HUS/TTP very unlikely.

    b. Autoimmune hemolytic anemia. Laboratory clues include spherocytes on smear and positive direct Coombs' test. It can be idiopathic, related to an autoimmune process (SLE), hematologic malignancy (CLL), prior blood trans-fusions or drugs.
  2. Hemorrhage. If hemorrhage is suspected, the source of the blood loss must be determined (e.g., the gastrointestinal tract).
B. Hypoproliferative normocytic anemia. Anemia accompanied by **low white blood cell (WBC)** and **platelet counts** indicates pancytopenia. A hypoproliferative normocytic anemia accompanied by normal or high WBC and platelet counts usually indicates ACD, renal disease or a pure RBC aplasia.

V TREATMENT

A. Symptomatic therapy. Patients who have acute symptoms because of their anemia may require **blood transfusions** (and perhaps hospitalization).

HOT KEY One unit of packed RBCs increases the hematocrit by approximately 3%. In patients with coronary artery disease (CAD), it is usually advisable to keep the hematocrit above 30%.

B. **Iron deficiency** is best treated with **ferrous sulfate** (325 mg orally, 3 times daily). The hematocrit should return to normal after 8 weeks. Patients who cannot tolerate or do not respond adequately to oral therapy can be referred to a hematologist for IV Iron therapy. Ferric gluconate and iron sucrose may be safer alternatives to iron dextran.

HOT KEY It is of utmost importance to determine the underlying cause of iron deficiency (i.e., excluding gastrointestinal malignancy via upper and lower endoscopy).

C. **Vitamin B$_{12}$ deficiency** as a result of **pernicious anemia** is treated with **intramuscular vitamin B$_{12}$** (100 μg daily for the first week, weekly for the next 3–4 weeks, and then monthly for life). Patients usually feel better within a few days of therapy, and the HCT should return to normal in 2 months.

D. **Folate deficiency** is treated with **folic acid** (1 mg orally daily). As with therapy for vitamin B$_{12}$ deficiency, therapy for folate deficiency usually results in rapid improvement in symptoms, followed by a return to normal HCT within 2 months.

HOT KEY In patients with concomitant vitamin B$_{12}$ and folic acid deficiencies, large doses of folic acid may produce an increase in the HCT but will allow the neurologic damage caused by the vitamin B$_{12}$ deficiency to progress.

E. **Sickle Cell Disease (SCD). Mainstay of therapy remains hydroxyurea. Some patients meet criteria to receive hematopoietic cell transplants. Other treatments include folate 1 mg/day, and treatment of pain crises with opiods and NSAIDS. Administration of (single or exchange) blood transfusions are given for specific indications but only in consultation with a hematologist.**

HOT KEY

Yearly ophthalmological exams in sickle cell disease patients are important to evaluate for retinopathy.

F. Autoimmune hemolytic anemia. This should be managed in consultation with a hematologist. Prednisone (1 mg/kg/day in divided doses) is usually the initial therapy for this disorder. Other therapies, such as blood **transfusions, azathioprine, intravenous immunoglobulin therapy,** or **splenectomy may be necessary, but only after consultation with a hematologist**.

VI FOLLOW-UP AND REFERRAL

A. Referral to a **hematologist** is advised if the cause of the anemia remains unclear after initial evaluation, or if bone marrow biopsy is being contemplated.
B. Consultation with a **gastroenterologist** is necessary if endoscopy is required to rule out a gastrointestinal cause of blood loss.

References
Claster S, Vichinsky EP. Managing sickle cell disease. *Br Med J* 2003;327:1151–1155.
Silverstein SB, Rodgers GM. Parenteral iron options. *Am J Hematol* 2004;76:74–78.
Weiss G, Goodnough L. Anemia of chronic disease. *N Engl J Med* 2005;352(10): 1011–1023.

70. Polycythemia

I **INTRODUCTION.** Polycythemia is an **abnormal increase in the red blood cell (RBC) mass.** It may be a secondary, physiologic response to another disorder, or it may herald a primary, more malignant disorder. **A hemoglobin >18.5 g/dL in men and >16.5 g/dL in women** (or hematocrit [Hct] greater than 52% in men and 48% in women) indicates polycythemia and requires further evaluation.

A. **Absolute polycythemia** is characterized by an increase in RBC mass, greater than 25% of normal.

B. **Relative polycythemia** is characterized by a decrease in plasma volume.

II **CLINICAL MANIFESTATIONS OF POLYCYTHEMIA**

A. Patients are **often asymptomatic if the Hct is lower than 60%.**

B. Higher Hcts may be associated with **vaso-occlusive episodes** resulting in **headaches, blurry vision, dizziness, strokes, cardiac ischemia,** and **peripheral thromboses.** A **"ruddy" cyanosis** may be found on physical examination.

C. **Polycythemia vera (PV) is** a myeloproliferative disorder characterized by prominent proliferation of the RBC line. It may present with **pruritus** and **peptic ulcers** in addition to the symptoms described in II B. The mechanisms for these symptoms are still unclear but theories include increased histamine levels or elevated prostaglandin production by platelet aggregation. Both **thrombosis** and **bleeding** may occur as a result of abnormal platelet function, and **splenomegaly** is common.

III **CAUSES OF POLYCYTHEMIA**

A. **Absolute polycythemia.** There are five common causes of absolute polycythemia. Remember, "Hypoxia May Cause Polycythemia Every Time."

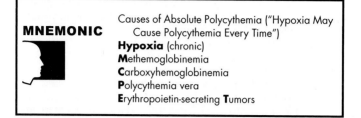

	Causes of Absolute Polycythemia ("Hypoxia May
MNEMONIC	Cause Polycythemia Every Time")
	Hypoxia (chronic)
	Methemoglobinemia
	Carboxyhemoglobinemia
	Polycythemia vera
	Erythropoietin-secreting **T**umors

1. **Hypoxia.** Chronic hypoxia, as a result of cardiopulmonary disease or high altitude, can lead to polycythemia.
2. **Carboxyhemoglobinemia** or **methemoglobinemia.** Carboxyhemoglobin, methemoglobin and other high-affinity variants cause a leftward shift of the hemoglobin dissociation curve, decreased oxygen delivery to the tissues, and a compensatory polycythemia. Smoking is a common cause of carboxyhemoglobinemia.
3. **PV** causes polycythemia by clonal proliferation of stem cells independent of erythropoietin.
4. **Erythropoietin-secreting tumors** are primarily renal cell carcinoma, hepatocellular carcinoma, cerebellar hemangioblastomas, pheochromocytoma or uterine fibroids.

B. **Relative polycythemia.** There are two main causes of relative polycythemia.
   1. **Dehydration** (e.g., from vomiting, diarrhea, excessive perspiration, or diuretics) can deplete plasma volume, leading to a relative polycythemia.
   2. **Stress erythrocytosis (Gaisböck's disease)** results from contraction of the plasma volume and is not a true erythrocytosis. This benign disorder is seen most often in hypertensive, obese men.

IV APPROACH TO THE PATIENT

A. **Rule out hypoxia and carboxyhemoglobinemia.** These are common causes of polycythemia and are easy to evaluate. If secondary causes are found that are significant enough to result in polycythemia, the need for additional work-up may be unecessary. Cooximetry of an **arterial blood gas with carboxyhemoglobin level** is necessary for all patients who smoke, and is more accurate than oxygen saturation measurements. If clinical suspicion is present, the methemoglobin level can also be checked.

B. **Look at the patient's Hct.**

1. A Hct greater than 60% in men or 56% in women suggests a primary cause. But, remember to rule out secondary causes of polycythemia first, as above.

   a. **PV.** The diagnostic criteria include:

      (1) Red cell mass >25% predicted.

      (2) Normal arterial oxygen saturation.

      (3) No elevation in serum erythropoietin.

      (4) Palpable splenomegaly.

      (5) Presence of JAK2 mutation. This tyrosine kinase mutation was recently discovered in many PV cases. But, it is also present in about half of all cases of essential thrombocytosis and idiopathic myelofibrosis. As a result, this test is not solely diagnostic for PV.

      (6) Other helpful clues include: thrombocytosis (plts >400 × 109/L), neutrophilia (neutrophils > 10 × 109/L), radiographic splenomegaly, low serum erythropoietin, or endogenous erythroid colonies.

   b. **Erythropoietin-secreting tumors.** In patients without a definitive diagnosis, the possibility of an erythropoietin-secreting tumor should be considered.

      (1) An **abdominal computed tomography (CT)** scan may help rule out renal pathology (including cancer) and hepatic malignancies.

      (2) **Brain imaging** [preferably magnetic resonance imaging) may be performed if there is any clinical suspicion of a cerebellar lesion.

2. A **Hct less than 60% in men** or **55% in women** suggests mild polycythemia, which is more common with secondary polycythemia. An **RBC mass study** should be ordered to rule out **decreased plasma volume,** which is responsible for the polycythemia in approximately 50% of cases.

V **TREATMENT.** Definitive therapy is aimed at the underlying disorder. Stress erythrocytosis requires no treatment. Supportive measures include the following.

A. **Oxygen therapy** is useful in patients with an arterial oxygen tension (Pao$_2$) lower than 60 mm Hg.

B. **Smoking cessation** is encouraged (especially in patients with carboxyhemoglobinemia).

C. **Hydration** is recommended for dehydrated patients.

D. **Phlebotomy** lowers the Hct, reducing blood viscosity, preventing thromboembolic complications, and improving oxygen delivery.

   1. Phlebotomy is the **treatment of choice for PV** and has been shown to dramatically prolong survival. The target Hct is in the mid to low 40s.

2. Because the risk of thrombotic complications increases dramatically with a Hct greater than 55%, phlebotomy is also recommended for other causes when the Hct remains elevated despite correction of the underlying disorder.

E. Aspirin. Low-dose aspirin is used to prevent thrombotic complications, as long as there are no contraindications to anti-platelet therapy. Avoid if platelet count $> 1000 \times 10^9/L$

F. Manage reversible thrombotic risk factors: hyperlipidemia, smoking, hypertension and obesity.

G. Cytoreduction therapy should be considered for polycythemia vera if: the patient is intolerant of phlebotomy or develops thrombocytosis or symptomatic/progressive splenomegaly. Options include hydroxyurea (first-line therapy), interferon alpha, anagrelide or 32P.

H. Allopurinol (300 mg daily in patients with normal renal function) is often indicated for patients who have hyperuricemia and gout, which often accompany the increased cell turnover that is characteristic of polycythemia vera.

VI FOLLOW-UP AND REFERRAL

A. A hematologist can help guide specific anti-platelet and myelosuppressive therapy; all patients with polycythemia vera should be managed in consultation with a hematologist.

B. Patients with marked polycythemia must be seen for phlebotomy every 1–3 days until the Hct is lowered to less than 55%; the target Hct can then be reached with weekly blood draws. Regular monitoring of the Hct (at least monthly) and phlebotomy are essential in order to prevent life-threatening complications.

References

Campbell PJ, Green AR. Management of polycythemia vera and essential thrombocythemia. *Hematology 2005, American Society of Hematology Education Program Book*. 2005;201–208.

Percy MJ et al. Disorders of oxidized hemoglobin. *Blood Reviews* 2005;19:61–68.

Landolfi R, Marchioli R, Kutti J, et al. Efficacy and safety of low-dose aspirin in polycythemia vera. *N Engl J Med* 2004;350:114–124.

71. Thrombocytopenia and Thrombocytosis

I **INTRODUCTION.** Thrombocytopenia and thrombocytosis are common disorders that may be discovered during an evaluation for bleeding or clotting disorders, or noted as a response to another illness.

A. **Thrombocytopenia** is defined as a **platelet count less than 150,000 cells/µL.**

B. **Thrombocytosis** is defined as a **platelet count greater than 450,000 cells/µL.**

II **THROMBOCYTOPENIA**

A. **Clinical manifestations.** Signs and symptoms are related to the degree of thrombocytopenia (in the absence of concomitant coagulopathy or platelet dysfunction).

1. **Platelet count of 50,000–150,000 cells/µL.** Clinical manifestations are usually absent.

2. **Platelet count of 20,000–50,000 cells/µL.** Patients may report **easy bruisability,** but spontaneous bleeding is usually not seen.

3. **Platelet count less than 20,000 cells/µL.** Patients are at increased risk for **spontaneous mucocutaneous bleeding** (e.g., **petechiae, epistaxis, gingival, conjunctival bleeding, and if severe, gastrointestinal bleeding).**

B. **Causes of thrombocytopenia.** Thrombocytopenia may occur via 3 different mechanisms: decreased production, splenic sequestration, or increased destruction (Figure 71-1).

1. **Decreased production.** Diseases of the bone marrow often involve a decrease in other cell lines as well. The causes of decreased platelet production are almost identical to those of pancytopenia ("PANCYTO"), with the exception of consumption ("C").

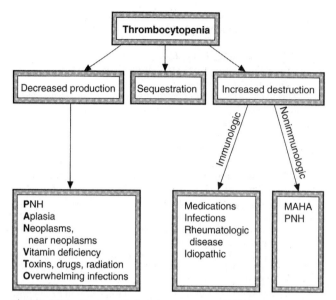

FIGURE 71-1. Causes of thrombocytopenia. *MAHA* = microangiopathic hemolytic anemia; *PNH* = paroxysmal nocturnal hematuria. (Reprinted from Saint S, Frances C. *Saint-Frances Guide to Inpatient Medicine, 2nd edition.* Baltimore: Williams & Wilkins, 2004, p 323.)

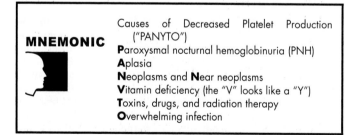

MNEMONIC

Causes of Decreased Platelet Production ("PANYTO")
Paroxysmal nocturnal hemoglobinuria (PNH)
Aplasia
Neoplasms and **N**ear neoplasms
Vitamin deficiency (the "V" looks like a "Y")
Toxins, drugs, and radiation therapy
Overwhelming infection

a. **PNH** is more commonly associated with increased destruction, but may be associated with a production defect.
b. **Aplasia. Aplastic anemia** usually causes pancytopenia but occasionally can result in isolated thrombocytopenia.
c. **Neoplasms** and **near neoplasms** include **leukemia, metastatic malignancies** and **myelodysplasia.**
d. **Vitamin deficiencies,** including **vitamin B$_{12}$** and **folate deficiency,** are rare causes of isolated thrombocytopenia.

   e. **Toxins, drugs** and **radiation therapy. (e.g., ethanol** and **chemotherapeutic agents** can lead to decreased platelet production.
   f. **Overwhelming infections,** including sepsis, tuberculosis, fungal infection, and HIV disease, can lead to decreased platelet production.
2. **Increased splenic sequestration** can result from **hypersplenism** of any cause, leading to thrombocytopenia.
3. **Increased destruction** is probably the most common cause of isolated thrombocytopenia. Disorders that cause increased destruction of platelets can be classified as nonimmunologic or immunologic.
   a. **Nonimmunologic** causes of platelet destruction include the following.
      (1) **Microangiopathic hemolytic anemia (MAHA)** may cause platelet destruction as a result of shearing in small vessels (see also Chapter 69 IV A 1 a). MAHA is often seen in the setting of disseminated intravascular coagulation (DIC) or hemolytic-uremic syndrome/thrombotic thrombocytopenic purpura (HUS/TTP).
      (2) **PNH** causes defects in all cell lines, which predisposes cells to complement-mediated lysis. Therefore, PNH is a **rare** cause of isolated thrombocytopenia.
   b. **Immunologic** causes of platelet destruction include:
      (1) **Drugs.** Heparin, clopidogrel, glycoprotein (Gp) IIb/IIIa inhibitors, and antibiotics (i.e., β-lactam or sulfa drugs) can induce production of antibodies that lead to platelet destruction and clearance.
         (a) There are two types of **Heparin induced thrombocytopenia (HIT)**. Type 1 HIT is a non-immune mediated mild thrombocytopenia with no clinical signs of bleeding or thrombosis. It is safe to continue heparin only in these cases. In **Type 2 immune-mediated HIT**, however, antibodies are produced that bind to platelet receptors, resulting in their activation and clearance. These thrombocytopenic patients paradoxically present with thromboembolic sequelae due to platelet activation. It is imperative to stop heparin in these cases and treat instead with direct thrombin inhibitors (e.g., lepirudin and argatroban).
      (2) **Infections (e.g., tuberculosis)**
      (3) **Rheumatic disease (e.g., systemic lupus erythematosus)**
      (4) **Idiopathic thrombocytopenic purpura (ITP).** An acquired autoimmune disorder in which antiplatelet

antibodies attack and destroy platelets. Children may present with an acute form, usually related to a viral illness, and resolves spontaneously over 3–6 months. In adults, ITP usually follows a chronic course.

C. Approach to the patient

1. **Exclude pseudothrombocytopenia.** Pseudothrombocytopenia is an artifact of platelet clumping in the test tube in EDTA-anticoagulated blood. Look for clumps of platelets in the peripheral blood smear. Sending a heparinized specimen corrects the clumping and confirms your suspicion.

2. **Try to determine the cause of the thrombocytopenia.**

   a. **Patient history.** Pay particular attention to the patient's medications, risk factors for HIV, or a history of substance abuse (e.g., alcohol). A review of systems and asking about "B symptoms" (i.e., fevers, night sweats, and weight loss) may help reveal an occult malignancy.

   b. **Physical examination.** A complete physical examination is always necessary.

      (1) **Splenomegaly** suggests sequestration.

      (2) **Lymphadenopathy** suggests an underlying malignancy or chronic infection.

   c. **Laboratory studies**

      (1) **Peripheral blood smear.** A peripheral blood smear is extremely helpful.

         (a) **Large platelets.** This finding implies increased destruction and early release of platelets from the bone marrow. Large platelets on the peripheral blood smear are a classic finding in ITP.

         (b) **Schistocytes.** The finding of fragmented red blood cells (RBCs) implies MAHA.

         (c) **Leukoerythroblastosis**

            (i) The finding of **early (nucleated) RBCs** and **early white blood cells (WBCs)** [e.g., **bands, metamyelocytes, and myelocytes**] on a peripheral smear implies marrow invasion by malignancy, fibrosis, or infection.

            (ii) **Teardrop cells** (i.e., RBCs shaped like teardrops as a result of being squeezed out of the bone marrow) may be seen in a leukoerythroblastic smear.

         (d) **Megaloblasts** imply vitamin B_{12} or folate deficiency.

         (e) **Neutrophils with bilobed nuclei** (i.e., the Pelger-Huët anomaly) are seen in patients with myelodysplasia.

      (2) The **prothrombin time (PT),** the **partial thromboplastin time (PTT),** and the **lactate dehydrogenase**

(LDH) level may be used to evaluate the possibility of MAHA. **Blood urea nitrogen (BUN)** and **creatinine levels** should be obtained when HUS/TTP is a consideration. (See also Chapter 69 IV A 1 a.)

(3) Serologic studies.

    (a) Antinuclear antibody (ANA) is sent to evaluate for a rheumatologic disorder, such as SLE.

    (b) An HIV and Hepatitis C antibody test is necessary in patients with risk factors.

    (c) Epstein-Barr virus, cytomegalovirus (CMV) and toxoplasmosis serologies are most useful when the patient has systemic symptoms, lymphadenopathy or splenomegaly on examination.

(4) Vitamin B$_{12}$ and folate levels and **tests for PNH** can be sent but are usually not helpful because these disorders are rarely associated with isolated thrombocytopenia.

(5) Antiplatelet antibody testing is usually not performed as it is **not** diagnostic for ITP (which is a diagnosis of exclusion).

(6) HIT antibody testing is performed to confirm a clinical diagnosis of heparin-induced thrombocytopenia. HIT antibodies are heparin-platelet-Factor 4 antibodies. Platelet activation assays are also used, specifically the serotoinin release assay.

d. Bone marrow biopsy is performed in many patients with thrombocytopenia. Pertinent findings include the following.

    (1) Decreased megakaryocytes are diagnostic of one of the production problems. Evidence of the specific cause of the decreased production may also be found (e.g., malignancy, infection).

    (2) Increased megakaryocytes are found when there is increased destruction or sequestration of platelets. Increased megakaryocytes on bone marrow biopsy **without** other identifiable causes of increased destruction or sequestration is usually diagnostic for ITP.

    (3) Evidence for myelodysplasia (e.g., hypercellularity, megaloblastic features, nuclear budding, multinucleated erythroblasts) can also be seen on bone marrow biopsy.

HOT **KEY** If the cause of the patient's thrombocytopenia is identifiable (e.g., clopidogrel), a trial of removing the inciting agent may be both diagnostic and therapeutic, and obviates the need for a bone marrow biopsy.

D. Treatment
1. General treatment
a. Discontinue medications that may cause thrombocytopenia. Usually, the platelet count returns to normal in 7–10 days.

HOT KEY HIT can be caused by any heparin exposure, including heparin flushes for indwelling lines. It is imperative to search for and discontinue all heparin exposures if a diagnosis of HIT Type 2 is made and switch to a direct thrombin inhibitor.

---

b. Platelet transfusions
  (1) Contraindications
   (a) Platelet transfusions are not indicated for patients with platelet counts greater than 20,000 cells/μL and no evidence of bleeding.
   (b) In general, patients with TTP should not receive platelet tranfusions because transfusions may exacerbate the TTP.
  (2) Indications. Platelet transfusions are indicated in the following situations:
   (a) Prior to surgery. The platelet count is usually maintained above 50,000 cells/μL for surgery. Although in patients with ITP, this may be both impossible and unnecessary. When neurosurgery is to be performed, the platelet count is usually maintained above 90,000 cells/μL.
   (b) In a patient with active bleeding
    (i) Severe bleeding. The platelet count is always maintained above 50,000 cells/μL.
    (ii) Mild bleeding or **petechiae.** The platelet count should be maintained above 20,000 cells/μL.
   (c) To prevent spontaneous bleeding. The platelet count is usually kept above 10,000–20,000 cells/μL, depending on physician preference.

HOT KEY Unnecessary platelet transfusions should be avoided because they may induce immune resistance; if this complication occurs, human leukocyte antigen (HLA)-matched platelets can be administered.

---

2. Treatment of ITP
a. Observation is appropriate for patients with platelet counts greater than 20,000 cells/μL and no evidence of bleeding.

    b. Pharmacologic therapy
- **(1) Steroids** (e.g., prednisone, 1 mg/kg/day) benefit approximately two thirds of patients, leading to a significant increase in platelet count in 3 to 7 days. Once platelet response is achieved, steroids should be tapered slowly. Unfortunately, counts often fall again when steroids are being tapered or stopped.
- **(2) Intravenous gammaglobulin** can increase the platelet count faster than steroids, with a significant increase in 1–2 days. It is therefore useful for actively bleeding patients and those with extremely low counts in the "window" before steroids take effect.
- **(3) Anti-D (WinRho) is only effective in Rh positive patients.**
- **(4) Immunosuppressive agents, including rituximab (anti-CD20),** can also be used for patients with ITP.
- **(5) Danazol** is sometimes useful for patients with refractory ITP.

    c. Splenectomy is indicated when steroid therapy fails or relapse occurs following a steroid taper.

E. Follow-up and referral. Consultation with a hematologist is indicated when the cause of the thrombocytopenia cannot be identified despite a thorough evaluation, or when the thrombocytopenia is severe, prolonged, or complicated by bleeding or abnormal clotting.

III THROMBOCYTOSIS

A. Clinical manifestations
1. **Primary thrombocytosis.** If the thrombocytosis is caused by a myeloproliferative disorder, the platelets are frequently abnormal and the patient may be prone to both bleeding and clotting events.
2. **Secondary (reactive) thrombocytosis.** If the thrombocytosis is secondary to another disorder, patients are usually asymptomatic. This is true even with extremely high platelet counts (e.g., greater than 1,000,000 cells/μL).

B. Causes of thrombocytosis
1. **Primary thrombocytosis** is caused by **myeloproliferative disorders,** which increase the platelet count through clonal proliferation of stem cells. The four myeloproliferative disorders are:
   - **a. Essential thrombocytosis,** characterized by prominent proliferation of platelets.
   - **b. Chronic myelogenous leukemia (CML),** characterized by prominent proliferation of the WBC line.

    c. Polycythemia vera, characterized by prominent proliferation of the RBC line.

    d. Myelofibrosis, characterized by prominent proliferation of fibroblasts.

  2. Secondary thrombocytosis is more common than primary thrombocytosis. Causes include:

    a. Malignancies

    b. Infections

    c. Connective tissue disorders

    d. Iron deficiency anemia

    e. Splenectomy

C. Approach to the patient

  1. Patient history

    a. A history of **gastrointestinal bleeding** may imply iron deficiency.

    b. Fevers, night sweats, or **weight loss** may implicate malignancy or chronic infection.

    c. A history of recent **splenectomy** may provide a simple explanation for the thrombocytosis.

  2. Physical examination. Perform a thorough physical examination, including pelvic and rectal examinations. Pay special attention to the spleen and lymph nodes because enlargement may signal malignancy or infection.

  3. Laboratory studies can further narrow the differential diagnosis.

    a. Serum ferritin level. The serum ferritin level helps to evaluate the possibility of iron deficiency anemia.

    b. Hematocrit and **WBC count.** The hematocrit and WBC count are often elevated in patients with myeloproliferative disorders, although essential thrombocytosis may result in an isolated elevation of the platelet count.

    c. Other tests may be performed if a reactive thrombocytosis is suspected [e.g., a purified protein derivative (PPD) test for possible tuberculosis].

D. Treatment

  1. Primary thrombocytosis. Hydroxyurea should be considered for patients with marked thrombocytosis (i.e., a platelet count greater than 700,000 cells/μL), or if symptomatic thromboses occur.

  2. Secondary thrombocytosis. Most patients with reactive thrombocytosis do not require treatment. The platelet count usually returns to normal following treatment of the underlying disorder.

E. Follow-up and referral

  1. A hematologist can provide recommendations concerning long-term therapy for patients with thrombocytosis that is caused by a myeloproliferative disorder.

2. Most other cases of thrombocytosis respond to treatment of the underlying disorder, and platelet counts should be followed every 1–4 weeks until they return to normal. Patients with persistent abnormalities require referral.

References

Chong BH, Ho SJ. Autoimmune thrombocytopenia. *J Thromb Haemos* 2005;3:1763–1772.

Davoren A, Aster RA. Heparin induced thrombocytopenia and thrombosis. *Am J Hematol* 2006;81:36–44.

George JN. Thrombotic thrombocytopenic purpura. *NEJM* 2006;354(18):1927–1935.

72. Leukocytosis

I INTRODUCTION

A. The **circulating pool of white blood cells** (WBCs, leukocytes) consists of:
1. **Neutrophils**
2. **Lymphocytes**
3. **Monocytes**
4. **Eosinophils**
5. **Basophils**

B. Definitions
1. **Leukocytosis.** In leukocytosis, the total WBC count **exceeds 11,000 cells/mm³ (11 × 10⁹/L).**
2. **Leukemoid reaction.** A leukemoid reaction is said to occur when the leukocyte count **exceeds 30,000 cells/mm³** and there is no evidence of immature WBCs or nucleated red blood cells (RBCs) on the peripheral smear. This process reflects a healthy bone marrow that is reacting to some type of stress (e.g., trauma, inflammation, infection, malignancy).
3. **Leukoerythroblastosis.** This term is used when there is evidence of immature WBCs or nucleated RBCs on the peripheral smear, regardless of the total WBC count. Leukoerythroblastosis usually implies bone marrow infiltration (e.g., from tumor or marrow fibrosis).

C. Because each cell type can be increased in response to various stimuli, determining the predominant cell type in patients with leukocytosis may offer some insight into the cause.

II TYPES OF LEUKOCYTOSIS

A. Neutrophilia is defined as a neutrophil count that **exceeds 7700 cells/mm³.**
1. **Causes of neutrophilia.** Neutrophilia can be caused by many of the major disease categories listed in Chapter 1 II B 2 (Table 72-1).
2. **Approach to the patient**
   a. When evaluating patients with neutrophilia (especially with a left shift), the most important initial consideration should be **infection.**

TABLE 72-1. Common Causes of Neutrophilia

Category of Disease	Specific Causes
Hematologic	Hemolytic anemia, splenectomy
Pregnancy-related	Pregnancy-induced neutrophilia
Drugs/toxins	Corticosteroids, lithium, catecholamines, GM-CSF
Metabolic/endocrine	Hyperthyroidism, ketoacidosis
Inflammatory	Rheumatoid arthritis, vasculitis, gout
Infectious	Bacteria, viruses, fungi, parasites
Neoplastic	Myeloproliferative disorders, myelodysplastic syndromes, gastrointestinal or renal malignancy, melanoma, Hodgkin's disease
Trauma	Insect bites, jellyfish stings, crush injuries, electric shock

   b. If this and other benign disorders are excluded, a search for **malignancy** (which may necessitate a bone marrow biopsy) is usually warranted.

HOT KEY

Acutely infected or injured patients have elevated levels of endogenous glucocorticoids, which, in turn, lead to low levels of eosinophils and basophils. The presence of eosinophils and basophils in critically ill patients with neutrophilia may indicate relative adrenal insufficiency, a granulocyte-macrophage colony-stimulating factor (GM-CSF)—secreting tumor, or a hematologic malignancy.

B. Lymphocytosis is defined as a lymphocyte count that **exceeds 4000 cells/mm^3**.
   1. Causes of lymphocytosis. The severity of the lymphocytosis is usually indicative of the cause (Table 72-2).
   2. Approach to the patient. Look for leukoerythroblastosis on the peripheral smear.
      a. If **leukoerythroblastosis** is **present, malignancy** is likely and bone marrow biopsy is necessary.
      b. If **leukoerythroblastosis** is **not present, infection** is likely. A bone marrow biopsy is necessary if the diagnosis remains unclear.
C. Monocytosis is defined as a monocyte count that **exceeds 800 cells/mm^3**. Monocytes play an important role in **killing obligate**

TABLE 72-2. Common Causes of Lymphocytosis

Type of Lymphocytosis	Specific Causes
Mild to moderate (4000–15,000/mm^3)	Viral illness (mononucleosis, hepatitis)
	Secondary to other infections (e.g., tuberculosis, toxoplasmosis, syphilis)
	Malignancy (e.g., Hodgkin's disease, early CLL)
Severe (>15,000/mm^3)	Mononucleosis
	Hepatitis
	Pertussis
	Late CLL
	ALL
	LGL

ALL = acute lymphocytic leukemia; CLL = chronic lymphocytic leukemia; LGL = large granulocytic leukemia.

intracellular parasites and are associated with granulomatous inflammation.

1. **Causes of monocytosis** are given in Table 72-3.
2. **Approach to the patient.** If the levels of monocytes are extremely high, a hematologic malignancy should be suspected.

D. Eosinophilia. Eosinophils normally dwell in the tissues. Eosinophilia is defined as an eosinophil count that exceeds 600 cells/mm^3. Counts are highest in the morning and fall during the day as glucocorticoid levels increase. Causes of eosinophilia include the following.

1. **Pulmonary disease.** Many primary lung disorders can lead to eosinophilia, including **Löffler's syndrome, hypersensitivity pneumonitis,** and **eosinophilic pneumonia.**

TABLE 72-3. Common Causes of Monocytosis

Category of Disease	Specific Causes
Infectious	Tuberculosis, endocarditis, brucellosis, syphilis, fungal or protozoal infections, listeriosis
Neoplastic	Hodgkin's disease, leukemia, carcinoma
Inflammatory	Inflammatory bowel disease, sarcoidosis

2. **Helminthic infections**. Eosinophils play a major role in defending the host against multicellular, helminthic parasites. Examples of helminthic infections include:
   a. **Filariasis**
   b. **Ascariasis**
   c. **Schistosomiasis**
   d. **Trichinosis**
   e. *Strongyloides* **infection**

HOT KEY

Disseminated *Strongyloides* infection sometimes does not cause eosinophilia because of the superimposed bacterial infection that may accompany parasitic dissemination.

3. **Other infections** may also be associated with eosinophilia.
   a. **Allergic bronchopulmonary aspergillosis**

HOT KEY

Invasive aspergillosis does not cause eosinophilia.

   b. **Coccidioidomycosis**
   c. **Tuberculosis,** especially chronic tuberculosis
4. **Although rarely seen now, contaminated L-tryptophan** can cause eosinophilia-myalgia syndrome.
5. **Immunologic disorders,** such as vasculitis (especially Churg-Strauss syndrome), severe rheumatoid arthritis, and eosinophilic fasciitis, can cause eosinophilia.
6. **Addison's disease (corticosteroid deficiency)** can be associated with eosinophilia.
7. **Cutaneous disorders** associated with eosinophilia include **bullous pemphigoid, scabies,** and **eosinophilic cellulitis.**
8. **Allergic disorders.** Eosinophils induce the release of allergic mediators by mast cells and basophils. Therefore, eosinophilia is often seen in **asthma, allergic rhinitis, atopic dermatitis, drug reactions, acute urticaria,** and other allergic disorders.
9. **Hematologic and neoplastic disorders.** Solid tumors of epithelial origin, mucus-secreting tumors, lymphoma, leukemia, myeloproliferative disorders, and hypereosinophilic syndrome can lead to eosinophilia.

	Causes of Eosinophilia
	P H I L I A → C A N
	A C T→F A S T
	Pulmonary disease
	Helminthic infections
	Filariasis
	Ascariasis
MNEMONIC	**S**chistosomiasis or **S**trongyloides infection
	Trichinosis
	Infections, in general
	Allergic bronchopulmonary aspergillosis
	Coccidioidomycosis
	Tuberculosis (especially chronic)
	L-Tryptophan
	Immunologic disorders
	Addison's disease
	Cutaneous disorders, **C**hurg-Strauss syndrome
	Allergic disorders
	Neoplasms

III FOLLOW-UP AND REFERRAL

A. Follow-up. During the process of evaluation, the patient should be seen every 2–4 weeks.

B. Referral. A referral to a hematologist can be helpful when the diagnosis remains unclear after a preliminary evaluation. Referral to a hematologist is necessary when a hematologic malignancy or bone marrow biopsy is being contemplated.

References

Zander DS. Allergic Bronchopulmonary aspergillosis. *Arch Pathol Lab Med* 2005; 129:924–928.

Cottin V, Cordier JF. Eosinophilic pneumonias. *Allergy* 2005;60:841–857.

73. Bleeding Disorders

I **INTRODUCTION.** A predisposition to bleeding can result from **problems with platelets** (either number or function) or **problems with coagulation** (factor deficiency or factor inhibitors).

II **CLINICAL MANIFESTATIONS OF BLEEDING DISORDERS**

A. **Inherited problems. Recurrent bleeding since childhood** or a **family history of bleeding** implies an inherited coagulation factor deficiency or an inherited problem with platelet function.

B. **Platelet problems** usually cause **mucocutaneous petechiae** or **ecchymoses.**

C. **Coagulation problems** are suspected in patients with **spontaneous deep bleeding** into hematomas or joints (hemarthroses) or **delayed bleeding** after surgery or trauma.

III **APPROACH TO THE PATIENT.** Figure 73-1 summarizes the general approach to a patient with a bleeding disorder.

A. **Platelet count.** Check the platelet count first. If the patient has a normal or mildly decreased count, the patient may have a platelet function disorder. Bleeding time is now rarely used to test platelet function. Newer techniques, involving semi-automated platelet function analyzers, are being developed and validated to better assess platelet functionality.

B. **Prothrombin time (PT)/partial thromboplastin time (PTT).** There are three types of PT/PTT abnormalities: increased PT/ normal PTT, increased PT and PTT, and normal PT/increased PTT.

   1. **Increased PT/normal PTT**

      a. **Differential diagnoses**

         (1) Early disseminated intravascular coagulation (DIC)

         (2) Liver disease

         (3) Warfarin therapy

         (4) Vitamin K deficiency

         (5) Factor VII deficiency (rare)

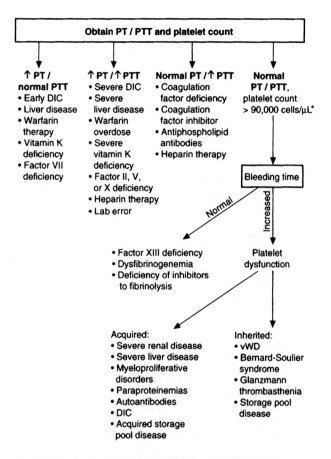

Obtain PT / PTT and platelet count

↑ PT / normal PTT	↑ PT / ↑ PTT	Normal PT / ↑ PTT	Normal PT / PTT, platelet count > 90,000 cells/μL*
• Early DIC	• Severe DIC	• Coagulation factor deficiency	
• Liver disease	• Severe liver disease	• Coagulation factor inhibitor	
• Warfarin therapy	• Warfarin overdose	• Antiphospholipid antibodies	
• Vitamin K deficiency	• Severe vitamin K deficiency	• Heparin therapy	
• Factor VII deficiency	• Factor II, V, or X deficiency		
	• Heparin therapy		
	• Lab error		

Bleeding time

Normal / *Increased*

• Factor XIII deficiency
• Dysfibrinogenemia
• Deficiency of inhibitors to fibrinolysis

Platelet dysfunction

Acquired:
• Severe renal disease
• Severe liver disease
• Myeloproliferative disorders
• Paraproteinemias
• Autoantibodies
• DIC
• Acquired storage pool disease

Inherited:
• vWD
• Bernard-Soulier syndrome
• Glanzmann thrombasthenia
• Storage pool disease

* A platelet count less than 90,000 cells/μL may result in an increased bleeding time and a bleeding disorder. Patients with platelet counts greater than 90,000 cells/μL may still be thrombocytopenic (i.e., a platelet count less than 150,000 cells/μL), but this level of thrombocytopenia is usually not the cause of a bleeding disorder; therefore, other causes should be considered.

FIGURE 73-1. Approach to the patient with a bleeding disorder. *DIC* = disseminated intravascular coagulation; *PT* = prothrombin time; *PTT* = partial thromboplastin time; *vWD* = von Willebrand's disease.

   b. Recommended work-up
      (1) Patient history. Ask about medications and note factors that may predispose a patient to vitamin K deficiency (e.g., malnutrition, alcoholism, pancreatic

insufficiency, recent antibiotic use). DIC is associated with predisposing conditions including sepsis, burns, trauma, malignancies, and pregnancy-related conditions (i.e., HELLP and placental abruption).

  (2) **DIC panel** and **peripheral smear.** Evidence for DIC may include a low **fibrinogen** level, elevated **D-dimers** or **schistocytes** on the peripheral blood smear. Keep in mind that D-dimers may also be elevated in patients with liver or renal disease or with bleeding, and hypofibrinogenemia may occur with severe liver dysfunction. Schistocytes may be the only distinguishing feature of DIC.

  (3) **Liver function tests** (bilirubin, albumin, and transaminase levels) are also obtained.

  (4) A **factor VII level** is rarely necessary but obtained if the cause of an increased PT is still unknown.

2. **Increased PT and PTT**

  a. **Differential diagnoses.** Generally, more severe versions of the same conditions that cause an isolated elevated PT cause an increase in both the PT and PTT.

  (1) DIC

  (2) Severe liver disease

  (3) Warfarin overdose

  (4) Severe vitamin K deficiency

  (5) Factor II, V, or X deficiency (rare)

  (6) Heparin therapy (usually the PT is only mildly increased)

  (7) Laboratory error: **if the test tube is underfilled.**

  b. **Recommended work-up.** First, repeat the test. The recommended evaluation is the same as that for increased PT/normal PTT. But on the rare occasion of a completely negative work-up, different factor levels need to be tested.

3. **Normal PT/increased PTT**

  a. **Differential diagnoses.** After excluding **heparin** therapy as an obvious cause, there are three main possibilities to consider.

  (1) Coagulation factor deficiency

  (2) Coagulation factor inhibitor

  (3) Antiphospholipid antibodies

HOT

KEY
Moderate to severe von Willebrand's disease disease may lead to elevated PTT due to FVIII deficiency. The lack of adequate vWF to bind and protect FVIII from clearance can lead to low FVIII levels.

b. Recommended work-up

(1) Patient history. If the patient has a history of bleeding, a factor deficiency or a factor inhibitor is likely. If the patient has a history of clotting, an antiphospholipid syndrome is implicated.

(2) 50:50 mixing study. Only 30% factor activity is needed to have a normal PTT. By mixing the patient's blood with an equal amount of blood with normal coagulation (i.e., blood with a normal PTT), enough factor will be provided to correct any factor deficiency.

(a) If the PTT corrects (and stays corrected on later testing) a **factor deficiency** is diagnosed. The most common factor deficiencies are **factor VIII** (hemophilia A), **factor IX** (hemophilia B), and **factor XI** deficiencies. Send these factor levels first.

(b) If the PTT does not correct with mixing, an **antiphospholipid antibody** or a **factor inhibitor** is present. Send laboratory tests for lupus anticoagulant and anticardiolipin antibody.

(c) If the PTT initially corrects, but prolongs on later testing, a **factor inhibitor** is probably present (i.e., the added factor has been consumed by the inhibitor). **Factor VIII inhibitor is the most common and FVIII assays should be checked first.**

C. Bleeding time

1. Bleeding time starts to prolong when the platelet count is less than 100,000 cells/μl. Therefore, if the platelet count is only mildly decreased or normal and the bleeding time is prolonged, a concurrent problem of platelet function or coagulation must exist. Bleeding time is now rarely used, as it is poorly sensitive to mild platelet function abnormalities and a poor predictor of surgical bleeding risk. It is also dependent on technical expertise and an imprecise endpoint. Instead, semi-automated platelet function analyzers are now being developed to better test platelet function.

a. Differential diagnoses for acquired platelet disorders. These are usually systemic.

(1) Severe renal disease leading to uremia can cause platelet dysfunction.

(2) Severe liver disease. Liver disease not only leads to factor deficiencies, it causes coagulopathy via platelet dysfunction.

(3) Malignancy. Multiple myeloma, Waldenström's macroglobulinemia and myeloproliferative disorders can lead to platelet dysfunction.

(4) Autoantibodies [from β-lactam antibiotic therapy or idiopathic thrombocytopenic purpura (ITP)] can coat platelets and increase the bleeding time even with a normal platelet count.

(5) DIC. The fibrin split products produced in DIC inhibit platelet function.

(6) Acquired storage pool disease. Cardiopulmonary bypass surgery or vasculitis can cause platelets to release all of their granules, resulting in dysfunctional platelets.

(7) Aspirin irreversibly inhibits platelet function for the life of the platelet (7–10 days); other nonsteroidal anti-inflammatory drugs (NSAIDs) reversibly inhibit platelet function and the effect is more transient.

(8) Gp IIb/IIIa inhibitors are used in the management of patients with acute coronary syndromes. They bind to the Gp IIb/IIIa receptor preventing platelet aggregation.

   (a) Clopidogrel and ticlopidine irreversibly inhibit the binding of ADP to its receptor on the platelet membrane, ultimately leading to decreased platelet aggregation.

(9) Recommended work-up

   (a) Patient history. A medication history—(including all over-the-counter drugs) should always be obtained. Also ask for a history of ITP.

   (b) A **complete blood count (CBC) with differential** will help evaluate the possibility of a myeloproliferative disorder.

   (c) Obtain a **DIC panel** to evaluate for DIC.

   (d) Liver function tests and **blood urea nitrogen (BUN)** and **creatine levels** help exclude liver and renal disease, respectively.

   (e) Protein electrophoresis may be used to detect a paraproteinemia.

b. Inherited platelet dysfunction. Normally, platelets first adhere to the endothelium during injury, and then aggregate by binding fibrinogen.

   (1) Differential diagnoses. The first two disorders involve **problems with platelet adherence,** and the second two involve **problems with platelet aggregation.**

   (a) von Willebrand's disease (vWD). vWD is the most common inherited bleeding disorder. von Willebrand's factor (vWF) is made by megakaryocytes and endothelial cells. It circulates in the plasma in multimers of varying size and binds factor VIII, protecting it from clearance. vWF binds to the glycoprotein Ib receptor on platelets, and helps platelets adhere to each other and to the endothelium.

  (i) In **type 1 vWD** (80% of cases), there is a decreased quantity of vWF.

 (ii) In **type 3 vWD,** there is a complete absence of vWF.

(iii) In **type 2 vWD,** there are qualitative abnormalities in the vWF molecule. Type 2A vWD involves a decrease in the formation of the large multimers of vWF. Type 2B vWD involves abnormal vWF binding to platelets that results in decreased formation of the large multimers of vWF. Type 2M vWD involves a defect in the binding of vWF to the platelet receptor (glycoprotein Ib). Finally, Type 2N vWD results from decreased binding of FVIII to vWF.

(b) Bernard-Soulier syndrome results from a reduced or abnormal expression of the platelet receptor for vWF (glycoprotein Ib).

(c) Glanzmann's thrombasthenia results from qualitative or quantitative abnormalities in Gp IIa/IIIb glycoprotein platelet receptor expression. This defect leads to decreased fibrinogen binding and, therefore, decreased platelet aggregation.

(d) Storage pool disease is caused by the defective release of platelet granules, which results in decreased platelet aggregation.

(2) Recommended work-up

(a) Patient history. Obtain any family history regarding bleeding disorders.

(b) vWD panel. Screen for vWD first because it is the most common inherited disorder of platelet function. A vWD panel includes the following tests.

  (i) **vWF antigen level**

 (ii) **Ristocetin cofactor activity test** measures the activity level of vWF. The patient's plasma is mixed with normal platelets and ristocetin. Ristocetin should cause plasma vWF to bind to the platelet surface, resulting in platelet aggregation. Lack of aggregation implies vWD.

(iii) **Factor VIII activity** may be decreased with a decrease in vWF level resulting in a prolonged PTT (mainly in moderate to severe disease).

(iv) **vWF multimer assay.** Detects distribution of vWF multimers via electrophoresis.

(v) **Ristocetin-induced platelet agglutination (RIPA) test** detects Type 2B vWD, where lower than normal levels of ristocetin aggregate the patient's platelet-rich plasma.

> **HOT**
> ▶
> **KEY**
>
> Type 1 vWD often causes a parallel decrease in all parts of the panel, while type 3 vWD demonstrates no activity in any part of the panel. In type 2 vWD, there will be decreased ristocetin cofactor activity out of proportion to the decreased factor VIII antigen level.

(c) **Platelet aggregation tests** involve the addition of agonists (ADP, thrombin, collagen, or ristocetin) to the patient's plasma and platelets. **Bernard-Soulier syndrome** is diagnosed by an abnormal ristocetin aggregation test but normal platelet aggregation tests with the other agonists. The ristocetin aggregation test in Bernard-Soulier patients is corrected with the addition of normal platelets. On the other hand, in vWD patients this test only corrects with the addition of normal plasma, which contains vWF.

(d) **Platelet aggregometry** is used to diagnose **Glanzmann's thrombasthenia** and **storage pool diseases.**

(3) If platelet function is normal (via bleeding time or platelet function analyzer tests) in a patient with a normal PT/PTT and platelet count, but there is still clinical suspicion of a bleeding diathesis, rare disorders that involve a defect in cross-linking of fibrin should be considered. These disorders include:

   a. Dysfibrinogenemia
   b. Factor XIII ("fibrin-stabilizing factor") deficiency
   c. Deficiency of inhibitors to fibrinolysis (i.e., plasminogen activator inhibitor or α_2 plasmin inhibitor)

IV TREATMENT

A. Platelet problems
   1. Quantitative problems. Patients may require platelet transfusions (see Chapter 71 II D 1 b).
   2. Qualitative problems are usually only treated when the patient is bleeding or surgery is planned. The use of aspirin and NSAIDs should be avoided.

    a. Desmopressin (DDAVP), 0.3 μg/kg per day, works by increasing the release of stored vWF and FVIII from endothelial cells. This drug can be used for disorders of platelet function (e.g., uremia or Type 1 vWD).

       (1) Stores of vWF are depleted in 2–3 days, so desmopressin is only a short-term treatment.

       (2) Desmopressin is ineffective in type 3 vWD. In type 2B vWD, large multimers of vWF are already stuck to platelets, and exposure to desmopressin can trigger paradoxical thromboses and thrombocytopenia (from splenic removal). Therefore, the use of desmopressin should be avoided in patients with these subtypes.

    b. Cryoprecipitate and **platelet transfusions** may be necessary for patients who have been hospitalized as a result of refractory bleeding.

    c. vWF concentrates are used in vWD when bleeding is not controlled with DDAVP.

    d. Humate P contains vWF and is labeled with vWF ristocetin cofactor units.

    e. Adjunctive agents include **antifibrinolytic agents (Amicar)** and topical agents **(fibrin sealant).**

    f. Specific therapies may include dialysis for uremia, myelosuppression for myeloproliferative disorders, or steroids for immune disorders.

B. Coagulation problems

  1. Vitamin K (10 mg subcutaneously or PO, daily for 3 days) should be administered routinely, in case vitamin K deficiency has a primary or contributing role.

  2. Warfarin. If the PT is higher than desired, the **warfarin dose** is usually **decreased** or **withheld,** and the PT is rechecked daily. Vitamin K can be administered at low doses (1 mg IV or PO) to gradually lower the PT in patients with marked PT elevations (INR > 9). Remember, there is approximately a 3-day lag between the changes in warfarin dose and the changes in the PT.

  3. Factor replacement

    a. Factor deficiencies. Hemophilia A and B are treated with **factor VIII** and **IX concentrates** respectively; other factor deficiencies are replaced with **fresh frozen plasma.**

    b. Factor inhibitors. Aggressive factor replacement (to "overwhelm" the inhibitor) can be tried. Activated factor VII can be used for patients with factor VIII inhibitors, thereby bypassing the point in the coagulation pathway where factor VIII is needed.

  4. Plasmapheresis can be used to remove factor inhibitors.

5. **Steroids** and **other immunosuppressants** (e.g., **cyclophos-phamide)** are used for chronic therapy in patients with factor inhibitor disorders.
6. **Fresh frozen plasma** and **cryoprecipitate** may be helpful for hospitalized patients with bleeding.

References

DiMichele DM. Management of Factor VIII Inhibitors. *Intern J Hematol* 2006;83(2):119–125.

Sadler EJ. New Concepts in von Willebrand Disease. *Annu Rev Med* 2005;56:173–191.

74. Lymphadenopathy

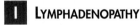

LYMPHADENOPATHY

A. Introduction

1. In lymphadenopathy, the lymph nodes are enlarged or have an abnormal consistency. Lymphadenopathy can be regional (i.e., affecting one group or a few contiguous groups of nodes) or generalized. Lymphadenopathy usually signals the presence of regional or systemic disease and therefore warrants medical evaluation.

2. Lymphadenopathy must not be confused with lymphangitis or lymphadenitis.

   a. **Lymphangitis** is inflammation of the lymphatics. Generally, red streaks that pass from a wound toward the draining lymph node are seen in lymphangitis.

   b. **Lymphadenitis,** a subtype of lymphadenopathy, is inflammation of the lymph node. The affected node is red, enlarged and tender.

HOT

KEY

Both lymphangitis and lymphadenitis are classically caused by streptococcal or staphylococcal infection.

B. Causes of lymphadenopathy.
There are numerous causes of lymphadenopathy; fortunately, four factors help guide the work-up and narrow the differential.

1. **Location of the lymphadenopathy**

   a. **Generalized lymphadenopathy.** If the lymphadenopathy involves more than two separate sites, the most likely causes can be remembered with the mnemonic, "SHE HAS CUTE LAN (lymphadenopathy)."

	Causes of Generalized Lymphadenopathy ("SHE HAS CUTE LAN")
MNEMONIC	**S**yphilis **H**epatitis **E**pstein-Barr virus **H**istoplasmosis **A**IDS/HIV **S**erum sickness **C**ytomegalovirus (CMV) **U**nusual drugs (e.g., phenytoin, carbamazepine, antithyroid medications, isoniazid) **T**oxoplasmosis, tuberculosis (TB) (including miliary) **E**rythrophagocytic lymphohistiocytosis **L**eishmaniasis **A**utoimmune (rheumatoid, SLE) **N**eoplasms (i.e., leukemia, lymphoma)

  b. Localized lymphadenopathy. Causes of localized lymphadenopathy are given in Table 74-1.
  2. HIV status of the patient. HIV status must always be considered whenever a patient has lymphadenopathy, regional or generalized. The lymphadenopathy can be caused by HIV itself or by other systemic diseases that are common in HIV-infected patients. In primary HIV, generalized lymphadenopathy usually occurs in the second week of an acute symptomatic HIV infection.
  3. Clinical scenario
    a. Patient age. Lymphadenopathy in patients younger than 30 years is usually benign and caused by an infection, whereas in patients older than 30 years, malignancy becomes a more worrisome possibility.
       As many as 50% of patients younger than 50 years have palpable cervical lymphadenopathy. Significant cervical, axillary, or inguinal lymphadenopathy in patients older than 60 years usually represents a serious underlying disorder.
    b. Associated findings
       (1) Symptoms of **fever, chills, night sweats,** and **weight loss** ("B" symptoms) usually imply a serious systemic infection or malignancy.
       (2) Symptoms or signs of a **local infection** or **trauma** usually imply a non-malignant etiology.
       (3) Exposures (e.g., cigarette smoke, cats, STDs, undercooked meats) should also be ascertained.

TABLE 74-1. Causes of Localized Lymphadenopathy	
Location of Lymphadenopathy	Potential Causes
Cervical nodes	Head or neck malignancy or infection Mononucleosis Tuberculosis Lymphoma
Supraclavicular nodes	Lung or gastrointestinal malignancy Lymphoma
Axillary nodes	Hand or arm infection or trauma (including bites) Cat-scratch disease Lymphoma Brucellosis Breast cancer
Epitrochlear nodes	Unilateral: hand infections, lymphoma, tularemia Bilateral: sarcoidosis, syphilis
Inguinal nodes	Leg or foot infections Pelvic malignancy Lymphoma Sexually transmitted diseases (STDs)
Hilar or mediastinal nodes	Sarcoidosis Tuberculosis Lymphoma Fungal infection Lung cancer
Abdominal nodes	Lymphoma Tuberculosis *Mycobacterium avium-intracellulare* infection Metastatic malignancy

4. **Characteristics of the node on palpation.** The physical attributes of the affected lymph nodes may assist in narrowing the differential diagnosis, although physical examination findings can be misleading. The following correlations tend to be true:

   a. **Infections** are associated with rapid growth of the node, causing **tender nodes** from capsular stretching. In addition, the nodes tend to be **asymmetric** and the overlying skin tends to be **erythematous.**

   b. **Lymphoma** classically leads to **large, firm, rubbery, non-tender nodes.**

    c. Metastatic cancer usually results in **very firm ("rock hard") non-tender nodes** that are **immobile** (i.e., fixed to the underlying tissue).

C. Approach to the patient

1. **Ensure that the lymph nodes are truly abnormal.** Certain lymph nodes [e.g., the submandibular nodes (in young adults) and the inguinal nodes] are commonly palpable. The submandibular and inguinal nodes should measure less than 1 and 2 centimeters, respectively.

2. **Generate a differential diagnosis** based on the location of the lymphadenopathy, the HIV status of the patient, the clinical scenario, and the physical attributes of the node. The differential will help you determine which laboratory and imaging studies to order initially.

3. **Laboratory testing may include a** complete blood count (CBC), peripheral blood smear, monospot test, hepatitis serologies, HIV test, serum lactate dehydrogenase (LDH) level, sedimentation rate, and Venereal Disease Research Laboratory (VDRL) test.

4. Perform fine needle aspiration (FNA) or an excisional biopsy of the node if lymphoma or metastatic malignancy is likely. FNA is good for diagnosing metastatic malignancies and infections. With the advent of flow cytometry, FNA has also been increasingly used to diagnose lymphomas, but its sensitivity and specificity are still inferior to excisional biopsy. If lymphoma is a strong possibility, obtain an excisional biopsy. With a biopsy, pathologists avoid sampling error and inadequate material, and they can evaluate the lymph node architecture and better distinguish reactive versus malignant cells.

5. **Consider a period of observation if the most likely diagnosis is infection.** In those with a likely bacterial cause (e.g., *Streptococcus, Staphylococcus*), a trial of antibiotics for the suspected organism is appropriate. If there is no evidence of resolution after 2–3 weeks, fine needle aspiration, an excisional biopsy, or both is usually required.

D. Treatment depends on the underlying cause.

E. Follow-up and referral

1. **Follow-up.** It is important to follow patients every 1–2 weeks until a diagnosis is made or the lymphadenopathy resolves.

    a. Lymphadenopathy as a result of infection or inflammation resolves within 3 weeks in most patients.

    b. Follow-up is essential for patients with lymphadenopathy of unclear etiology, because a small but significant percentage of these patients develop lymphoma within 1 year.

2. **Referral.** If the patient has lymphoma or another malignancy, prompt referral to a hematologist-oncologist is necessary.

TABLE 74-2. Comparison of Hodgkin's Disease and Non-Hodgkin's Lymphoma (NHL)

	Hodgkin's Disease	NHL
Cause	Unknown; viral cause suspected	Unknown, although Burkitt's lymphoma is associated with Epstein-Barr virus infection
Malignant cell line	B cell	B cell: 90% T cell: 10%
Site of origin	Nodal	Extranodal (in as many as 40% of cases)
Spread	Contiguous	Non-contiguous
Mediastinal involvement	Common	Rare
Bone marrow involvement	Rare	Very common in low grade NHL; unusual in high-grade NHL
Systemic or "B" symptoms	Very common	Seen in fewer than 50% of patients
Best prognostic indicator	Stage*	Grade*

*"Stage" refers to the extent of spread of the tumor, while "grade" refers to the degree of differentiation (i.e., histopathology).

II **Lymphoma** is a malignant disorder of the lymphoreticular system. When patients first notice lymphadenopathy, they are usually most concerned about lymphoma. It is important for primary care providers to have an overview of lymphoma in order to counsel their patients appropriately.

A. Introduction. Lymphoma is classified as belonging to one of two groups. Distinguishing the two is important because the treatment and prognosis depend on the type of lymphoma.
  1. The classification is based on the histologic presence or absence of Reed-Sternberg cells (bilobed, double or multinucleated large cells with prominent nucleoli).
    a. Hodgkin's lymphoma. Reed-Sternberg cells are present.
    b. Non-Hodgkin's lymphoma (NHL). Reed-Sternberg cells are absent.
  2. Hodgkin's disease and NHL are compared in Table 74-2.
B. Hodgkin's lymphoma (HL)
  1. Epidemiology

    a. Incidence. Fewer than 10,000 cases of Hodgkin's disease are diagnosed in the United States each year.

    b. Patient profile

        (1) HL has a **bimodal age distribution.** Patients are most often between the ages of 20 and 30 years or older than 55 years.

        (2) **Men** are affected more often than women.

        (3) **Caucasians** are affected more often than African-Americans.

        (4) In developed countries, HL of the nodular sclerosis subtype in young adults is often associated with **middle- to upper-class socioeconomic status, advanced educational status,** and **small family size.** This association is inverted for HL of other subtypes, such as the mixed cellularity subtype.

2. Clinical manifestations

    a. Painless, superficial lymphadenopathy (usually involving the cervical or supraclavicular nodes) may be noted on physical examination, or **mediastinal lymphadenopathy** may be seen on a chest radiograph.

    b. Constitutional ("B") symptoms (i.e., fever, night sweats, and weight loss) and **severe pruritus** are common patient complaints.

    c. Immunologic dysfunction develops with the onset of the lymphoma and is key in its pathogenesis. It is manifested as:

        (1) A loss of cell-mediated immunity (with cutaneous anergy)

        (2) A decrease in the ratio of T helper cells to T suppressor cells

        (3) Lymphopenia and an increased susceptibility to infection as the disease progresses

---

HOT KEY An increased incidence of Hodgkin's lymphoma is seen in HIV (at least seven-fold) and organ transplant patients. This can be seen in the setting of near normal CD4 counts. The risk for non-Hodgkins lymphoma is even greater.

---

3. Disease progression. Unlike NHL, Hodgkin's disease progresses in an **orderly** fashion.

    a. Initially, the tumor spreads to the anatomically adjacent lymph tissues.

    b. Hematogenous spread to the liver, bone marrow, and other viscera occurs in advanced disease.

C. NHL

1. Epidemiology

a. Incidence. The incidence of NHL is four times that of Hodgkin's lymphoma. With HIV/AIDS, the incidence of NHL has only increased further.

b. Patient profile

(1) Men are affected more often than women.

(2) Caucasians are affected more often than African-Americans.

(3) NHL is more common in **immunocompromised patients** (e.g., patients with AIDS, congenital immunodeficiencies, or autoimmune disease; those receiving immunosuppressive therapy).

2. Clinical manifestations.

The presentation depends on the site and subtype of tumor (over 20 different subtypes). Common complaints include:

a. Asymptomatic superficial lymphadenopathy

b. Constitutional ("B") symptoms (much less common than in Hodgkin's disease and with less prognostic significance)

c. Abdominal complaints (e.g., fullness, discomfort). The GI tract is the most common extranodal site for NHL.

d. Bone pain or pathologic fractures

e. Symptoms related to pancytopenia

f. Acute emergencies (e.g., superior vena cava syndrome, spinal cord compression, airway compression)

3. Disease progression.

Unlike Hodgkin's disease, the spread of tumor in NHL is **not contiguous.**

D. Treatment.

Both types of lymphoma are treatable; patients should be referred to a hematologist-oncologist for therapy.

References

Navarro WH, Kaplan LD. AIDS-related lymphoproliferative disease. *Blood* 2006;107(1):13–20.

Poppema S. Immunobiology and Pathophysiology of Hodgkin Lymphomas. *Hematology (Am Soc Hem Education Educ Prog)* 2005;231–238.

PART XI

ENDOCRINOLOGY

• •

75. Diabetes Mellitus
....

I INTRODUCTION

A. Diabetes mellitus (DM) affects over 9% of the United States population (more than **19 million Americans).** The disease is the leading cause of adult blindness, end-stage renal disease, and nontraumatic amputation, and it is a major risk factor for cardiovascular disease (CVD) and stroke.

B. **Classification of Diabetes** according to the American Diabetes Association (ADA) criteria.

1. **Type 1.** 5–10% of patients with DM have type 1 DM, which usually presents in childhood or early adulthood. The disorder is caused by autoimmune destruction of the insulin-secreting beta cells in the pancreas. Patients develop an absolute deficiency of insulin and ultimately require daily injections to prevent severe hyperglycemia and diabetic ketoacidosis.

   a. Some patients with type 1 DM (usually of African or Asian ancestry) have **idiopathic diabetes** with no evidence of autoimmunity and an intermittent absolute requirement for insulin therapy.

   b. Controversy exists regarding the distinction between type 1 diabetes initially presenting in adulthood and **latent autoimmune diabetes in adults (LADA),** which is also characterized by the presence of typical circulating autoantibodies (e.g. anti-glutamic acid dehydrogenase [anti-GAD], anti-islet cell antibody [anti-ICA]) and is often optimally treated with insulin.

2. **Type 2.** Most diabetic patients (90–95%) have type 2 DM. Obesity is a risk factor for this type of diabetes. Hyperglycemia in these patients is attributable to a combination of factors: impaired pancreatic insulin secretion, insulin resistance in peripheral tissues, and increased hepatic glucose production.

3. **Other specific types of diabetes**.
   a. **Maturity-onset diabetes of the young** (MODY) comprises several single-gene defects of the beta cell, characterized by impaired insulin secretion and normal insulin action. These disorders are inherited in an autosomal dominant pattern, and patients usually develop hyperglycemia before 25 years of age.
   b. **Genetic defects in insulin action** are a rare cause of diabetes and may be associated with other characteristic abnormalities.
   c. **Diseases of the exocrine pancreas** that cause extensive pancreatic destruction including pancreatitis, trauma, infection, carcinoma, cystic fibrosis, hemochromatosis, and surgical resection.
   d. **Endocrinopathies** that involve excess secretion of a hormone that antagonizes insulin (e.g. Cushing's syndrome, acromegaly, pheochromocytoma).
   e. **Drug- or chemical-induced** (e.g. pentamidine, glucocorticoids, niacin).
   f. **Infections** that cause significant beta cell destruction (e.g. congenital rubella, coxsackievirus B, cytomegalovirus).
   g. **Uncommon immune-mediated forms** (e.g. "stiff-man" syndrome, anti-insulin receptor antibodies).
   h. **Other genetic syndromes** that are associated with increased incidence of DM (e.g. Down's, Klinefelter's. Turner's, Wolfram's syndromes).
4. **Gestational** DM (GDM). GDM affects about 4% of pregnancies and is defined as glucose intolerance first detected during pregnancy, regardless of the treatment (diet changes or insulin therapy) required. Even if hyperglycemia resolves after delivery, GDM is a strong risk factor for the subsequent development of type 2 DM.

II **CLINICAL MANIFESTATIONS.** Many patients are asymptomatic at the time of diagnosis; however, the following are classic presenting symptoms:

A. **Polyuria, polydipsia,** and **polyphagia (the 3 "poly"s).** Hyperglycemia leads to glycosuria, which is responsible for this classic triad of symptoms.
B. **Weight change, fatigue, blurred vision,** and **vaginitis** or **balanitis** are also commonly reported.
C. **Diabetic ketoacidosis** (usually seen in patients with type 1 DM) or **hyperglycemic hyperosmolar nonketotic state** (seen in patients with type 2 DM). Some patients with previously undiagnosed DM present with these serious conditions.

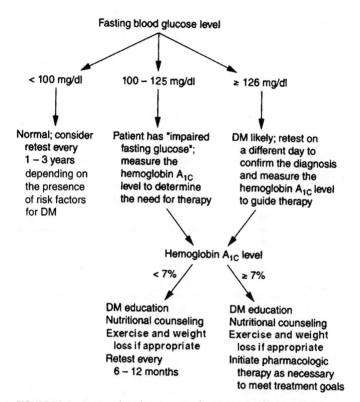

FIGURE 75-1. Approach to the patient with signs and symptoms of diabetes mellitus (DM).

III APPROACH TO THE PATIENT (FIGURE 75-1)

A. **Blood glucose levels.** In patients who present with symptoms suggestive of DM, the diagnosis can be established with **laboratory testing.** Diagnosis is based on finding **persistent hyperglycemia,** characteristic of all forms of DM. According to the ADA, DM can be diagnosed by any of the following criteria demonstrated on two separate days.

1. A **random blood glucose level** greater than or equal to 200 mg/dL in a patient with classic symptoms of DM.

2. A **fasting blood glucose level** (i.e., one taken 8 or more hours after eating) greater than 126 mg/dL.

3. During an **oral glucose tolerance test** (OGTT), a 2-hour blood glucose level greater than or equal to 200 mg/dL after a standard 75 gm glucose load.

4. Some authors have suggested using an elevated **hemoglobin A1C** level for diagnosis, but this is not currently recommended by the ADA.

HOT

▶

KEY

Some patients do not meet the definition of DM but have abnormal laboratory test results: (1) a fasting blood glucose level of 100–125 mg/dl defines **"impaired fasting glucose"**; and (2) a 2-hour post-load glucose level of 140–199 mg/dL during a standard OGTT defines **"impaired glucose tolerance."** These patients with **"pre-diabetes"** are at high risk for developing DM and warrant lifestyle interventions.

B. Hemoglobin A_{1c} level. Although this test is not officially used for the diagnosis of DM, it is the mainstay for monitoring control of DM and response to therapy. The hemoglobin A_{1c} level indicates the amount of glucose attached to hemoglobin in red blood cells (RBCs). Higher hemoglobin A_{1c} levels occur with higher blood glucose levels over time; therefore, the hemoglobin A_{1c} level reflects the average degree of glucose control over the preceding 2–3 months.

1. Check hemoglobin A_{1C} at least twice per year in patients with stable glycemic control meeting treatment goals.

2. Check hemoglobin A_{1C} every 3 months in patients not meeting treatment goals or if there has been a change in therapy.

IV TREATMENT

A. General considerations

1. **Goal of therapy.** The goals of therapy are to **minimize symptoms** and **prevent complications.**

2. **Team approach.** DM is best managed when the patient and the health care team share the responsibility for diabetes care. All new patients should be offered a DM education program that addresses diet, exercise, monitoring of blood glucose levels, warning signs, potential complications, and the importance of establishing emergency contacts.

3. **Intensity of therapy.** Intensive insulin therapy reduces the risk of developing complications from DM (e.g., retinopathy, nephropathy, neuropathy) by 50%–75%. However, intensive treatment is associated with an increased incidence of hypoglycemia. Therefore, the decision to initiate intensive

TABLE 75-1. Target Blood Glucose and Hemoglobin A_{1c} Levels* for Nonpregnant Adults

	Target†	Normal‡
Fasting blood glucose level (mg/dl)	90–130	60–110
Peak postprandial blood glucose level (mg/dl)§	<180	<140
Hemoglobin A_{1c} level (%)	<7	<6

*In patients with complicating medical problems, higher blood glucose and hemoglobin A_{1c} levels may be appropriate to avoid the risk of hypoglycemia.
†In patients with diabetes mellitus (DM).
‡In patients without DM.
§Postprandial glucose measured 1–2 hours after meal initiation.

treatment depends on the patient's risk profile and preferences.

a. Patients who are poorly compliant, who experience recurrent episodes of severe hypoglycemia, or who have multiple comorbidities may not be appropriate candidates for intensive treatment.

b. Table 75-1 shows target blood glucose and hemoglobin A_{1c} levels that can be used to help guide therapy in nonpregnant adults. Note that therapy should always be individualized and that certain populations (e.g. pregnant women, children, elderly) require special consideration.

HOT KEY

Patients treated with intensive insulin therapy are likely to have a higher incidence of hypoglycemia and may require more training, frequent contact, and follow-up.

B. Type 2 DM

1. Weight loss and **exercise** have been shown to reduce and even correct insulin resistance in patients with type 2 DM. Patients who lose weight may be able to reduce their need for medications.

2. Oral medications. Patients with type 2 DM who are unable to adequately lower their hemoglobin A_{1c} levels or who remain symptomatic despite diet and exercise should be started on oral medication.

a. Biguanides act by decreasing hepatic glucose production and improving insulin sensitivity. The only biguanide available in the United States is **metformin**.

(1) Dose. The starting dose is 500 mg or 850 mg daily, taken with a meal. The dose can be increased gradually as necessary every 2 weeks (to a maximum daily dose of 2550 mg, divided in two or three doses).

(2) Side effects. Lactic acidosis is the most serious side effect. **Gastrointestinal side effects** (e.g., diarrhea, nausea) are common, but usually diminish over time and are less common with gradual dose titration.

(3) Contraindications. Metformin therapy should be avoided under any of the following circumstances:

   (a) Decreased renal function (i.e., a serum creatinine level greater than 1.4 in women or 1.5 in men)

   (b) Acute or chronic liver disease

   (c) Significant alcohol use

   (d) 48 hours before and after radiologic studies using contrast agents

   (e) Congestive heart failure

   (f) Acute illness, such as sepsis, myocardial infarction, shock, or hypoxia

(4) Monitoring. Periodic serum creatinine levels should be obtained in all patients.

b. Sulfonylureas (Table 75-2) act by increasing pancreatic insulin release. The first-generation agents (e.g., **tolbutamide**) have shorter half-lives than the second generation agents (e.g., **glyburide, glipizide**).

(1) Doses of the commonly used sulfonylureas are shown in Table 75-2.

(2) Side effects. Hypoglycemia is the most important side effect; patients taking longer-acting agents who skip meals or have comorbidities are at higher risk.

TABLE 75-2. Characteristics of Selected Sulfonylureas

Agent	Starting Dose	Maximum Dose	Half-Life (hrs)
First generation			
Tolbutamide	500 mg daily	1000 mg three times daily	6–12
Second generation			
Glipizide	2.5–5 mg daily	20 mg twice daily*	12–24
Glyburide	1.25–2.5 mg daily	20 mg daily	16–24

*Must be administered twice daily if the total dose is greater than 15 mg/day.

(3) **Contraindications.** Use cautiously in elderly patients and those with renal or hepatic impairment due to the increased risk of prolonged hypoglycemia. Given the chemical similarity, patients with documented severe allergic reactions to other "sulfa" drugs should not receive sulfonylureas.

(4) **Monitoring** for hypoglycemia and adequacy of glucose control is recommended.

HOT KEY

All of the sulfonylureas can cause hypoglycemia, so patients should be aware of the characteristic signs and symptoms (dizzyness, lightheadedness, fatigue, hunger, sweats, shakes, blurred vision).

---

c. **Thiazolidinediones (TZDs)** act by increasing insulin sensitivity in muscle and fat.

(1) **Dose.** Rosiglitazone (2–8 mg per day, may be divided in two doses) and pioglitazone (15–35 mg per day) are currently available.

(2) **Side effects** include weight gain, fluid retention, macular edema, and hypoglycemia (only when used in conjunction with insulin or sulfonylureas). Unlike the first-generation agent (troglitazone) that caused fatal hepatic failure and was withdrawn from the market, the newer TZDs have only rarely been associated with abnormal liver function.

(3) **Contraindications.** The Food and Drug Administration (FDA) recommends baseline assessment of liver function, and patients with alanine aminotransferase (ALT) levels greater than 2.5 times normal are not candidates for therapy. Those with less severe elevations in ALT should be treated cautiously and monitored closely. Since these agents may exacerbate fluid retention, they are not recommended in patients with CHF.

(4) **Monitoring.** Periodic monitoring of liver function should be performed based on clinical judgment, taking into account baseline values, comorbidities, and signs or symptoms of hepatic toxicity.

d. **Meglitinides**, like sulfonylureas, augment insulin release by beta cells, but they are structurally different and act through a different receptor. These short-acting agents are marketed as leading to fewer hypoglycemic episodes.

(1) **Dose. Repaglinide** (0.5–4 mg) and **nateglinide** (60–120 mg) are both dosed up to three times daily before meals.

    (2) Side effects, contraindications, and monitoring recommendations are similar to those for sulfonylureas.

  e. Exenatide is the first FDA-approved agent in a new class of medications that take advantage of the "incretin effect," the stimulatory effect of gut hormones on endogenous insulin release. Exenatide binds to the **glucagon-like peptide-1** (GLP-1) receptor and is resistant to degradation by **dipeptidyl peptidase IV** (DPP-IV), another target of drug action currently under investigation. Exenatide also causes weight loss in some patients, although it is not FDA-approved for this indication.

    (1) Dose. Exenatide is currently available in pre-filled syringes containing either 5 or 10 mcg doses, to be administered subcutaneously twice daily before breakfast and dinner.

    (2) Side effects. The most commonly reported side effect is **nausea**. Hypoglycemia can occur when used in combination with sulfonylureas; thus, the dose of concurrent sulfonylureas should be reduced preemptively.

    (3) Contraindications. Patients with severe **gastroparesis** (or other gastrointestinal disease) or severe renal impairment should not be treated with exenatide. It is only approved for use with metformin, sulfonylureas, or the combination of these agents.

    (4) Monitoring. As with other medications for diabetes, monitoring for hypoglycemia and adequacy of glucose control is recommended.

  f. Acarbose and miglitol are **alpha-glucosidase inhibitors** that delay the breakdown of ingested complex carbohydrates, decreasing postprandial glucose concentrations.

    (1) Dose. Both agents are administered in doses of 50–100 mg three times per day with meals.

    (2) Side effects. The major side effects are gastrointestinal, including **flatulence and diarrhea**, which may hinder compliance. Elevations of transaminases have also been reported.

    (3) Contraindications. Patients with significant gastrointestinal disease, impaired digestion or absorption should not receive these agents.

    (4) Monitoring. In addition to glucose and hemoglobin A1C, transaminases should be checked every 3 months during the first year of treatment and periodically after that.

3. Insulin therapy.

  a. In type 2 diabetics without severe hyperglycemia or symptoms, it is usually appropriate to try diet, exercise, and/or oral agents prior to initiating insulin therapy.

b. If the patient's DM is still not controlled, consider continuing the oral agents and adding a **once-daily injection of long-acting insulin** (either NPH, glargine, or detemir) at bedtime. Insulin-sensitizing medications may enable therapy with lower total daily doses of insulin. In order to simplify therapy, some providers prefer to discontinue all oral therapy for DM and rely only on insulin. Titrate the dose to control the fasting (morning) glucose level. If more insulin is required, use the four-step approach described in IV C 3.

HOT KEY

When patients with type 2 DM require insulin, they usually require higher doses than those required by patients with type 1 DM who are generally more insulin sensitive.

C. Type 1 DM. These patients require **insulin therapy.**
   1. Insulin preparations (Table 75-3). Insulin preparations vary in the time to maximum effect and duration of action; therefore, the clinical situation dictates the choice of insulin. Many practitioners prefer using the newer analog insulins (i.e. glargine and a rapid-acting insulin) in type 1 diabetics in order

TABLE 75-3. Characteristics of Commonly Used Insulin Preparations

Type*	Class	Onset of Action	Time to Maximum Effect (hrs)	Duration (hrs)
Lispro	Rapid-acting	10–30 minutes	0.5–1.5	3–4
Glulisine	Rapid-acting	10–30 minutes	0.5–1.5	3–4
Aspart	Rapid-acting	10–30 minutes	1–3	3–5
Inhaled	Rapid-acting	10–20 minutes	0.5–1.5	6–8
Regular	Short-acting	30 minutes	2–4	6–8
NPH	Intermediate-acting	1–2 hours	6–12	14–24
Detemir	Long-acting	3–4 hours	6–8	6–23
Glargine	Long-acting	3–4 hours	None	24

*Mixtures of NPH and regular insulin are also available in 70%/30% and 50%/50% combinations. Mixtures of an intermediate-acting insulin (like NPH) and a rapid-acting insulin are also available (75%/25% lispro and 70%/30% aspart). Glargine cannot be mixed with any other insulin because of its low pH.

to achieve tight glucose control with fewer hypoglycemic episodes, although they are more expensive.

2. **General approach.** Insulin requirements can be separated into two components: (1) **"Basal"** needs that maintain euglycemia and prevent ketosis even when the patient is not eating; and (2) **"Bolus" or "nutritional"** needs to cover the carbohydrates consumed in meals or snacks.

 HOT KEY Patients with type 1 diabetes require exogenous **insulin at all times**, even if they are not eating (e.g. prior to surgery, in the setting of gastroenteritis), to avoid development of ketosis.

---

3. **Approximating initial insulin requirements.** There are many strategies for achieving optimal glucose control in patients with DM who are taking insulin. Two effective, simple strategies are presented (using either NPH and regular insulin or glargine and a rapid-acting insulin):
   a. Calculate the total daily insulin dose based on the patient's weight.
      (1) **Newly diagnosed type 1 DM.** These patients often have a "honeymoon" period during which only small doses of insulin are required (e.g., 0.3 units/kg/day).
      (2) **Established type 1 DM.** These patients usually require approximately 0.5 units/kg/day (if they do not have coexisting insulin resistance).
   b. **Divide the dose** (Figures 75-2 and 75-3).

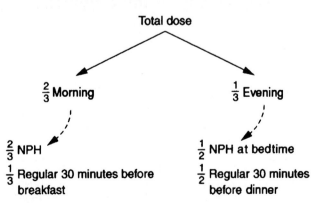

FIGURE 75-2. One simple strategy for insulin therapy in a patient with diabetes using NPH and regular insulin.

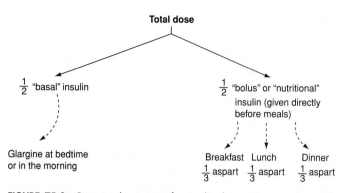

FIGURE 75-3. One simple strategy for insulin therapy in a patient with diabetes using glargine and a rapid-acting insulin.

    (1) When **NPH and regular insulin** are used, give two thirds of the total daily dose before breakfast and one third before the evening meal. Given regular insulin's onset of action, it should be given about 30 minutes before meals.

        (a) The morning dose should be two thirds NPH insulin and one third regular insulin.

        (b) The evening dose should be one half NPH insulin (administered at bedtime) and one half regular insulin (administered 30 minutes before dinner).

    (2) When **glargine and a rapid-acting insulin** (e.g. aspart, lispro, glulisine) are used, give one half of the total daily dose as glargine (basal) insulin and the other half as rapid-acting (bolus or nutritional) insulin.

        (a) **Glargine insulin** can be administered either at bedtime or in the morning.

        (b) The **rapid-acting insulin** can initially be divided in thirds and administered directly before meals. For optimal insulin dosing, patients can be taught to **count carbohydrates** and adjust their insulin dose based on the carbohydrate content of the meal. Patients may also have varying insulin sensitivity throughout the day.

    (3) Note that the different types of insulins can be "mixed and matched" according to the particular clinical situation (e.g. NPH and aspart insulin used together) and that several pre-mixed insulin preparations are commercially available (see Table 75-3).

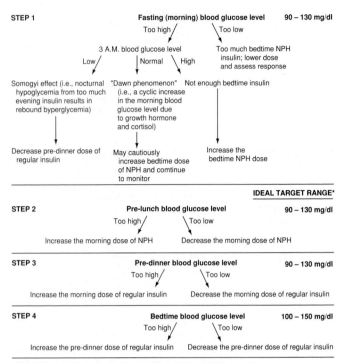

STEP 1   **Fasting (morning) blood glucose level**   90 – 130 mg/dl

Too high / \ Too low

3 A.M. blood glucose level   Too much bedtime NPH insulin; lower dose and assess response

Low / | Normal \ High

Somogyi effect (i.e., nocturnal hypoglycemia from too much evening insulin results in rebound byperglycemia)   "Dawn phenomenon" (i.e., a cyclic increase in the morning blood glucose level due to growth hormone and cortisol)   Not enough bedtime insulin

Decrease pre-dinner dose of regular insulin   May cautiously increase bedtime dose of NPH and comtinue to monitor   Increase the bedtime NPH dose

IDEAL TARGET RANGE*

STEP 2   **Pre-lunch blood glucose level**   90 – 130 mg/dl

Too high / \ Too low

Increase the morning dose of NPH   Decrease the morning dose of NPH

STEP 3   **Pre-dinner blood glucose level**   90 – 130 mg/dl

Too high / \ Too low

Increase the morning dose of regular insulin   Decrease the morning dose of regular insulin

STEP 4   **Bedtime blood glucose level**   100 – 150 mg/dl

Too high / \ Too low

Increase the pre-dinner dose of regular insulin   Decrease the pre-dinner dose of regular insulin

* Higher blood glucose levels may be acceptable in patients at risk for hypoglycemia.

FIGURE 75-4. A step-wise approach to monitoring insulin therapy in patients treated with NPH and regular insulin. Once the fasting (morning) blood glucose level is within the target range, move on to the pre-evening meal blood glucose level, the pre-lunch blood glucose level, and the bedtime blood glucose level. A pattern of hypoglycemia requires immediate attention.

    4. Monitoring therapy. A simple way to monitor therapy is to use a step-wise approach based on blood glucose measurements at four times of the day, before meals and at bedtime (Figures 75-4 and 75-5).

        a. NPH and glargine, intermediate- and long-acting insulins that act as the patient's basal insulin, should be adjusted first. In general, the **morning blood glucose level** is used to adjust the previous evening's bedtime insulin dose. For regimens containing NPH, **pre-evening meal blood glucose levels** reflect the action of NPH administered in the morning.

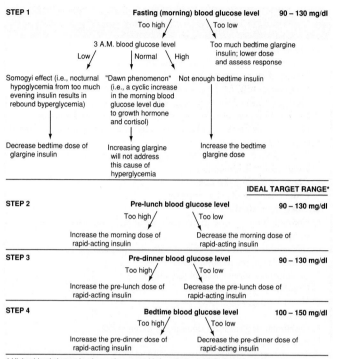

FIGURE 75-5. A step-wise approach to monitoring insulin therapy in patients treated with glargine at bedtime and a rapid-acting insulin before meals. Once the fasting (morning) blood glucose level is within the target range, move on to the pre-lunch blood glucose level, the pre-dinner blood glucose level, and the bedtime blood glucose level. A pattern of hypoglycemia requires immediate attention.

   b. Regular (a short-acting insulin) **and rapid-acting insulins** (e.g. aspart, lispro, and glulisine), are used as bolus or nutritional insulin and are adjusted based on the following **pre-meal blood glucose level** (or the **bedtime glucose level** for the dose given before dinner).

   c. If the patient's pre-meal and bedtime blood glucose values are in the ideal range but the HgA1c is still not at goal, then it may be useful to measure and target **peak postprandial blood glucose levels** (1–2 hours after meal initiation) (see Table 75-1).

TABLE 75-4. Areas to Address During Follow-Up Visits with Patients with Diabetes

Patient history
☐ Symptoms of hypo- or hyperglycemia
☐ Results of home monitoring
☐ Symptoms of complications of diabetes mellitus (e.g., visual changes, chest pain, shortness of breath, neuropathy)
☐ Medication history, including any adjustments in insulin therapy
☐ Lifestyle issues (e.g., smoking, exercise, diet, psychosocial concerns)

Physical examination
☐ Evaluation of vital signs (i.e., weight and blood pressure)
☐ Fundoscopic examination
☐ Cardiovascular examination
☐ Examination of the skin and feet

Laboratory studies
☐ Hemoglobin A_{1c} level (biannually if stable therapy, otherwise quarterly)
☐ HDL and LDL levels (annually if normal, more often if patient is being treated for hypercholesterolemia)
☐ Urinary microalbumin level (annually)
☐ Creatinine level (annually)
☐ Consider a baseline EKG

Referrals
☐ Ophthalmologist for an annual eye examination
☐ Podiatrist (as needed)

EKG = electrocardiogram; HDL = high-density lipoprotein; LDL = low-density lipoprotein.

 FOLLOW-UP AND REFERRAL. Patients with DM require ongoing monitoring (Table 75-4). The frequency of visits varies, depending on the need for medication adjustments, co-morbidities, and the patient's understanding of DM. The goal at each follow-up visit is to maximize the effectiveness of treatment and prevent the progression of complications.

A. Monitoring for complications. The patient should be evaluated for symptoms and signs of all major long-term complications at each follow-up visit. The **patient history** should be reviewed and a **physical examination** should be performed at each visit, as well as appropriate **laboratory testing**.

1. **Neuropathy.** The skin, particularly that of the feet, should be examined for signs of neuropathy. Patients with evidence of skin breakdown or loss of sensation to light touch (detected by monofilament testing) should be educated about preventive foot care and may be referred to a podiatrist. **Specialized footwear** may be indicated.

2. **Cardiovascular** and **peripheral vascular disease.** Signs and symptoms suggestive of vascular disease should be sought at each visit. Providers should try to reduce the diabetic patient's already high risk of CVD by identification and treatment of other known **cardiac risk factors**. Recommended treatment goals are often more aggressive in diabetics than in the general population.

   a. **Hypertension.** Target blood pressure is lower than 130/80; this often requires multiple anti-hypertensive medications.

   b. **Dyslipidemia.** The primary goal is a low-density lipoprotein (LDL) cholesterol level less than 100 mg/dL, although a lower LDL goal of less than 70 mg/dL is appropriate for very high-risk patients (e.g. those with known CVD). Secondary goals include a triglyceride level less than 150 mg/dL and a high-density lipoprotein (HDL) cholesterol level greater than 40 mg/dL (greater than 50 mg/dL in women).

   c. **Aspirin therapy** (75–162 mg/day) is recommended for secondary prevention in all diabetic patients with known CVD. It may also be used as primary prevention in diabetics older than 40 years or those with additional cardiac risk factors.

   d. **Smoking cessation** should be discussed at each visit, and patients should be offered any adjunctive services available (e.g. nicotine replacement methods, counseling, pharmacologic therapies).

   e. **Avoidance of sedentary lifestyle and maintenance of healthy body weight** should be a treatment goal for all diabetics.

HOT KEY

Because **angiotensin-converting enzyme (ACE) inhibitors and angiotensin receptor blockers (ARBs)** are known to prevent diabetic nephropathy, these classes of drugs should be used in patients with DM and hypertension. Note that ACE-inhibitors and ARBs are contraindicated during pregnancy.

HOT KEY

Hydroxymethylglutaruly CoA (HMG-CoA) reductase inhibitors ("statins") have been shown in multiple clinical trials to reduce the risk of CVD in diabetics and should be used to achieve 30–40% LDL reduction in diabetics older than 40 years (regardless of baseline LDL levels) and in all diabetics with known CVD. Note that statins are contraindicated during pregnancy.

3. **Retinopathy.** An annual **dilated retinal examination** by a skilled practitioner is necessary to monitor for retinopathy.
   a. **Treatment** may include laser therapy to reduce the risk of vision loss if high-risk lesions are present.
4. **Nephropathy.** A **spot urine for microalbuminuria**, an early sign of diabetic nephropathy, should be performed yearly in patients who have had type 1 diabetes for at least 5 years and in those with type 2 diabetes beginning at diagnosis. Serum creatinine should be checked at least annually.
   a. **Treatment** includes optimization of glucose control and hypertension, therapy with an ACE-I or ARB (in non-pregnant patients), and protein restriction (0.8 g/kg) in those with chronic kidney disease (CKD).

HOT KEY

A urine dipstick for protein can be normal in patients with microalbuminuria.

B. **Patient education**
1. The **importance of diet** and **exercise** should always be emphasized because weight loss can improve glucose sensitivity in overweight patients with DM.
2. **Psychosocial** and **lifestyle issues** should also be addressed, especially in patients with a new diagnosis or in those who have had a deterioration in their clinical condition.

HOT KEY

To reduce the risk of maternal and fetal complications, women with DM who wish to have children should consult with an endocrinologist before becoming pregnant. Contraception must therefore be discussed with all women with DM who are of reproductive age. Note that only aspart, lispro, regular, and NPH insulins are approved for use during pregnancy.

References

American Diabetes Association. Diagnosis and classification of diabetes mellitus. *Diabetes Care* 2006;29(S1):S43–S48.

American Diabetes Association. Standards of medical care in diabetes-2006. *Diabetes Care* 2006;29(S1):S4–S42.

Cowie CC, Rust KF, Byrd-Holt DD, et al. Prevalence of diabetes and impaired fasting glucose in adults in the U.S. population. *Diabetes Care* 2006;29(6):1263–1268.

76. Hypothyroidism

I. INTRODUCTION

A. Hypothyroidism is the clinical state in which the availability of thyroid hormone is diminished.
1. **Primary hypothyroidism** (99% of cases) refers to thyroid gland failure.
2. **Secondary (central) hypothyroidism** (1% of cases) is caused by a disorder of the pituitary gland, hypothalamus, or hypothalamic-pituitary portal circulation.
B. Hypothyroidism is five to seven times **more common in women** than in men. The condition is seen in as many as 10% of women older than 50 years.

II.

Causes of Hypothyroidism are summarized in Table 76-1. **Chronic autoimmune thyroiditis (Hashimoto's disease)** is the most common cause of hypothyroidism.

 HOT KEY Autoimmune thyroid disease may be associated with other autoimmune conditions, including primary adrenal insufficiency, type I diabetes mellitus (DM), pernicious anemia, and Sjögren's syndrome.

III. CLINICAL MANIFESTATIONS OF HYPOTHYROIDISM.

Most of the clinical manifestations of hypothyroidism result from **slowing of metabolic processes,** which is caused by thyroid hormone deficiency, and can be nonspecific and insidious.

A. **Symptoms** include fatigue, generalized weakness, cold intolerance, hair loss, dry skin, myalgias, paresthesias, constipation, menstrual irregularities, weight gain, and cognitive decline.

 HOT KEY Hypothyroidism leads to cold intolerance.

B. **Signs** include bradycardia, diastolic hypertension, hoarseness, doughy skin, and mucinous edema (myxedema). The relaxation phase of the skeletal muscle reflexes may be delayed.

TABLE 76-1. Causes of Hypothyroidism

Primary hypothyroidism
Thyroiditis
  Chronic autoimmune thyroiditis (Hashimoto's disease)
  Subacute thyroiditis
  Postpartum thyroidiis
  External irradiation
Iatrogenic
  Radioiodine ablation (iodine 131 treatment)
  Thyroidectomy
Infiltrating disorders
  Infection
  Granulomatous disease
  Malignancy
Drugs
  Antithyroid agents (e.g., methimazole, propylthiouracil)
  Lithium
  Iodide
  Amiodarone
  Cytokin
  Perchlorate
Iodine deficiency
Congenital disorders
  Thyroid dysgenesis
  Defects in thyroid hormone synthesis
Idiopathic
  Thyroid gland atrophy (probably autoimmune)
Secondary hypothyroidism (central)
TSH deficiency due to pituitary disease
  Postpartum infarction
  Tumor infiltration (e.g., pituitary macroadenoma)
  Granulomatous disease
  Infection
  Irradiation
  Idiopathic
TRH deficiency due to hypothalamic disease
  Tumor (e.g., craniopharyngioma)
  Irradiation
  Transient occurrence in nonthyroidal illness

TRH = thyroid-releasing hormone; TSH = thyroid-stimulating hormone.

HOT **KEY**   If hypothyroidism occurs early in life, the patient may experience mental and growth retardation.

IV **APPROACH TO THE PATIENT.** If hypothyroidism is suspected on the basis of the patient's clinical presentation, **laboratory studies should be ordered.** Typically, the biochemical profile consists of an **increased serum thyroid-stimulating hormone (TSH) level** and **decreased peripheral thyroid hormone** [i.e., **free thyroxine (FT$_4$)** and **free triiodothyronine (FT$_3$)] levels.**

A. A **TSH level** is the best test to obtain in the outpatient setting if primary hypothyroidism is suspected. TSH elevation is caused by the loss of negative feedback effects (as a result of low thyroid hormone levels) on pituitary thyrotrophs. A peripheral FT$_4$ level, rather than a serum TSH level, is helpful if pituitary dysfunction (i.e., secondary hypothyroidism) is suspected.

B. A **FT$_4$ level** should be obtained to confirm the diagnosis. If the peripheral FT$_4$ level is normal but the serum TSH level is elevated, then the patient has subclinical hypothyroidism.

HOT **KEY**   Triiodothyronine (T$_3$) levels are generally not used to diagnose hypothyroidism because the T$_3$ value may be transiently decreased by nonthyroidal illness or malnutrition.

C. **Antithyroid antibodies** [i.e., **antithyroid peroxidase** (TPO) and **antithyroglobulin] titers** should be obtained in patients diagnosed with hypothyroidism.
   1. If positive, underlying autoimmune thyroid disease is confirmed. Approximately 90% of patients with autoimmune thyroiditis have positive antithyroid antibodies on testing.
   2. If negative, then the patient probably has a nonautoimmune thyroiditis and may have a transient hypothyroid state (e.g., subacute thyroiditis).

HOT **KEY**   The practice of screening for hypothyroidism in asymptomatic patients is controversial, but screening should be considered for women older than 60 years and for patients with hypercholesterolemia, elevated creatinine kinase levels, hyponatremia, hyperprolactinemia, or a family history of thyroid disease.

Ⅴ TREATMENT

A. Clinical hypothyroidism. Treatment is the same for all patients, regardless of the cause of the hypothyroidism.

1. **Levothyroxine (T_4) therapy** (thyroid hormone replacement)*

   a. In **otherwise healthy young adults,** treatment can be initiated at a near-total replacement dose of **75–100 μg daily.** The usual levothyroxine requirement is 1.6 μg/kg/day, but the dose may need to be increased for patients with conditions associated with malabsorption or increased serum levels of thyroid-binding globulin (e.g., pregnancy).

HOT KEY

Patients with a history of thyroid carcinoma may be given higher doses of levothyroxine in an attempt to keep the serum TSH level at a lower value. Because TSH can promote thyroid growth and possibly tumor genesis, keeping the TSH level low may decrease the patient's risk of cancer recurrence or growth.

---

   b. In **elderly patients** or **those with risk factors for heart disease,** it is prudent to initiate treatment at a dose of **25–50 μg daily,** unless the patient is markedly symptomatic. The dose can then be increased in 25 μg increments each month, as tolerated. This approach decreases the risk of precipitating an untoward cardiac event. ("Start low, go slow")

HOT KEY

Multivitamins with iron, sucralfate, cholestyramine, fiber, calcium, and other similar substances can interfere with the absorption of levothyroxine. Patients should be advised to take their levothyroxine separate from other medications and preferably on an empty stomach.

---

2. **Monitoring**

   a. **Ongoing evaluation of thyroid status.** Thyroid hormone requirements may decrease with aging; therefore, the patient's thyroid status should be evaluated at least annually, even when the patient has become euthyroid.

---

* There is little evidence to support therapy with mixtures of T_3 and T_4 or T_3 alone in the outpatient setting (except when preparing a patient for iodine 131 therapy in the setting of a well-differentiated thyroid carcinoma).

(1) In patients with **primary hypothyroidism,** a **TSH level** can be used to follow thyroid status. The TSH level should be checked 6–8 weeks after any dosage adjustment.

HOT

▶

KEY

It often takes approximately 6 weeks for the serum TSH level to equilibrate after an adjustment in thyroid hormone dose.

---

(2) In patients with **secondary hypothyroidism,** a **FT$_4$ level** (rather than a serum TSH level) and assessment of clinical symptoms should be used to evaluate thyroid status.

b. Monitoring for adrenal insufficiency. In some instances, initiation of thyroid hormone replacement therapy unmasks underlying adrenal insufficiency secondary to increased metabolism of cortisol. Therefore, signs and symptoms of adrenal insufficiency need to be monitored, especially in patients with severe hypothyroidism, pituitary disease, or a polyglandular autoimmune syndrome.

B. Subclinical hypothyroidism. Treatment with levothyroxine should be considered if the patient is only midly symptomatic, but has a TSH level greater than normal, or if the patient has a goiter or positive antithyroid antibody status.

VI FOLLOW-UP AND REFERRAL

A. Follow-up. Patients should see their primary care physician annually for clinical evaluation, or sooner if they experience a change in clinical status.

B. Referral to an endocrinologist is indicated in the following circumstances:

1. Thyroid function tests continue to be abnormal, despite what appear to be appropriate changes in dose.

2. The hypothyroidism is determined to be secondary rather than primary.

References

Lindsay RS, Toft AD. Hypothyroidism. *Lancet* 1997;349(9049):413–4177.

Weetman AP. Hypothyroidism: screening and subclinical disease. *BMJ* 1997;314(7088): 1175–1178.

77. Hyperthyroidism

I INTRODUCTION

A. Hyperthyroidism is the clinical state in which the availability of thyroid hormone is increased.

    1. Excessive production of thyroid hormone by the thyroid gland is responsible for most cases of hyperthyroidism.

    2. Ectopic production of thyroid hormone or exogenous sources account for the diagnosis in a small number of cases.

B. Hyperthyroidism is **more common in women.** The overall incidence of hyperthyroidism is 0.2%–0.4%.

II CAUSES OF HYPERTHYROIDISM

A. **Graves' disease,** the most common cause of hyperthyroidism, is an autoimmune process in which an abnormal immunoglobulin (thyroid-stimulating immunoglobulin) stimulates the thyroid gland to produce excess hormone. Graves' disease is most common in women between the ages of 20 and 40 years.

B. **Toxic multinodular goiter** and **toxic adenoma of the thyroid** result in autonomous thyroid hormone production.

C. **Iodine exposure (Jodbasedow phenomenon).** Some patients may become overtly hyperthyroid after ingesting or being exposed to iodine (e.g., radiographic contrast agents). The iodine serves as a substrate for thyroid hormone production.

D. **Subacute thyroiditis** (e.g., as a result of viral infection) and **certain drugs** (e.g., amiodarone) can lead to injury and disruption of the thyroid follicles, causing preformed thyroid hormone to be released into the circulation.

E. **"Hashitoxicosis"** describes rare patients with autoimmune thyroid disease who initially present with hyperthyroidism due to TSH-receptor stimulating antibodies, but later develop hypothyroidism due to chronic lymphocytic thyroiditis (Hashimoto's thyroiditis).

F. **Exogenous hyperthyroidism** may be caused by inappropriate ingestion of thyroid hormone by patients (e.g., as a weight-loss aid) or by inadvertent overdose of prescribed medication.

G. **Struma ovarii** (teratoma of the ovary containing thyroid tissue) may be associated with ectopic production of thyroid hormone.

H. **Hydatidiform moles** produce chorionic gonadotropin, which has intrinsic TSH-like activity, and may rarely cause overt thyrotoxicosis.

I. Pituitary adenomas can rarely produce thyroid-stimulating hormone (TSH), leading to hyperthyroidism.

J. Pituitary resistance to thyroid hormone is a rare cause of clinical hyperthyroidism and is characterized by goiter, elevated levels of T4 and T3, with normal or elevated TSH.

K. Thyroid carcinoma, even though it often concentrates radioactive iodine, only very rarely produces functional thyroid hormone that can cause hyperthyroidism.

III **CLINICAL MANIFESTATIONS OF HYPERTHYROIDISM.** Most of the clinical manifestations of hyperthyroidism result from the **acceleration of metabolic processes** caused by thyroid hormone excess.

A. Symptoms. Palpitations, tremulousness, irritability or anxiety, heat intolerance, diaphoresis, hyperdefecation, menstrual irregularities, hair loss, increased appetite, and weight loss are common.

B. Signs include tachycardia, atrial fibrillation, fine tremor, hyperreflexia, proximal muscle weakness, thyromegaly, moist skin, lid lag, and gynecomastia. Patients with Graves' disease may have associated ophthalmopathy (i.e., proptosis and conjunctival irritation) and dermopathy (e.g., pretibial myxedema).

HOT KEY

Elderly patients may have very subtle or no symptoms despite overt biochemical evidence (apathetic hyperthyroidism).

IV **APPROACH TO THE PATIENT**

A. Patient history. Typical symptoms are described in III A.

B. Physical examination
  1. A **diffusely but symmetrically enlarged thyroid gland** is suggestive of Graves' disease, especially when associated with ophthalmopathy or dermopathy.
  2. An **irregularly enlarged thyroid gland** is suggestive of either a toxic multinodular goiter or a toxic adenoma.
  3. A **tender thyroid gland** suggests thyroiditis.

C. Laboratory studies are useful to confirm a clinical diagnosis of hyperthyroidism and to determine the cause.
  1. **Confirming the clinical diagnosis.** Typically, the biochemical profile consists of a **decreased serum TSH level** and **increased peripheral thyroid hormone** [i.e., **free thyroxine (FT_4)** and **free triiodothyronine (FT_3)**] **levels.**

TABLE 77-1. Narrowing the Differential Using Thyroid Scan Results

| Radioiodine Uptake | | Likely Cause of Hyperthyroidism |
Amount	Distribution	
Increased	Homogeneous	Graves' disease
Increased	Multiple focal "hot spots"	Toxic multinodular goiter
Increased	One focal "hot spot"	Toxic adenoma
Decreased ("white out")	—	Thyroiditis or exogenous hyperthyroidism

    a. Subclinical hyperthyroidism. Patients have a decreased TSH level but normal FT$_4$ and FT$_3$ levels.

HOT KEY Because chronic exposure to excess thyroid hormone may lead to decreased bone density and cardiac abnormalities (e.g., left ventricular hypertrophy, atrial fibrillation), most experts now agree that treatment of subclinical hyperthyroidism is indicated.

    b. T$_3$ thyrotoxicosis is characterized by a low TSH level, a normal FT$_4$ level, and an elevated FT$_3$ level.

    c. TSH-producing pituitary adenomas or **thyroid resistance hormone syndrome** may result in increased FT$_4$ and FT$_3$ values but normal or elevated serum TSH levels.

  2. Determining the underlying cause

    a. Radioiodine uptake and scan. A radioiodine tracer (i.e., iodine 123) is administered and then the uptake at 24 hours is determined (sometimes a 6-hour measurement is also made), and thyroid gland imaging may be performed. The degree and distribution of radioiodine uptake usually suggests the cause of the hyperthyroidism (Table 77-1).

HOT KEY Radioiodine thyroid scans are not useful in patients who have recently been exposed to iodine (e.g., by consumption of shellfish or seaweed or by administration of iodine-containing radiocontrast agents). Thyroid ultrasound may be a useful alternative for these patients, who usually must wait several months before demonstrating increased radioiodine uptake .

b. **Antithyroid antibody titers** are positive in the majority of patients with Graves' disease.

c. **Thyroid-stimulating immunoglobulin** is specific for Graves' disease, but less sensitive, and may be useful for diagnosis when radioiodine uptake and scan is not performed. TSI-negative patients with Graves' Disease may be more likely to experience clinical remission.

d. **Thyroglobulin levels** are decreased in patients with exogenous hyperthyroidism and are increased in patients with thyroiditis.

e. **Erythrocyte sedimentation rate (ESR).** The ESR is increased in patients with thyroiditis.

f. **Alpha subunit levels** are elevated in patients with TSH-producing pituitary adenomas.

HOT **KEY** Laboratory abnormalities seen in many patients with hyperthyroidism include hypercalcemia and elevated alkaline phosphatase (AP) levels, which are indicative of increased bone turnover.

 TREATMENT. When possible, treatment should be tailored to the cause; however, treatment should not be deferred while awaiting the results of a pending study if the patient is moderately or severely ill.

A. Pharmacologic therapy

1. **Thionamide agents** (e.g., **methimazole, propylthiouracil**) inhibit thyroid hormone synthesis. Propylthiouracil has the theoretical benefit of inhibiting peripheral conversion of T_4 to T_3 (T_3 is the more biologically active form), while methimazole has the advantage of less frequent dosing.

   a. **Indications**

   (1) **Graves' disease.** Thionamide agents are often the first choice for therapy of Graves' disease because these patients may experience clinical remission.

HOT **KEY** Patients who take thionamides for Graves' disease optimize their chances for full remission if they continue treatment for at least 1 year after becoming euthyroid.

---

(2) **Toxic multinodular goiter** or **toxic adenoma.** Methimazole or propylthiouracil may be used to treat toxic

multinodular goiter or toxic adenoma when radioiodine ablation or surgery is not desired by the patient; however, this approach is not preferred since these patients do not remit and life-long therapy will generally be required.

b. Doses. Typical starting doses are:

    (1) Propylthiouracil, 150–600 mg daily in two or three divided doses

    (2) Methimazole, 10–40 mg daily in two doses, which can later be changed to once-daily dosing

c. Side effects most commonly include an allergic reaction and gastrointestinal distress. Rarely, PTU can cause severe, irreversible hepatic necrosis and methimazole can cause a reversible cholestasis. Both medications cause idiosyncratic agranulocytosis in about 1/300 treated patients. Upon initiation of therapy, patients should be cautioned about these side effects and instructed to discontinue the medication immediately if they experience concerning symptoms.

d. Pregnancy. PTU is the preferred anti-thyroid drug in pregnant women, as methimazole may be associated with aplasia cutis congenita in offspring of treated mothers. Lowest-tolerated doses (less than 300 mg/day of PTU) that maintain thyroid hormones levels in the upper normal or slightly hyperthyroid range should be used to avoid fetal hypothyroidism and/or goiter.

HOT KEY

If a patient taking a thionamide agent develops a sore throat or a fever, then blood should be drawn immediately for a complete blood count (CBC) to rule out agranulocytosis.

---

2. Sodium ipodate and iopanoic acid, two oral iodine-containing cholecystographic agents no longer available in the United States, inhibit both thyroid hormone synthesis and release, as well as potently inhibit peripheral T_4 conversion.

a. Because sodium ipodate acts quickly (i.e., within 1–2 days of initiating therapy), it can be used to rapidly restore euthyroidism in moderate or severe presentations of hyperthyroidism (e.g. thyroid storm or in preparation for thyroidectomy).

b. Since these agents saturate the thyroid gland with iodide, they should not be used before radioiodine therapy.

     c. These agents should not be used without co-administration of thionamides in patients with toxic adenoma or toxic multinodular goiter, since the iodine may provide substrate for thyroid hormone synthesis and exacerbate hyperthyroidism.

     d. Lugol's solution or saturated solution of potassium iodide (3 drops twice daily) is used pre-operatively in patients with Graves' disease to reduce the vascularity of the thyroid gland. Potassium perchlorate is another alternative used to acutely block thyroid hormone synthesis and release.

3. Beta Blockers decrease tissue response to catecholamines and, to a lesser degree, decrease peripheral conversion of T_4 to T_3. Therefore, they provide symptomatic relief and are usually used as an adjunct to other treatments.

4. Glucocorticoids are used to treat several different thyroid disorders.

     a. The use of systemic glucocorticoids to decrease peripheral conversion of T4 to T3 should be reserved for patients with severe hyperthyroidism refractory to other treatments or "thyroid storm."

     b. Glucocorticoids are used for their immunosuppressive effects in the acute treatment of Graves' ophthalmopathy.

     c. Topical steroids have a role in the local treatment of Graves' dermopathy.

     d. If symptoms are disabling and unresponsive to symptomatic treatments, then a short course of glucocorticoids may be used in the acute phase of thyroiditis to reduce inflammation.

5. Nonsteroidal anti-inflammatory drugs (NSAIDs) or **acetaminophen** are used to relieve neck discomfort in patients with thyroiditis.

6. Cholestyramine may be used as adjunctive therapy in thyroid storm to reduce levels of T4 rapidly by binding T4 in the gut during its enterohepatic circulation.

B. Radioiodine ablation (iodine 131 treatment) takes advantage of the thyroid gland's relatively selective uptake of iodine. One dose of iodine 131 can significantly decrease the size and function of the thyroid gland.

1. Indications. Radioiodine ablation is most often used to treat toxic multinodular goiter, toxic adenoma, and Graves' disease.

2. Side effects. The treatment is generally well tolerated when given in doses appropriate for the treatment of benign thyroid disease.

3. Levothyroxine replacement. Thyroid gland ablation usually occurs over the course of weeks to months with the doses of radioiodine typically administered in the United States, resulting in post-ablation hypothyroidism and the requirement for life-long thyroid hormone replacement.

HOT KEY

Radioiodine ablation should be used with caution in elderly patients, who may develop a transient post-treatment thyroiditis leading to temporary thyrotoxicosis and possible cardiac complications (e.g., angina, atrial fibrillation). Careful monitoring of symptoms and thyroid hormone status, as well as judicious use of beta-blockers and anti-thyroid drugs, may avoid these complications.

C. Surgery is a last resort. Possible indications include:
1. Failure of primary treatment
2. Significant local or obstructive symptoms as a result of an enlarged thyroid gland
3. Pregnancy, when the patient's hyperthyroidism cannot be controlled with medication (radioiodine ablation is absolutely contraindicated in pregnant women)

VI FOLLOW-UP AND REFERRAL

A. Follow-up. Frequent visits (i.e., every 1–2 months) are necessary during the initial treatment phase. Once the patient is euthyroid, the frequency of visits can be reduced to once every 3–4 months for 1 year after the onset of euthyroidism.
1. Periodic thyroid function tests are critical to monitor response to treatment.
   a. Because patients who have undergone radioiodine ablation are at increased risk over time for developing hypothyroidism, thyroid function should be monitored in these patients.
   b. Remember that the TSH level may remain suppressed for several months after the patient becomes euthyroid (either as a result of treatment with anti-thyroid drugs or radioiodine ablation); therefore, measurement of peripheral FT_4 level may be more helpful.

B. Referral
1. Given the complexity of diagnosing and treating hyperthyroidism and the potentially rapid dynamics of the patient's clinical status, you should have a low threshold to refer the patient to an endocrinologist.
2. Patients with significant ophthalmopathy warrant referral to an ophthalmologist, and those with dermopathy warrant evaluation by a dermatologist.

3. Some patients (e.g., those with very large goiters) may need to be referred to a surgeon for evaluation.

> Any patient with suspected **thyroid storm** (an acute exacerbation of thyrotoxicosis usually associated with a specific precipitant and characterized by high fever, marked tachycardia such as rapid atrial fibrillation, mental status changes, nausea, vomiting, and seizures) requires inpatient intensive care and immediate consultation with an endocrinologist since it can be fatal.

HOT KEY

References

Cooper DS. Antithyroid drugs for the treatment of hyperthyroidism caused by Graves' disease. *Endocrin Metab Clin North Am* 1998;27(1):225–247.

Gittoes NJ, Franklyn JA. Hyperthyroidism. Current treatment guidelines. *Drugs* 1998;55(4):543–553.

Lazarus JH. Hyperthyroidism. *Lancet* 1997;349(9048):339–343.

78. Solitary Thyroid Nodule

I INTRODUCTION

A. Thyroid nodules are common, and palpable nodules are found in 4%–7% of the population of the United States. Improved imaging techniques (e.g., ultrasound) have led to an increase in the number of incidentally discovered thyroid nodules; in surveys using ultrasound and autopsy studies, up to 70% of those screened may have at least one thyroid nodule.

B. Women are affected four times more often than men.

II DIFFERENTIAL DIAGNOSIS

A. Benign colloid nodule
B. Benign follicular adenoma
C. Malignancy
D. Cyst
E. Inflammatory condition
F. Developmental abnormality (i.e., thyroglossal duct cyst)

III APPROACH TO THE PATIENT.

The goals of evaluation are to determine if the nodule is malignant, assess compression of nearby structures (e.g., the trachea and esophagus), and determine the patient's thyroid functional status.

HOT **KEY**

Most solitary thyroid nodules are benign (approximately 5% are malignant).

A. Patient history. Patients are typically euthyroid and asymptomatic. Important questions to ask include:

1. Does the patient have **local symptoms** (e.g., dysphagia, difficulty breathing, chronic irritative cough, hoarseness) as a result of compression of adjacent structures?

2. Are there any **symptoms of hyper-** or **hypothyroidism?**

3. Does the patient have a **history of external radiation exposure to the neck region** (e.g., as a result of treatment for cancer, acne, or an enlarged thymus)?

481

4. Does the patient have a **family history of papillary thyroid carcinoma, medullary thyroid carcinoma** or **multiple endocrine neoplasia, type II (MEN-II)?**

B. Physical examination. Palpate the neck to assess the size and firmness of the nodule, adherence to surrounding tissue, lymphadenopathy, and tracheal deviation. Be sure to note any tenderness.

HOT KEY Factors that increase the chance of malignancy are age younger than 20 years or older than 60 years; history of head and neck irradiation; male gender; rapidly growing or firm nodule; hoarseness; surrounding lymphadenopathy; and a family history of thyroid carcinoma or MEN-II.

HOT KEY A sudden increase in size, pain, or both in a preexisting nodule is usually caused by an acute hemorrhage and is less concerning for malignancy.

C. Laboratory studies

1. A **thyroid-stimulating hormone (TSH) level** should be obtained to evaluate the functional status of the thyroid gland.

2. A **calcitonin level** should be considered if the patient has a family history of medullary thyroid carcinoma or MEN-II.

3. A **serum thyroglobulin level** should be measured if the nodule turns out to be a well-differentiated thyroid carcinoma. After thyroidectomy is performed, thyroglobulin is a useful tumor marker for thyroid cancer.

D. Fine needle aspiration biopsy is the mainstay of evaluation. When performed by an experienced practitioner, the false-negative rate is less than 5% and the false-positive rate is approximately 1%.

1. The diagnostic accuracy, convenience, and minimal risk associated with fine needle aspiration biopsy has significantly reduced the role of radioiodine thyroid scanning in the diagnostic work-up of a solitary thyroid nodule.

2. Four basic results can be seen. These results, which guide further work-up and treatment, are:

a. Benign

b. Malignant or suspicious for malignancy

c. Insufficient for diagnosis

d. Follicular neoplasm

E. Imaging studies have little use during the early stages of evaluation because they cannot rule out or confirm a diagnosis of malignancy. However, in certain situations, imaging studies may be indicated.

1. **Ultrasound** can determine the size and consistency of the nodule. In addition, ultrasound can be used to help guide fine needle aspiration biopsy of a nodule that is difficult to palpate. Certain nodule characteristics observed on ultrasound, such as microcalcifications, are associated with malignancy.

2. **Computed tomography (CT)** and **magnetic resonance imaging (MRI)** may help determine the degree of local compression of neighboring structures.

3. **Radioiodine thyroid scan**
   a. Radioiodine thyroid scanning is helpful when the TSH level is suppressed, because it can determine if the nodule in question is "hot," possibly obviating the need for fine needle aspiration biopsy.
      (1) "Hot" nodules function autonomously and suppress the uptake of iodine by the surrounding thyroid tissue on a radioiodine scan. **"Hot" nodules are rarely malignant.**
      (2) "Cold" and "warm" nodules may be malignant.
   b. Some advocate thyroid scanning when fine needle aspiration biopsy results reveal a follicular neoplasm. It is believed that if the nodule takes up iodine, then the risk of malignancy is decreased.

IV TREATMENT

A. Approach to management. Management primarily depends on the patient's TSH level and results of fine needle aspiration biopsy (Figure 78-1). However, if a nodule is rapidly increasing in size or causing local compressive symptoms, then surgical evaluation is warranted independent of the results of TSH evaluation and fine needle aspiration biopsy.

1. **TSH level**
   a. If the TSH level is **normal** or **high,** then the results of fine needle aspiration biopsy dictate the approach to management (see IV A 2).
   b. If the TSH level is **low,** then a radioiodine thyroid scan may be performed. If the nodule is "hot," then radioiodine ablation should be considered because these nodules are rarely malignant.

2. **Fine needle aspiration biopsy results**
   a. **Benign.** The patient should be reassured and subsequently monitored to ensure that the nodule does not increase in size or lead to the development of local symptoms.

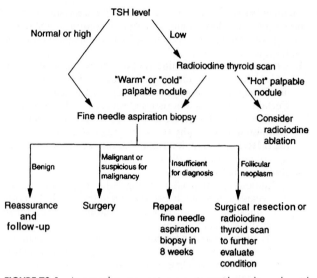

FIGURE 78-1. Approach to managing a patient with a solitary thyroid nodule. TSH = thyroid-stimulating hormone.

    b. Malignant or suspicious for malignancy. The patient should be referred for surgery unless the diagnosis is primary lymphoma, in which case chemotherapy may be indicated. If the results are suggestive of medullary thyroid carcinoma, then the patient and other family members need to be evaluated for MEN-II.

    c. Insufficient for diagnosis. This finding warrants a repeat fine needle aspiration biopsy. Because inflammatory changes from the previous biopsy can confuse results on subsequent biopsies, adequate time (e.g., 8 weeks) should be allowed between biopsies.

    d. Follicular neoplasm. Cytologic evaluation cannot determine the exact nature of this lesion. Either capsular or vascular invasion is required to diagnose malignancy. Approximately 10%–20% of follicular neoplasms are found to be malignant at surgery. Many physicians recommend surgery given this risk, although some advocate a radioiodine scan to further evaluate the patient's risk of malignancy (see III E 3 b).

B. Treatment modalities

    1. Thyroid hormone administration. The underlying rationale is that thyroid nodules will shrink in response to thyroid hormone, which suppresses TSH secretion.

    a. Recent prospective studies have demonstrated that fewer than 15% of nodules respond to this therapy. In addition, long-term risks are associated with thyroid hormone suppression (e.g., decreased bone density, tachyarrhythmias).

    b. For these reasons, the role of thyroid hormone suppression in the management of thyroid nodules is controversial and should be used only in selective situations. A means of objectively documenting change in nodule size (e.g., serial ultrasounds) should be used to determine whether the therapy is effective .

2. Near-total thyroidectomy. Many experts recommend near-total thyroidectomy (without fine needle aspiration biopsy) for patients with a history of neck irradiation and a solitary nodule, due to the high incidence of malignancy in this population (30%–50%).

V **FOLLOW-UP AND REFERRAL.** Referral to an endocrinologist or surgeon should be considered when the TSH level is decreased or results of fine needle aspiration biopsy are inconclusive or indicate malignancy.

References

Boigon M, Moyer D. Solitary thyroid nodules. Separating benign from malignant conditions. *Postgrad Med* 1995;98(2):73–74, 77–80.

Hermus AR, Huysmans DA. Treatment of benign nodular thyroid disease. *New Engl J Med* 1998;338(20):1438–1447.

79. Calcium Disorders

I **INTRODUCTION.** At any given time, 99% of the body's calcium stores is within the skeleton. Of the remaining 1% in the circulation, 40% is bound to albumin, 10% is complexed (citrate, phosphate), and 50% is free (ionized). It is the free (ionized) component that is biologically active and thus of primary clinical importance.

A. The **serum ionized calcium level** is maintained within a relatively narrow range (1.0–1.3 mmol/L), primarily via regulation by parathyroid hormone (PTH) and vitamin D.

B. The **total serum calcium level** is normally 8.4–10.6 mg/dl (exact reference range may depend on the assay used). Measurements of the total serum calcium level need to be interpreted with caution because they depend on the concentration of other proteins in the serum (e.g., albumin). For every 1 mg decrease in the serum albumin level (normally 4 mg/dl), you must increase the total serum calcium level by 0.8 mg/dl. For example, if the total serum calcium level is 7.5 mg/dl and the serum albumin level is 2 mg/dl, then the corrected total serum calcium level is 9.1 mg/dl (and the patient is normocalcemic). However, this rule is an approximation and loses validity at extremes of albumin levels. Thus, the serum ionized calcium level is the preferred laboratory test for determining calcium status in this setting.

II **HYPOCALCEMIA**

A. Clinical manifestations of hypocalcemia. The severity of signs and symptoms depends on both the degree and the acuity of the hypocalcemia. Patients with chronic hypocalcemia may be asymptomatic, whereas patients who experience a sudden decrease in calcium may have severe symptoms. Because hypocalcemia leads to enhanced excitation of the nervous system and muscle cells, the symptoms and signs primarily involve the neuromuscular and cardiovascular systems.

   1. Symptoms
      a. Mild symptoms include **muscle cramps** and **paresthesias of the lips and extremities.**
      b. More severe symptoms include **tetany, stridor,** (as a result of laryngospasm), **seizures,** and **altered mental status.**

2. **Signs** may include:
   a. **Chvostek's sign** (tapping the facial nerve leads to contraction of the facial muscles)
   b. **Trousseau's sign** (occlusion of the brachial artery with a blood pressure cuff leads to carpal spasm)
   c. **Extrapyramidal signs**
   d. **Hypotension,** signs of **congestive heart failure (CHF),** or **prolongation of the QT interval** or **atrioventricular (AV) block** on an electrocardiogram (EKG)
   e. **Cataract formation** (in patients with chronic hypocalcemia)

B. Causes of hypocalcemia

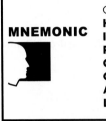

MNEMONIC

Causes of Hypocalcemia ("HIPOCAL")
Hypoparathyroidism
Infection
Pancreatitis
Overload States
Chronic renal failure
Absorption abnormalities
Loop diuretics and other drugs

1. **Hypoparathyroidism**
   a. Causes of hypoparathyroidism include **parathyroid damage** (e.g., as a result of surgery, irradiation, or ischemia), **autoimmune destruction, congenital abnormalities (e.g. DiGeorge syndrome), and infiltrative disorders**.
   b. Functional hypoparathyroidism (i.e., impaired secretion and action of PTH) may occur secondary to **magnesium deficiency.**
2. **Infection.** As many as 20% of patients with Gram-negative sepsis are hypocalcemic due to acquired—defects in the parathyroid-vitamin D axis. This hypocalcemia may cause hypotension that is responsive to calcium replacement.
3. **Pancreatitis.** A serum calcium level of less than 8 mg/dl is one of Ranson's criteria; the calcium level may correlate with the severity of acute pancreatitis.
4. **Overload states.** Occasionally, hypocalcemia may be seen in cases of rapid intravascular volume expansion.
5. **Chronic renal failure.** The metabolism of 25-hydroxyvitamin D to 1,25-dihydroxyvitamin D occurring in the kidney is impaired, leading to decreased intestinal calcium absorption and subsequent hypocalcemia.

6. **Absorption abnormalities.** Patients with malabsorption of calcium, magnesium, or vitamin D (from any cause) may have hypocalcemia.

7. **Loop diuretics and other drugs.** Unlike thiazide diuretics (which can cause hypercalcemia), furosemide and other loop diuretics lead to enhanced renal excretion of calcium. Other drugs (e.g., foscarnet, citrate, bisphosphonates) or blood transfusions may also lead to hypocalcemia.

C. **Approach to the patient**

1. Obtain a **serum ionized calcium level** to confirm the clinical diagnosis of hypocalcemia.

2. Obtain a **concomitant serum magnesium level** to rule out hypomagnesemia, which, if corrected, may correct the hypocalcemia and obviate the need for additional work-up or intervention.

3. Obtain the following **serum levels:**
   a. **PTH**
   b. **25-Hydroxyvitamin D** and **possibly 1,25-dihydroxyvitamin D**
   c. **Phosphate**
   d. **Creatinine**
   e. **Amylase** and **lipase** (if pancreatitis is suspected)

4. Obtain an **EKG** to evaluate for QT prolongation.

HOT KEY

Because hypocalcemia due to hypoparathyroidism can be associated with an autoimmune polyglandular syndrome, consider evaluation for other endocrine deficiencies (e.g., adrenal insufficiency).

D. **Treatment**

1. **Severe symptoms.** If the patient has tetany, arrhythmias, or seizures, immediate referral to the emergency department (ED) is indicated.
   a. **Calcium gluconate.** An initial bolus of 1–2 ampules (each containing 93 mg elemental Ca) should be administered intravenously, followed by continuous calcium infusion at a rate of 0.5–1.5 mg/kg/hr.
   b. **Magnesium sulfate** (2 g over 10 minutes) should be administered to most patients. If the patient is hypomagnesemic, then the magnesium deficiency must be corrected before the serum calcium level will normalize.

2. **Mild symptoms.** If the patient is relatively asymptomatic, then oral administration of elemental calcium and vitamin D is usually all that is required. In order to minimize hypercalciuria, which can lead to nephrolithiasis or nephrocalcinosis,

the doses of calcium and vitamin D should be titrated to keep the serum ionized calcium level in the low-normal range.

   a. Elemental calcium. The dose is usually 2–4 g/day in two or three divided doses.

   b. Vitamin D. Because of its relatively short half life, greater potency, and greater bioavailability, **calcitriol** (1,25-dihydroxyvitamin D) is used most commonly. The dose ranges from 0.25–0.5 μg, administered once or twice daily. However, high doses of ergocalciferol (vitamin D_2) may also be effective and less expensive.

HOT KEY

Patients with hypoparathyroidism usually require larger doses of calcium and vitamin D.

E. Follow-up and referral

  1. Follow-up

    a. The **serum ionized calcium level** should be measured **every 6 months** once levels have normalized.

    b. Consider obtaining a **24-hour urine collection for calcium annually** to ensure that the patient is not developing hypercalciuria (defined as >400 mg calcium/24 hours).

  2. Referral to an endocrinologist should be made when patients have fluctuating serum calcium levels, unusual calcium or vitamin D requirements, or concomitant endocrine dysfunction.

III HYPERCALCEMIA

A. Clinical manifestations of hypercalcemia. As with hypocalcemia, both the degree and acuity of the hypercalcemia influence the severity of the patient's signs and symptoms.

  1. Symptoms are usually nonspecific and tend to occur when the serum calcium level exceeds 12 mg/dl. "**Abdominal MOAN, psychiatric GROAN, kidney STONE,** and **urination ZONE** (i.e., the bathroom)" is an easy way to remember the common symptoms of hypercalcemia.

    a. Gastrointestinal symptoms include constipation, nausea, vomiting, and anorexia.

    b. Central nervous system (CNS) symptoms include confusion, depression, lethargy, and weakness. Symptoms can progress to coma and death.

    c. Renal complications include nephrolithiasis, polyuria and polydipsia as a result of decreased concentrating ability of the kidney, and renal failure.

2. **Signs** of hypercalcemia include hypertension, hypotonia, decreased deep tendon reflexes, and a shortened QT interval on the EKG.

B. **Causes of hypercalcemia.** In 80%–90% of cases, hypercalcemia is caused either by malignancy or hyperparathyroidism. In the hospital setting, malignancy is the more common cause, while in the ambulatory setting, hyperparathyroidism predominates.

MNEMONIC

Causes of Hypercalcemia ("**My Favorite MISHAP**")
Medications (e.g., lithium, thiazide diuretics)
Familial hypocalciuric hypercalcemia (FHH)
Malignancy
Intoxication (vitamin D or A overdose) or **I**mmobilization
Sarcoidosis (and other granulomatous diseases or lymphoma)
Hyperparathyroidism or **H**yperthyroidism
Addison's disease or milk-**A**lkali syndrome
Paget's disease or **P**heochromocytoma

---

1. **Medications**
   a. **Lithium.** Chronic exposure to lithium can alter the set point for PTH secretion, resulting in a hyperparathyroid state.
   b. **Thiazide diuretics** result in increased renal reabsorption of calcium.
2. **FHH** is a benign autosomal dominant disorder characterized by mild hypercalcemia, hypocalciuria, and occasional hypermagnesemia. A defect in the calcium sensors in the kidneys and the parathyroid glands results in altered set points for renal calcium reabsorption and PTH secretion, respectively. PTH may be mildly elevated in this disorder; thus, it is important to distinguish FHH from primary hyperparathyroidism.
3. **Malignancy.** Several mechanisms can be responsible for the hypercalcemia of malignancy.
   a. Some tumors (e.g., breast, lung, renal cell) produce PTH-related peptide. This is the most common underlying mechanism.
   b. Other malignancies (e.g., multiple myeloma, possibly some lymphomas) produce osteoclast-activating factors, which stimulate osteoclastic bone resorption.
   c. Hypercalcemia can result from local osteolysis (seen with extensive bone involvement).

    d. Some lymphomas cause increased conversion of 25- hydroxyvitamin D to 1,25-hydroxyvitamin D.

4. Intoxication. Some patients take large amounts of vitamin D for unclear reasons. Vitamin A intoxication can also occur, but is much less common than vitamin D intoxication.

5. Immobilization is a diagnosis of exclusion. Hypercalcemia (as a result of increased bone resorption) is usually only seen in children or young adults or patients with Paget's disease who have been immobilized for a significant amount of time, and is often accompanied by hypercalciuria.

6. Sarcoidosis, other granulomatous diseases (e.g., tuberculosis, berylliosis), and lymphoma. Hypercalcemia results from increased conversion of 25-hydroxyvitamin D to 1,25-hydroxyvitamin D within macrophages or lymphoid tissue.

7. Hyperparathyroidism

    a. Primary hyperparathyroidism caused by a solitary adenoma accounts for more than 80% of cases of hyperparathyroidism.

    b. Four-gland hyperplasia (10% of cases) which is sometimes associated with multiple endocrine neoplasia, type 1 or type 2 (MEN-1, MEN-2), multiple adenomas (fewer than 5% of cases), and carcinoma (1–2% of cases) can also cause hyperparathyroidism.

    c. Tertiary hyperparathyroidism occurs in the setting of long-standing secondary hyperparathyroidism (usually in patients with end-stage renal disease) when hyperplastic parathyroid tissue becomes autonomous and leads to hypercalcemia.

8. Hyperthyroidism. Hypercalcemia occurs in 15%–20% of hyperthyroid patients and is most likely related to increased osteoclastic bone resorption.

9. Addison's disease. The mechanism by which adrenal insufficiency induces hypercalcemia is unclear and may be multifactorial. One contributing aspect may be significant volume depletion and resultant hemoconcentration.

10. Milk-alkali syndrome. Hypercalcemia occurs secondary to excess calcium carbonate ingestion (often seen in patients with peptic ulcer disease or chronic renal insufficiency who are treated with oral calcium).

11. Paget's disease (osteitis deformans), is characterized by both excessive resorption and formation of bone, which leads to disruption of bone architecture and sometimes skeletal deformities (e.g., kyphosis, bowing of the tibias, enlargement of the skull with occasional deafness). At least two thirds of patients are asymptomatic. Hypercalcemia may occur in the setting of prolonged immobilization.

12. Pheochromocytoma. In some cases, parathyroid hormone–related peptide (PTHrP) may be released, but the mechanism of hypercalcemia is not entirely clear.

C. Approach to the patient. As with hypocalcemia, a **serum ionized calcium level** should be obtained to confirm the clinical diagnosis. Once it is determined that hypercalcemia is present, an effort should be made to determine its cause.

1. Patient history. Inquire about calcium, vitamin D, or vitamin A ingestion and thiazide diuretic or lithium use.

2. Laboratory studies may be helpful.

    a. Obtain the **serum PTH, alkaline phosphatase (AP),** and **phosphate levels** to evaluate for **hyperparathyroidism,** which is characterized by elevated serum PTH, and AP levels and a low phosphate level.

HOT KEY

The serum PTH level is often slightly increased in patients with FHH, which can lead to a mistaken diagnosis of hyperparathyroidism. A "normal" PTH level in the setting of hypercalcemia is inappropriate and either represents hyperparathyroidism or FHH.

HOT KEY

The serum AP level is usually elevated in patients with active Paget's disease.

---

    b. A **24-hour urine collection** to evaluate calcium and creatinine clearance is helpful because if calcium excretion is low (<50 mg/24 hours), then FHH is a strong possibility. The creatinine clearance also helps determine if there is any renal impairment.

    c. If the serum PTH is suppressed and does not explain the hypercalcemia, the following tests may be useful in establishing the cause:

1. Serum PTHrP level. An elevated PTHrP level suggests occult malignancy.

2. Serum vitamin D levels

    a. The **25-hydroxyvitamin D level** screens for vitamin D toxicity.

    b. The **1,25 hydroxyvitamin D level** screens for granulomatous processes and lymphoma as the cause of hypercalcemia.

3. Thyroid function tests should be performed to rule out hyperthyroidism.

4. **Serum protein electrophoresis** may be indicated to evaluate for multiple myeloma.

5. A **morning serum cortisol level** or an **adrenocorticotropic hormone (ACTH) stimulation test** may be performed to rule out adrenal insufficiency if clinical suspicion warrants.

D. Treatment focuses on lowering the serum calcium level and treating the underlying cause of hypercalcemia.

1. **Acute therapy.** Patients with altered mental status, arrythmia, or other unstable medical problems should be hospitalized for aggressive treatment of hypercalcemia.

   a. **Hydration with normal saline** (1–2 L initially, followed by infusion at a rate of 250 ml/hour as tolerated by the patient's volume status) usually initiates calciuresis.

   b. **Loop diuretics** (e.g. furosemide) may be given once the patient is euvolemic. If these agents are given while the patient is hypovolemic, they may exacerbate the hypercalcemia.

   c. **Bisphosphonates** administered intravenously also decrease the serum calcium level, independent of the cause of the hypercalcemia. **Pamidronate** given as an infusion of 60–90 mg over 2–4 hours or zoledronic acid 4 mg over at least 15 minutes may be used.

      (1) The onset of action of IV bisphosphonates is at least 24–48 hours after administration, so repeat doses should not be prematurely administered.

      (2) The effects of pamidronate may last several weeks, and zoledronic acid may last even longer.

HOT KEY

Osteonecrosis of the jaw has been recently reported in patients receiving bisphosphonates. Risk factors include prolonged duration of exposure to potent IV bisphosphonates (especially zoledronic acid), concomitant therapy with chemotherapy and/or radiation, and oral trauma or underlying dental problems. Patients should be counseled about this risk and oral hygiene monitored during therapy.

---

   d. **Calcitonin** (4 IU/kg administered intramuscularly or subcutaneously) also may be used to decrease the serum calcium level to a modest degree, especially while waiting for IV bisphosphonates to take effect.

      (1) Due to tachyphylaxis, the effects are usually not long lasting.

      (2) Calcitonin can be effective for relieving acute pain associated with osteoporotic compression fractures.

  e. Cortisosteroids, which inhibit conversion of 25-hydroxy-vitamin D to 1,25 hydroxyvitamin D, may be especially useful in treating hypercalcemia associated with granulomatous diseases.

  f. Oral phosphates (250–500 mg four times daily) decrease calcium levels through binding. Their role is limited by the possibility of ectopic calcification and diarrhea.

  g. Other measures. In patients with resistant hypercalcemia, agents such as **gallium nitrate** and **mithramycin** can be considered, but these drugs are very toxic. As a last resort, either **peritoneal dialysis** or **hemodialysis** can be performed.

2. **Definitive therapy.** When the calcium is lowered to a reasonable level and the patient's symptoms have improved, treatment should focus on the underlying cause.

  a. Primary Hyperparathyroidism. In symptomatic patients, definitive therapy is usually **parathyroidectomy**. Consensus guidelines recommend surgery in asymptomatic patients with:

  (1) Ca > 1.0 mg/dL above the upper limit of normal
  (2) hypercalciuria (>400 mg/day while eating normal diet)
  (3) osteoporosis (T-score <-2.5 at the hip, spine, or distal radius)
  (4) creatinine clearance that is reduced by at least 30%
  (5) age less than 50 years
  (6) follow-up that is either not possible or not desirable

  Asymptomatic patients who do not undergo surgery should be monitored with a serum calcium level biannually, and a serum creatinine and bone mineral density measurements (hip, spine, and forearm) annually.

  b. Treatment should be targeted to the other underlying causes (e.g. malignancy, sarcoidosis) and is often associated with improvement or resolution of hypercalcemia.

HOT KEY

Patients with FHH do not require treatment.

E. Follow-up and referral

1. **Follow-up** depends on the underlying cause. For example, in cases of treated malignancies or parathyroid hyperplasia, periodic measurements of serum calcium are useful because hypercalcemia may herald recurrence of disease.

2. **Referral** should be sought in the following circumstances:

a. When acute hypercalcemia is refractory to conventional treatment
b. When the underlying cause is best treated by a specialist
c. When it is unclear whether surgery is the appropriate therapy for hyperparathyroidism
d. When MEN-1 or MEN-2 is suspected

References

Barri YM, Knochel JP. Hypercalcemia and electrolyte disturbances in malignancy. *Hematol Onc Clin North Am* 1996;10(4):775–790.

Bilezikian JP, Potts JT Jr, Fuleihan Gel-H, Kleerekoper M, Neer R, Peacock M, Rastad J, Silverberg SJ, Udelsman R, Wells SA. Summary statement from a workshop on asymptomatic primary hyperparathyroidism: a perspective for the 21st century. *J Clin Endocrinol Metab* 2002;87(12):5353–5361.

Bushinsky DA, Monk RD. Calcium. *Lancet* 1998;352(9124):306–311.

Reber PM, Heath H 3rd. Hypocalcemic emergencies. *Med Clin North Am* 1995;79(1):93–106.

Rude RK. Hypocalcemia and hypoparathyroidism. *Curr Ther Endocrinol Metab* 1997;6:546–551.

Woo SB, Hellstein JW, Kalmar JR. Systematic review: bisphosphonates and osteonecrosis of the jaws. *Annals of Internal Medicine* 2006;144(10):753–761.

80. Osteoporosis

I INTRODUCTION

A. Definition. In osteoporosis, bone resorption exceeds bone formation, resulting in low bone mass, disordered skeletal microarchitecture, and an increased risk of fracture.

1. The World Health Organization (WHO) has developed a classification scheme based on **bone mineral density (BMD)**, usually applied to the spine and hip in white postmenopausal women (Table 80-1).

2. Diagnostic criteria for osteoporosis in **men** are controversial. There is also disagreement about whether BMD measurements should be compared to a reference range that is sex-matched. Since men and women appear to have a similar risk for fracture at a given bone density, the same cut-offs have been used for men (Table 80-1).

B. Epidemiology

1. It is estimated that more than one half of all women and approximately one third of all men will experience at least one osteoporotic fracture at some point during their lifetimes.

2. In women, hip fractures lead to a 10–20% excess mortality within 1 year. The mortality associated with hip fractures is even higher in men.

C. Risk factors. Age is the primary risk factor for the development of osteoporosis. Other risk factors are summarized in Table 80-2.

HOT KEY

Although osteoporosis is a silent disease until a fragility fracture occurs, its complications can be prevented in many patients.

II APPROACH TO THE PATIENT

A. Screening

1. **Bone densitometry.** Osteoporotic fracture risk is directly correlated with bone mass, as measured using bone densitometry: the lower the BMD, the greater the fracture risk.

TABLE 80-1. World Health Organization Definition of Osteoporosis

Definition	BMD T Score* by DEXA
Normal	>-1
Low Bone Density (or osteopenia)	-1 to -2.5
Osteoporosis	<-2.5
Severe (or established) osteoporosis	<-2.5 in the presence of one or more fragility fractures

*T score = Number of standard deviations below the mean for young, healthy reference population.

   a. Method. Bone densitometry is a noninvasive method of measuring bone mass that has been shown to be accurate, safe, and predictive of fracture risk. The most common and accurate method in widespread use is **dual x-ray absorptiometry (DXA).**
   b. Indications. BMD testing should be performed in:
     (1) All women aged 65 years or older
     (2) Younger postmenopausal women with risk factors (see Table 80-2)
     (3) Women who demonstrate premature estrogen deficiency (e.g. menopause before the age of 45 years,

TABLE 80-2. Risk Factors for Osteoporosis and Related Fractures in White Postmenopausal Women*

Major risk factors
   History of fracture as an adult
   First-degree relative with fragility fracture
   Low body weight
   Current smoking
   Corticosteroid therapy for more than 3 months
Additional risk factors
   Impaired vision
   Premature estrogen deficiency (<45 years)
   Dementia
   Poor health/frailty
   Recent falls
   Low calcium or vitamin D intake
   Low physical activity
   Alcohol use (>2 drinks per day)

*Data from National Osteoporosis Foundation guidelines.

bilateral oophorectomy prior to a natural menopause, premenopausal women with amenorrhea or oligo-menorrhea)

(4) Patients currently receiving or planning to receive long-term glucocorticoid therapy

(5) Patients with primary hyperparathyroidism

(6) Patients who present with fragility fractures or radio-logic evidence of osteopenia

(7) Men with known risk factors for osteoporosis (e.g. hypogonadism) or who have lost more than 1.5 inches in height

---

HOT

KEY

Routine screening of men with DXA is not recommended at this time.

---

c. Interpretation. BMD results are expressed as the number of standard deviations between the patient's measurement and the mean of either a sex-matched reference group of "young normals" (**T score**) or an age- and sex-specific reference group (**Z score**). See Table 80-1 for definitions.

HOT

KEY

Degenerative changes in the posterior spinous processes may increase anterior-posterior spinal density, especially in elderly patients, and spuriously "normalize" BMD measurements. Lateral DXA, quantitative CT (QCT), and evaluation of alternate skeletal sites may all be useful in interpretation.

---

2. Laboratory studies. Currently, there are no generally accepted biochemical markers for establishing the diagnosis of osteoporosis. Markers of bone turnover such as N-telopeptide and osteocalcin may be useful in determining whether there is accelerated bone loss.

B. Assessment of patients with osteoporosis

1. Laboratory studies.

a. General studies.

Limited biochemical testing may be appropriate for all patients with osteoporosis:

(1) Complete blood count (CBC) and **routine chemistries** (renal and liver function tests) to exclude previously undiagnosed chronic disease.

TABLE 80-3. Medical Conditions and Medications That May Be Associated With an Increased Risk of Osteoporosis*

Medical Conditions

AIDS/HIV	Hemochromatosis	Malabsorption
Amyloidosis	Hemophilia	Mastocytosis
Ankylosing spondylitis	Hyperparathyroidism	Multiple myeloma
Chronic obstructive pulmonary disease	Hyperthyroidism	Multiple sclerosis
	Hypogonadism	Pernicious anemia
	Hypophosphatasia	PTHrP secretion by tumor
Congenital porphyria	Idiopathic scoliosis	
	Inflammatory bowel disease	Rheumatoid arthritis
Cushing's syndrome	Liver disease	Spinal cord transection
Diabetes mellitus	Lymphoma & leukemia	Sprue
Eating disorders		10 Stroke
Female athlete triad		
Gastrectomy		
Gaucher's disease		

Medications

Aluminum	Gonadotropin-releasing hormone agonists	Progesterone (depot form)
Anticonvulsants		Tamoxifen
Cytotoxic drugs		Thyroxine (supraphysiologic doses)
Glucocorticoids	Heparin (long-term use)	
	Immunosuppresants	
	Lithium	

*Data from National Osteoporosis Foundation guidelines.

    (2) Serum calcium and phosphate concentrations.
  b. Specific studies can help rule out medical conditions that are secondary causes of osteoporosis (Table 80-3) in patients with suggestive signs or symptoms. See Table 80-4 for diagnostic testing in selected disorders.
    (1) A serum **25-hydroxy-vitamin D** level should be considered in all patients, given the high prevalence of reversible, subclinical vitamin D deficiency.
    (2) A serum **thyroid-stimulating hormone** (TSH) should probably be obtained in all patients receiving exogenous thyroid hormone.

TABLE 80-4. Some Common Medical Conditions That May Be Secondary Causes of Osteoporosis

Medical Condition	Diagnostic Test
Celiac sprue	IgA endomysial and tissue transglutaminase antibodies
Chronic kidney disease	BUN, creatinine
Cushing's syndrome	24-hour urinary free cortisol or 1 mg dexamethasone suppression test
Eating disorders (e.g., anorexia nervosa)	History and physical examination
Hyperparathyroidism	Intact PTH
Hyperthyroidism	TSH
Hypogonadism	Testosterone (males), menstrual history (females)
Liver disease	Liver enzymes and function tests
Multiply myeloma	Serum protein and urine electrophoresis
Vitamin D deficiency	25-hydroxy-vitamin D

(3) Some authors recommend a **24-hour urine collection for calcium** (and creatinine) to detect hypocalciuria (<100 mg/day; suggestive of vitamin D deficiency or inadequate calcium intake) or hypercalciuria (>300 mg/day; suggestive of primary hyperparathyroidism or renal calcium leak).

HOT KEY

A Zscore of −2.0 is a clue to investigate for a secondary cause of osteoporosis.

2. **Plain film radiography** can be essential for the proper diagnosis of fractures and should be obtained whenever clinical suspicion warrants (e.g., after a fall).

III TREATMENT AND PREVENTION

A. **Lifestyle modifications.**
   1. **Fall Prevention**. Measures to minimize risk of falling include correcting visual and hearing impairments, evaluating balance and gait, avoiding medications that may affect

stability, and improving home safety (e.g. lighting and removing hazards such as throw rugs. **Hip protectors** may be considered in patients with significant fall risk.

2. **Tobacco Cessation** and **avoiding excessive alcohol** intake.
3. **Regular weight-bearing exercise**. Weight-bearing and muscle-strengthening exercise can reduce fall risk and may also increase BMD to some extent.

B. Nutritional therapy

1. **Calcium** is an essential component of bone; adequate calcium intake should be ensured throughout life.
   a. The National Academy of Sciences (NAS) recommends that individuals over age 50 consume at least 1200 mg/day of elemental calcium.
   b. Postmenopausal women in the United States typically consume approximately 600 mg/day of dietary calcium; therefore, supplementation is often necessary.
2. **Vitamin D** increases calcium absorption in the gastrointestinal tract. Vitamin D deficiency, which may lead to secondary hyperparathyroidism and osteoporosis, is common in many populations. The elderly, chronically ill patients, and those with darkly pigmented skin are at even greater risk.
   a. The NAS recommends that all adults older than 50 years consume 400–600 IU/day of vitamin D.
   b. Those at risk for deficiency should consume 800 IU/day of vitamin D.

HOT

A tablet containing both vitamin D and calcium is available and may improve patient compliance.

KEY

C. Pharmacologic therapy

1. **Who to treat**. The National Osteoporosis Foundation (NOF) recommends therapy to reduce fracture risk in women with:
   a. BMD T scores <-2.0 by hip DXA with no risk factors
   b. BMD T scores <-1.5 by hip DXA with at least one risk factor (see Table 80-2)
   c. Prior vertebral or hip fracture
2. **Available pharmacologic agents.**
   a. **Bisphosphonates** are anti-resorptive agents that inhibit osteoclastic activity.
      (1) **Indications.** Bisphosphonates, approved by the Federal Drug Administration (FDA) for the treatment and prevention of osteoporosis, are considered

first-line therapy for most patients and may reduce the risk of fracture by up to 50%.

b. **Administration.** Bisphosphonates must be taken with a full glass of water at least 30–60 minutes before eating or lying down.

    (1) Alendronate (70 mg weekly or 10 mg daily)

    (2) Risedronate (35 mg weekly or 5 mg daily)

    (3) Ibandronate (150 mg once monthly)

c. **Side effects** include dysphagia, esophagitis, and myalgias. Oral bisphosphonates have not been adequately studied in patients with chronic kidney disease.

HOT KEY

Osteonecrosis of the jaw has been reported in patients treated with bisphosphonates, although the vast majority were patients with cancer receiving intravenous bisphosphonates. Very rarely patients taking oral bisphosphonates for osteoporosis have been affected. Practitioners should encourage patients to receive regular dental care and discuss the risks and benefits of therapy.

---

d. **Monitoring** with BMD measurements every 2–3 years is recommended, although small changes in BMD may underestimate the actual reduction in fracture risk.

e. The optimal **duration of therapy** is not known; however, alendronate can be taken safely for at least seven years without compromising bone strength. When alendronate is discontinued after at least 5 years of therapy, there is minimal bone loss over the next 3–5 years.

f. **Intravenous bisphosphonates** (e.g. pamidronate and zoledronic acid) are not currently FDA-approved for the treatment of osteoporosis, but they are available off-label. Zoledronic acid is being studied for this indication.

3. **Estrogen/Hormone Therapy (ET/HT)** are anti-resorptive agents that suppress osteoclast activity.

a. **Indications.** Currently these agents are only FDA-approved for the prevention of osteoporosis, and other treatments should be considered first.

b. **Administration.** Multiple oral and transdermal preparations exist. Women who have not undergone hysterectomy should be prescribed HT containing a **progestin** to avoid the increased risk of uterine cancer.

c. **Side effects.** The Women's Health Initiative (WHI) found increased risks of myocardial infarction, stroke, breast cancer, and venous thromboembolism in postmenopausal women treated with combined HT for a mean of 5.2 years.

Although these results may not be generalizable to all populations, other doses and/or combinations of hormones, they should be discussed with patients prior to initiation of HT/ET.

4. **Calcitonin.** In limited studies, calcitonin has been shown to prevent bone loss (but not fractures) in patients with osteoporosis.
   a. **Indications**
      (1) Calcitonin, FDA-approved for women at least 5 years post-menopause, may be considered in those who cannot tolerate bisphosphonates or other therapies.
      (2) Calcitonin (50–100 IU/day) has been shown to be effective in treating pain due to vertebral fractures.
   b. **Administration.** Calcitonin may be administered by nasal spray (200 IU) or by subcutaneous injection.

5. **Parathyroid hormone [PTH(1-34), teriparatide]**, which stimulates bone formation, is the first anabolic agent to be approved by the FDA for the treatment of osteoporosis.
   a. **Indications.** Currently therapy is limited to treatment of moderate to severe osteoporosis.
   b. **Administration.** Teriparatide (20 mcg) is administered by daily subcutaneous injection for no longer than two years.
   c. **Side effects**. Hypercalcemia (usually asymptomatic), nausea, dizzyness, and leg cramps may occur. Due to concern regarding the development of osteosarcoma in rats treated with high doses, teriparatide should not be used in patients with Paget's disease, prior radiation therapy, skeletal malignancy or bone metastases.
   d. Upon **discontinuation**, treatment with an anti-resorptive agent such as a bisphosphonate should be initiated to maintain the BMD gains induced by parathyroid hormone.

6. **Raloxifene** is a selective estrogen receptor modulator, demonstrating estrogen-like actions in some tissues, but not in others.
   a. **Indications.**
      (1) FDA-approved for the treatment and prevention of osteoporosis in postmenopausal women.
      (2) Raloxifene also reduces the risk of invasive breast cancer, although it is not yet approved for this indication.
   b. **Administration.** Raloxifene (60 mg daily)
   c. **Side Effects** may include hot flashes, nausea, leg cramps. Although raloxifene does not increase the risk of cardiovascular disease or mortality, it increases the risk of venous thromboembolism and fatal stroke.

7. **Non-FDA approved medications** for osteoporosis include other bisphosphonates (etidronate, pamidronate,

tiludronate, zoledronic acid), calcitriol (a synthetic vitamin
D analog), sodium fluoride, strontium ranelate, and tibolone.

References
Barrett-Connor E, Mosca L, Collins P, et al. Effects of raloxifene on cardiovascular events and breast cancer in postmenopausal women. *New Engl J Med*
2006;355(2):125–137.
Deal CL. Osteoporosis: prevention, diagnosis, and management. *Am J Med*
1997;102(1A): 35S–39S.
Manson JE, Hsia J, Johnson KC, et al. Estrogen plus progestin and the risk of coronary
heart disease. *New Engl J Med* 2003;349(6):523–534.
National Osteoporosis Foundation. Physician's Guide to Prevention and Treatment
of Osteoporosis; 1999, Updated September 2005. (Accessed July 18, 2006 at
http://www.nof.org)
Rosen CJ. Postmenopausal osteoporosis. *New Engl J Med* 2005;353(6):595–602.

PART XII

INFECTIOUS DISEASES

• •

81. Sexually Transmitted Diseases

I **INTRODUCTION.** More than 18 million cases of sexually transmitted diseases (STDs) are reported in the United States each year. STDs may result in significant consequences such as an increased risk of HIV transmission, infertility, adverse pregnancy outcomes, and anogenital cancer.

II **PREVENTION OF STDS**

A. **Education and counseling about safe sex practices.**
   1. Encourage the use of **latex condoms,** since they have lower rates of breakage and slippage than those made with other materials. Condoms should ideally be used for all acts of sexual intercourse (oral, vaginal, and anal).
   2. **Spermicides are not effective** in preventing STDs or HIV.
   3. Encourage abstinence from sexual activity when persons or their partners have an STD.
B. **Identify asymptomatic persons with STDs by appropriate screening** in selected populations.
   1. See section VI-E for screening recommendations for *C. trachomatis* and *N. gonorrhoeae* in women.
   2. Men who have sex with men (MSM) should be routinely screened for HIV, syphilis, urethral gonorrhea and chlamydia, pharyngeal gonorrhea (in men with oral-genital exposure), and rectal gonorrhea and chlamydia (in men who have receptive anal intercourse).
C. Encourage and facilitate the evaluation, counseling, and treatment of the **sexual partners** of patients with STDs.
D. Give **pre-exposure immunizations** for vaccine-preventable STDs, i.e. hepatitis A and B (see section X).

III **GENITAL ULCER DISEASE.** In the United States, genital ulcers are most often caused by genital herpes, syphilis, and less commonly chancroid.

A. **Diagnostic evaluation of the patient with genital ulcer disease.**
History and physical examination alone are usually not enough
to differentiate one disease entity from another. In addition, patients may be coinfected with two types of ulcer-causing organisms. Therefore, **all patients with a genital ulcer should undergo
evaluation including a serologic test for syphilis and diagnostic
evaluation for herpes simplex virus (HSV)**; in settings where
chancroid is prevalent, culture for *Haemophilus ducreyi* should
be performed as well. **HIV testing** is recommended in all patients with syphilis or chancroid, and should be considered in
those with HSV as well.

HOT

▶

KEY

All patients with a genital ulcer should have a serologic test for
syphilis and a diagnostic evaluation for HSV.

B. **Genital herpes.**
1. **Etiology.** Most cases of genital herpes are caused by HSV-2,
   but about 20% of cases are due to HSV-1.
2. **Epidemiology and transmission.** 25% of persons over the age
   of 30 in the United States have HSV-2, although most do not
   realize they have been infected. Persons with asymptomatic
   HSV infection may still shed the virus in their genital tract,
   referred to as **asymptomatic shedding;** in fact, most genital
   herpes is transmitted in this way.
3. **Clinical manifestations**
   a. **Initial episode.** After an incubation period of 2–12 days,
      small macules and papules appear and then progress to
      vesicles and ulcers. The lesions may be painful, and pa-
      tients may also have tender regional lymphadenopathy.
      Systemic symptoms of **fever, myalgia,** and **malaise** are
      seen in many cases. The first episode usually lasts about
      12 days.
   b. **Recurrent episodes.** Afer primary infection, the virus be-
      comes latent in the dorsal root ganglion and can period-
      ically reactivate and cause recurrences, which are more
      commonly asymptomatic. The frequency of symptomatic
      outbreaks varies widely but the median is 4 outbreaks per
      year, and recurrence rates decrease over time. About half
      of patients will have **prodromal symptoms** of a tingling
      sensation or shooting pains within hours or days prior to
      the onset of the eruption. Most recurrences last 5–10 days
      and are less severe than the primary episode.

HOT KEY While the risk of HSV transmission is higher when genital lesions are present, most HSV transmission occurs from asymptomatic shedding.

4. **Diagnosis.**
   a. **Isolation of HSV in viral culture** from a swab of an ulcer is the gold standard for diagnosis of genital HSV. However, the sensitivity of culture declines rapidly as lesions begin to heal.
   b. **Type-specific serologic tests** for HSV-1 and HSV-2 may be helpful to confirm a clinical diagnosis of genital herpes (especially when culture is falsely negative).
5. **Treatment.** See Table 81-1 for treatment options for initial and recurrent episodes of genital HSV.
6. **Follow-up.** Patients should return if lesions do not resolve, and should then be seen every 6–12 months to monitor for recurrences.

C. **Chancroid**
   1. **Etiology.** Chancroid is caused by *Haemophilus ducreyi.*
   2. **Epidemiology.** In the United States, chancroid usually occurs in discrete outbreaks (e.g. related to sex work or drug use) or in persons who have recently returned from chancroid endemic areas (Africa, Asia, Caribbean). Patients with chancroid have high rates of HIV coinfection, and about 10% of patients are coinfected with *Treponema pallidum* or HSV.
   3. **Clinical manifestations.** *H. ducreyi* has an incubation period of 4–7 days. Patients usually present with at least one **painful, nonindurated ulcer with irregular borders;** multiple ulcers are common. **Buboes,** tender inflamed inguinal lymph nodes that may become supporative, are seen in approximately 50% of patients.
   4. **Diagnosis**
      a. A **definitive diagnosis** is made by culture of *H. ducreyi* from the ulcer, which requires special culture media and has a sensitivity of only 80% or less.
      b. A **probable diagnosis** can be made if all of the following criteria are met:
         (1) the patient has one or more painful genital ulcers and the clinical presentation is typical of chancroid
         (2) testing of the ulcer exudate is negative for HSV
         (3) there is no evidence of syphilis on darkfield examination of the ulcer exudate or by serology performed at least 1 week after symptom onset

TABLE 81-1. Treatment of Herpes Simplex Virus Infections[*]

Clinical Situation	Recommended Treatment Regimens[†]	Comments on Therapy	Management of Sex Partners
Initial episode	(1) acyclovir 400 mg PO tid or 200 mg orally 5x/day for 7–10 days (2) valacyclovir 1000 mg PO bid for 7–10 days (3) famciclovir 250 mg PO tid for 7–10 days	Therapy may decrease the severity and duration of symptoms by 2–4 days, but has no effect on the frequency or severity of recurrences.	Sex partners should be offered evaluation and counseling regarding the natural history and implications of genital HSV infection.
Episodic treatment of recurrences	(1) acyclovir 400 mg PO tid or 200 mg 5x/day or 800 mg PO bid for 5 days (2) valacyclovir 500 mg PO bid or 1 gm PO once daily for 5 days (3) famciclovir 125 mg PO bid for 5 days	Treatment may decrease the length of the outbreak by 1–2 days, but must be initiated during the prodrome or within 1 day of symptoms. The patient should be given a supply of the drug or a prescription with instructions to self-initiate treatment when symptoms begin.	same as for initial episode
Suppressive therapy of recurrences	(1) acyclovir 400 mg PO bid (2) valacyclovir 500–1000 mg PO once daily (3) famciclovir 250 mg PO bid	Suppressive therapy is appropriate if the patient is experiencing frequent outbreaks (≥6 per year). Treatment can reduce the frequency of recurrences by 70–80%, and reduce subclinical viral shedding by 80–94%.	same as for initial episode

PO = orally

[*]Patients should be counseled to abstain from sex during outbreaks and to use condoms at all times since transmission is possible even when asymptomatic.

[†]For each clinical situation, any one of the listed regimens can be used as first line therapy.

5. **Treatment.**
   a. **Antibitoic therapy** should be with one of the following recommended regimens:
      (1) ceftriaxone 250 mg intramuscularly in a single dose
      (2) azithromycin 1 g orally in a single dose
      (3) erythromycin 500 mg orally tid for 7 days
      (4) ciprofloxacin 500 mg orally bid for 3 days
   b. Fluctuant lymph nodes may require aspiration or incision and drainage for proper healing.
6. **Follow-up.** The patient should be seen within 3–7 days to ensure clinical improvement. Patients with HIV and those who are uncircumcised do not respond as well to therapy.
7. **Management of sex partners**. All of the patient's sexual contacts within the past 10 days should be treated.

D. **Syphilis**
   1. **Etiology.** Syphilis is caused by *Treponema pallidum.*
   2. **Epidemiology.** After reaching a nadir in 2000, rates of primary and secondary sphilis in the United States have been increasing, largely due to the increase in cases among MSM.
   3. **Clinical stages.** The stages of syphilis are outlined in Table 81-2. **Early syphilis** refers to the **infectious** stages of syphilis in the first year after infection: primary, secondary, and early latent syphilis. **Late syphilis** refers to the **noninfectious** stages of syphilis after the first year: late latent and tertiary syphilis.

HOT KEY

Although neurosyphilis is often a form of tertiary syphilis, it can occur at any stage of the disease.

---

   4. **Diagnosis**
      a. **Serologic tests.** See Table 81-3 for a comparison of nontreponemal and treponemal antibody tests. In general, screening is performed using nontreponemal tests, and positive results are confirmed with the more specific treponemal tests. Serologic testing is useful in all stages of syphilis.
      b. **Darkfield examination** or **direct fluorescent antibody testing** of ulcer exudate or tissue is the definitive method for diagnosing primary or secondary syphilis, although these tests are only about 80% sensitive.
      c. **Diagnosis of neurosyphilis** is made by a positive CSF VDRL test result. This test is highly specific but only 30–70% sensitive. Results of serologic tests may need to be taken into account when the CSF VDRL is negative. Other

TABLE 81-2. Natural History and Clinical Manifestations of the Different Stages of Syphilis

Stage	Time Course	Clinical Manifestations
Early Syphilis		
primary syphilis	Usually occurs about 3 weeks after exposure, and resolves spontaneously.	1. painless indurated clean-based ulcer (**chancre**) usually with regional lymphadenopathy 2. chancres occur at the site of inoculation (usually anogenital but may be oral) and are usually solitary
secondary syphilis	Develops 4–10 weeks after the appearance of a chancre, and resolves spontaneously.	1. maculopapular **rash** (can involve the palms and soles) 2. generalized lymphadenopathy, malaise , headache, fever 3. **condyloma lata** (papular lesions in the intertriginous areas that are very infectious)
early latent syphilis	This stage encompasses the remainder of the first year of infection, after the signs of secondary syphilis have resolved.	Asymptomatic, although 25% of patients will have a relapse of secondary syphilis, usually within the first year after infection.
Late Syphilis		
late latent syphilis	This stage follows the first year of infection, prior to tertiary syphilis, and may last for months or for the rest of the patient's life. Patients with latent disease of unknown duration should be assumed to have late latent syphilis.	Asymptomatic

tertiary syphilis	Develops in approximately one third of untreated patients.	1. **gummas** are granulomatous lesions that form in the skin or viscera (usually respiratory tract, gastrointestinal tract, liver, and bones) 2. **cardiovascular complications** include aortitis, aortic regurgitation, or aneurysms 3. **neurosyphilis** (see below)
neurosyphilis	Early neurosyphilis occurs within weeks to a few years after infection (may occur during any stage of syphilis). Late neurosyphilis occurs years to decades after infection (as part of tertiary syphilis).	1. **early neurosyphilis** may be asymptomatic, or may manifest as meningitis (with or without cranial nerve findings) or as meningovascular disease/stroke 2. **late neurosyphilis** may manifest as **general paresis** or **tabes dorsalis** 3. **ocular involvment** can occur at any stage of disease

*__General paresis__ is a rapidly progressive dementia with psychotic features. **Tabes dorsalis** is degeneration of the posterior columns of the spinal cord resulting in impaired position sense, loss of reflexes, and ataxia; it may be associated with optic atrophy resulting in Argyll-Robertson pupils (react to accommodation but not to light).

TABLE 81-3. Serologic Tests for Syphilis

Serologic Test	What it Measures	When it is Positive	Clinical Uses	Sensitivity				Specificity
				primary Syphilis	Secondary Syphilis	Latent Syphilis	Tertiary Syphilis	
Nontreponemal tests (VDRL, RPR)	These tests measure antibodies to cardiolipin antigens, which increase with treponemal activity but may also increase in other diseases (e.g., connective tissue disorders, chronic infections) leading to false positives. False positives are usually low titer (≤1:8)	These tests turn positive 1–4 weeks after the development of a chancre (so can have false negatives in primary syphilis). Their positivity diminishes in the later stages of disease, and they usually become nonreactive after treatment.	(1) screening for syphilis (must be confirmed by a treponemal test) (2) follow response to therapy (a fourfold change in titer is considered a significant change) (3) VDRL in the CSF is used for diagnosis of neurosyphilis	78%	100%	95%	71%	85–99%

| Treponemal tests (FTA-ABS, TP-PA) | These tests measure antibodies to *T. pallidum* antigens, so are more specific. | These tests turn positive slightly sooner in the course of syphilis than the nontreponemal tests. Once positive, they usually remain reactive for the remainder of the patient's life. | (1) confirmation of nontreponemal screening tests may be useful (2) for the primary diagnosis of tertiary syphilis, where the sensitivity of nontreponemal tests is low | 84% | 100% | 100% | 96% | 96% |

FTA-ABS = fluorescent treponemal antibody-absorbed, RPR=rapid plasma reagin, TP-PA = *Treponema. pallidum* particle agglutination, VDRL = Venereal Disease Research Laboratory

CSF findings consistent with neurosyphilis are an elevated protein level and lymphocytic pleocytosis.

A **lumbar puncture and CSF analysis** should be performed in the following situations:

(1) neurologic or ocular signs or symptoms

(2) other evidence of active tertiary syphilis

(3) treatment failure

(4) HIV infection with late latent syphilis or syphilis of unknown duration

(5) nontreponemal serologic test of $\geq 1{:}32$

5. **Treatment**. See Table 81-4 for treatment regimens for the different stages of syphilis. Neurosyphilis, syphilitic eye disease, and syphilis in pregnancy or HIV infection should be treated in consultation with an infectious disease specialist.

6. **Follow-up.** All patients should have repeat clinical and serologic evaluation at 6, 12, and 24 months after treatment. If titers fail to fall four-fold after 6 months (for early syphilis) or 12 months (for late syphilis), or if they increase four-fold at any time, patients should be evaluated for treatment failure. Unless reinfection is certain, these patients should be retested for HIV and have a lumbar puncture to evaluate for neurosyphillis. Retreatment may be necesssary.

IV GENITAL WARTS (CONDYLOMATA ACUMINATA)

A. Etiology. Genital warts are usually caused by **human papillomavirus (HPV)** types 6 and 11 (these are rarely associated with anogenital cancer)**.**

B. Clinical manifestations. Genital warts can occur on the external gentalia and also in the cervix, vagina, urethra, anus, and mouth. They are flesh-colored exophytic lesions which are often asymptomatic, but can become painful, friable, and pruritic.

C. Dignosis is usually made on clinical grounds alone. There is no indication for type-specific HPV nucleic acid testing. **Biopsy,** however, may be necessary in the following cases: (1) if the diagnosis is uncertain, (2) the lesions do not respond to standard therapy, (3) the patient is immunocompromised, or (4) the lesions are pigmented, indurated, or ulcerated.

D. Treatment can eradicate warts in most patients, although recurrences are common. Treatment options for external genital warts are shown in Table 81-5. Some general considerations for treatment are as follows:

1. Since in some cases warts may resolve spontaneously, it is an acceptable alternative to defer treatment and wait for spontaneous resolution.

2. Chemical treatments are usually more effective on moist, soft warts, while keratinized warts respond better to ablative

TABLE 81-4. Treatment of the Different Stages of Syphilis

Disease	Recommended Treatment Regimens	Comments on Therapy	Management of Sex Partners
early syphilis (primary, secondary, and early latent syphilis)	**(1)** benzathine penicillin G 2.4 million units IM in a single dose **(2)** doxycycline 100 mg PO bid for 14 days can be used for penicillin allergic patients*	The **Jarisch-Herxheimer reaction (JHR)** is an acute febrile reaction associated with headache and myalgia that can occur within the first 24 hours after therapy for syphilis, most commonly early syphilis. JHR is thought to be caused by an inflammatory reaction that results as the treponemes are killed.	Sex partners within the last 90 days should be evaluated and treated for syphilis even if seronegative (since serologies may be negative at this point). Sex partners exposed >90 days prior should be tested and treated accordingly.
late syphilis (late latent and tertiary syphilis without eye or neurologic disease)	**(1)** benzathine penicillin G 2.4 million units IM once weekly for 3 weeks **(2)** doxycycline 100 mg PO bid for 28 days can be used for penicillin allergic patients*		same as for early syphilis
neurosyphilis or syphilitic eye disease	aqueous crystalline penicillin G 3–4 million units IV every 4 hours for 10–14 days	Treatment should be undertaken in conjunction with an infectious disease expert.	same as for early syphilis

IM = intramuscularly, PO = orally, IV = intravenously

*There is only limited data to support the alternatives to penicillin in the treatment of syphilis. Therefore, if used, compliance and close follow-up should be assured. If compliance or follow-up is in question, consider penicillin skin testing and desensitization in conjunction with an expert.

515

TABLE 81-5. Treatment Options for External Genital Warts

Type of Treatment	Treatment Details	Comments
Patient Administered		
Podofilox 0.5% solution	Apply to lesions twice daily for 3 days. Patients should allow the solution to dry before moving around, in order to prevent local irritation.	Treatment can be repeated weekly for up to 4 weeks. Podofilox should be avoided in pregnancy.
Imiquimod 5% cream	Apply 3 times per week at bedtime; should be washed off 6–10 hours after application.	Imiquimod may be used for as long as 16 weeks, but should be avoided in pregnancy.
Provider Administered		
Cryotherapy	Apply liquid nitrogen topically.	May be repeated every 1–2 weeks.
Podophyllin resin 10–25%	Apply in a compound tincture of benzoin and allow to dry completely. It should be washed off by the patient in 1–4 hours to reduce local irritation. Application should be limited to ≤0.5 ml of podophyllin.	Treatment can be repeated weekly. Podophyllin should be avoided in pregnancy.
Trichloracetic acid (TCA) or bichloracetic acid (BCA) 80–90%	Apply in a small amount; if applied excessively the solution can spread and damage adjacent tissues.	Treatment can be repeated weekly.
Surgical removal by scissor or shave excision, curettage, or electrosurgery.	Should be performed by a trained provider.	Most beneficial for patients who have a large number or area of warts.

therapies. For chemical treatments, consider starting with patient-applied therapy, then switch to physician-applied therapy if there is no response.

3. If there is no response after three cycles of treatment and the diagnosis is certain, change to a new modality.

4. **Treatment of warts in other locations** (cervix, urethra, anus, vagina) may require consultation with a specialist. For example, neoplastic lesions must be excluded prior to treatment of **cervical warts**.

E. **Follow-up.** Patients should be seen at 3 months after treatment to monitor for recurrences, which are most common during this time frame. Closer follow up may be useful to monitor for treatment complications.

HOT ▶ **KEY**

Visible genital warts are usually caused by HPV types 6 and 11, which are rarely associated with anogenital cancer.

F. **Management of sex partners.** Sex partners should be counseled regarding the natural history of genital HPV infection.

V URETHRITIS IN MEN

A. **Etiology. Gonococcal urethritis (gonorrhea)** is caused by *Neisseria gonorrhoeae*. **Nongonococcal urethritis (NGU)** is caused by *Chlamydia trachomatis* in 15–55% of cases. The etiology of most cases of non-chlamydial NGU remains unknown, but some are caused by *Ureaplasma urealyticum, Mycoplasma genitalium, Trichomonas vaginalis,* and HSV.

B. **Clinical manifestations.** The incubation period for gonococcal urethritis is 2–5 days, while for NGU it is 1–5 weeks. Symptoms include urethral discomfort and pruritis, dysuria, and mucopurulent urethral discharge, but asympomatic infections are common. Clinical manifestations alone cannot differentiate between gonorrhea and NGU.

C. **Diagnosis.** Figure 81-1 shows the approach to diagnosis and treatment of urethritis in men. Table 81-6 lists the characteristics of the different diagnostic tests for gonorrhea and chlamydia. In general, for *N. gonorrhoeae,* culture is still the gold standard, although nucleic acid amplification tests (NAATs) of urethral swabs, cervical swabs, or urine are as sensitive as culture (although urine from women may have slightly lower sensitivity). For *C. trachomatis,* NAATs from urethral swabs, cervical swabs, or urine are now the standard of care due to their superior sensitivity when compared to culture.

TABLE 81-6. Diagnostic Tests for Urethritis and Cervicitis

Diagnostic Test	Sensitivity	Specificity	Key Features
N. gonorrhoeae			
Gram stain of urethral discharge	90–95%	95–100%	-rapid diagnosis -not always readily available, requires training
culture from cervix, urethra	95%	100%	-can provide antibiotic susceptibilities -is still considered the **diagnostic method of choice** for gonorrhea
NAAT from urethra, cervix, first-void urine	92–99%	92–100%	-urine tests are noninvasive -sensitivity is as good if not better than culture (except for female urine specimens, for which sensitivity is only 85–90%)
C. trachomatis			
culture from cervix, urethra	70–85%	100%	less sensitive than NAAT
NAAT from urethra, cervix, first-void urine	90–97%	94–99%	-urine tests are noninvasive -is the **diagnostic method of choice** for chlamydia due to its better sensitivity

NAAT = nucleic acid amplification test.

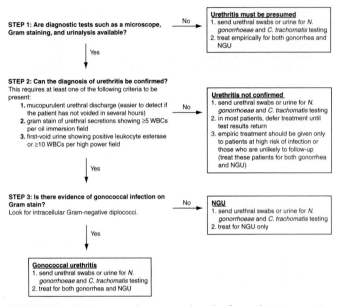

STEP 1: Are diagnostic tests such as a microscope, Gram staining, and urinalysis available? — No →

Urethritis must be presumed
1. send urethral swabs or urine for *N. gonorrhoeae* and *C. trachomatis* testing
2. treat empirically for both gonorrhea and NGU

Yes ↓

STEP 2: Can the diagnosis of urethritis be confirmed?
This requires at least one of the following criteria to be present:
1. mucopurulent urethral discharge (easier to detect if the patient has not voided in several hours)
2. gram stain of urethral secretions showing ≥5 WBCs per oil immersion field
3. first-void urine showing positive leukocyte esterase or ≥10 WBCs per high power field

— No →

Urethritis not confirmed
1. send urethral swabs or urine for *N. gonorrhoeae* and *C. trachomatis* testing
2. in most patients, defer treatment until test results return
3. empiric treatment should be given only to patients at high risk of infection or those who are unlikely to follow-up (treat these patients for both gonorrhea and NGU)

Yes ↓

STEP 3: Is there evidence of gonococcal infection on Gram stain?
Look for intracellular Gram-negative diplococci.

— No →

NGU
1. send urethral swabs or urine for *N. gonorrhoeae* and *C. trachomatis* testing
2. treat for NGU only

Yes ↓

Gonococcal urethritis
1. send urethral swabs or urine for *N. gonorrhoeae* and *C. trachomatis* testing
2. treat for both gonorrhea and NGU

FIGURE 81-1. Diagnostic and treatment algorithm for urethritis in men. See text for a discussion of the diagnostic testing options for *N. gonorrhoeae* and *C. trachomatis*. NGU = nongonococcal urethritis; WBC = white blood cell.

D. Treatment. See the diagnostic and treatment algorithm in Figure 81-1, and the specific treatment regimens in Table 81-7. Some general points are as follows:

1. **Patients with gonococcal urethritis** are often coinfected with chlamydia, and so must be treated for both infections.

2. **Patients with definitive NGU** do not need to be treated for gonorrhea as well. Note that the treatment for NGU is directed at *C. trachomatis,* but also covers most of the non-chlamydial causes of NGU as well.

E. Follow-up. Patients should be instructed to return if symptoms persist or recur after completion of therapy. A test of cure is not necessary.

HOT **KEY**   Persistent or recurrent NGU may be caused by *T. vaginalis* or doxycycline-resistant *U. urealyticum*. These patients should be treated with metronidazole (2 g orally in a single dose) and erythromycin (500 mg qid for 7 days).

TABLE 81-7. Treatment of Urethritis and Cervicitis*

Treatment of Gonococcal Urethritis or Cervicitis†	Treatment of NGU or Chlamydial Cervicitis	Management of Sex Partners with Urethritis or Cervicitis
cefixime 400 mg PO in a single dose ceftriaxone 125 mg IM in a single dose ofloxacin 400 mg PO in a single dose‡ levofloxacin 250 mg PO in a single dose‡ ciprofloxacin 500 mg PO in a single dose‡	azithromycin 1 gm PO in a single dose doxycyline 100 mg PO bid for 7 days	All sex partners within the preceding 60 days should be treated. If a patient's last sexual activity was >60 days prior, the most recent partner should be treated.

PO = orally, IM = intramuscularly
*Patients should abstain from sexual intercourse until 7 days after therapy is initiated. Any one of the listed regimens can be used for first line therapy.
†Recall that all patients diagnosed with gonococcal urethritis or cervicitis should be treated for chlamydial infection as well, with one of the regimens shown in the middle portion of this table.
‡Due to increased resistance, fluoroquinolones should not be used to treat gonococcal infections acquired in Asia, the Pacific, Hawaii, or California.

VI CERVICITIS

A. Etiology. Cervical infections are usually caused by *C. trachomatis* and *N. gonorrhoeae,* but may also be caused by other STDs including HSV and HPV. Cervicitis also may be caused by, or coexist with, vaginal infections such as trichomoniasis. If cervicitis is accompanied by a mucopurulent discharge, it is referred to as **mucopuulent cervicitis (MPC)** – this is often caused by *C. trachomatis* or *N. gonorrhoeae,* although in most cases no organism is identified.

HOT
KEY
Chlamydial and gonococcal cervicitis are important to recognize because they can lead to complications such as pelvic inflammatory disease and infertility. Because these infections are often asymptomatic, screening for *C. trachomatis* and *N. gonorrhea* is recommended in all asymptomatic women with risk factors for these infections.

B. Clinical manifestations. Patients may have symptoms of abnormal vaginal discharge or bleeding (e.g. after sexual intercourse), dyspareunia, dysuria, or lower abdominal pain. However, asymptomatic infection from either *C. trachomatis* or *N. gonorrhoeae* is common.

C. Physical examination. There may be a mucopurulent endocervical discharge (i.e. MPC), and the cervix may be inflamed, edematous, and have areas of bleeding. However, cervicitis may be present even in the absence of physical findings.

D. Diagnosis. See Table 81-6 and section V-C for a comparison of available diagnostic tests for *C. trachomatis* and *N. gonorrhoeae.*

E. Screening of asymptomatic women with risk factors. Current guidelines recommend screening all sexually active women ≤25 years old or any woman with new or multiple sex partners, a previous STD, or inconsistenet condom use.

F. Treatment, in general, should be guided by test results. As for urethritis in men, all patients with gonorrhea should also be treated for chlamydia. Treatment regimens for chlamydial and gonoccal cervicitis are shown in Table 81-7. Empiric treatment of gonorrhea and chlamydia in patients with MPC may be considered if the local prevalence of disease is high or the patient is unlikely to return for follow-up.

G. Follow-up. Patients should be instructed to return if symptoms persist or recur after completion of therapy. A test of cure is not necessary. However, due to the high prevalence of *C. trachomatis* infection in women who have had chlamydia in the preceding several months, all women with chlamydia should be rescreened at 3–4 months after treatment.

VII PELVIC INFLAMMATORY DISEASE IS DISCUSSED IN CHAPTER 47

VIII VAGINAL INFECTIONS ARE DISCUSSED IN CHAPTER 48

IX EPIDIDYMITIS IS DISCUSSED IN CHAPTER 42

X HEPATITIS

A. Hepatitis A.
  1. Epidemiology and transmission. Hepatitis A virus (HAV) is transmitted by the fecal-oral route, which may occur during sexual activity. Outbreaks have occurred in MSM and illicit drug users.
  2. Clinical manifestations.

   a. **Acute hepatitis.** The incubation period is 2–6 weeks. Symptomatic infection is more common in adults compared to children, with >80% of adults manifesting symptoms. Initially, symptoms are nonspecific and flu-like, but as the disease progresses the patient may develop fever, jaundice, and right upper quadrant pain. Fulminant hepatitis occurs in only about 0.3% of patients.

   b. **Chronic infection** does not occur from HAV.

3. **Diagnosis.**

   a. **Transaminases** are usually elevated, and levels may be >1000 IU/mL.

   b. **Serology.** The presence of **IgM antibodies against HAV** is diagnostic of HAV infection. A positive test for total anti-HAV antibodies cannot differentiate between acute and prior infection.

4. **Treatment** is with supportive care only. Medications that are metabolized by the liver or that are potentially hepatotoxic should be avoided.

5. **Follow-up.** Patients should be seen in 1–2 weeks to ensure that their symptoms have resolved and that transaminases have returned to normal.

6. **Management of sex partners.** Previously unvaccinated sex-partners of patients with HAV should receive **postexposure prophylaxis** with HAV immune globulin if within 2 weeks of exposure. Testing for prior immunity can be considered if it won't delay treatment beyond the 2 week window. These patients should also be considered for long term protection with HAV vaccine.

7. **Prevention.** HAV vaccine should be offered to MSM and illicit drug users (injection and non-injection). Prevaccination serologic testing to detect prior immunity may be cost-effective in areas of high prevalence.

B. **Hepatitis B.**

1. **Epidemiology and transmission.** Hepatitis B virus (HBV) can be transmitted by exposure to infectious body fluids. Sexual transmission accounts for most cases of HBV in the United States: heterosexual transmission accounts for about 40%, and MSM about 15%.

2. **Clinical manifestations.**

   a. **Acute hepatitis.** The incubation period for HBV is 6 weeks to 6 months. Symptomatic infection occurs in 50% of adults. The clinical features are similar to those of HAV. Fulminant liver disease occurs in about 1% of cases.

   b. **Chronic infection** can develop following acute infection, and the risk is higher in younger patients: 90% of infants, 60% of children <5 years old, and only 2–6% of infected

TABLE 81-8. Serologic Markers at Different Stages of Hepatitis B Infection

Stage of Hepatitis B Infection	Hepatitis B Surface Antigen (HBsAg)	Antibody against Hepatitis B Surface Antigen (anti-HBs)	Antibody against Hepatitis B Core Antigen (anti-HBc)
Acute infection	+	−	IgM
Chronic infection	+	−	IgG
Past infection, resolved	−	+	IgG
Immunization	−	+	−

adults will become chronically infected. Chronic HBV predisposes to cirrhosis and hepatocellular carcinoma.

3. **Diagnosis.**
   a. **Transaminases** are usually elevated, and may be >1000 IU/mL.
   b. **Serology**. See Table 81-8 for the patterns of serologic markers in different stage of HBV infection.
4. **Treatment**
   a. **Acute hepatitis** is treated with supportive care, as described for HAV infection.
   b. **Chronic infection.** Patients may respond to α-interferon and other antiviral drugs (e.g., lamivudine) and should be referred to a liver disease specialist for further evaluation.
5. **Follow-up.** Patients should be seen in 1–2 weeks to ensure that their symptoms have resolved and that liver function tests have returned to normal. Patients with chronic hepatitis B should be referred to a liver specialist.
6. **Management of sex partners**. Previoulsy unvaccinated sex partners of patients with acute HBV should receive **post-exposure prophylaxis** with HBV immune globulin if within 2 weeks of exposure. Testing for prior immunity can be considered if it will not delay treatment beyond the 2 week window. These patients should also be offerred the HBV vaccine for long term protection. Partners of patients with chronic HBV infection should be offered vaccination.
7. **Prevention.** HBV vaccine should be offered to all patients being evaluated for an STD. Prevaccination serologic testing to detect prior immunity may be cost-effective in areas of high prevalence.

HOT KEY

HAV and HBV are preventable by vaccination. All MSM and illicit drug users should be offered the HAV vaccine. All patients being evaluated for an STD should be offered the HBV vaccine.

C. Hepatitis C.

1. **Epidemiology and transmission.** Hepatitis C virus (HCV) is transmitted by exposure to infected blood, usually via injection drug use. HCV can also be transmitted via blood products, although this has been substantially decreased by screening of donated blood products. The role of sexual activity in the transmission of **HCV** is controversial. Sexual transmission between monogamous partners is rare, but may occur in persons with multiple sexual partners or with preexisting STDs.

2. **Clinical manifestations.**
   a. **Acute hepatitis.** The incubation period is about 8–9 weeks. Most acute infections are asymptomatic.
   b. **Chronic infection** develops in 75–85% of those infected. These patients tend to be asymptomatic until the complications of chronic hepatitis develop.

3. **Diagnosis.**
   a. **Transaminases** may be elevated intermittently in chronic infection.
   b. **Serology**. The diagnosis is made by detecting antibodies to HCV.

4. **Treatment of chronic infection.** Patients may benefit from therapy with α-interferon and ribavirin, and should be referred to a liver disease specialist for further evaluation.

5. **Follow-up.** Consider referral of patient with chronic HCV infection to a liver specialist, especially if treatment is being considered.

6. **Management of Sex Partners.** Sex partners should be encouraged to be tested for HCV, but there is no effective post-exposure prophylaxis. Long term partners should be counseled regarding the low but present risk of sexual transmission.

7. **Prevention**. There is no effective vaccine against HCV.

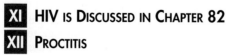

XI HIV is Discussed in Chapter 82

XII Proctitis

A. Etiology. Sexually acquired proctitis is usually caused by *N. gonorrhoeae*, *C. trachomatis*, *T. pallidum*, or HSV.

B. Transmission. Proctitis can be acquired sexually via receptive anal intercourse.

C. Clinical manifestations include rectal pain, tenesmus, and rectal discharge.

D. Diagnosis. Patients should undergo anoscopy, and rectal swabs should be sent for *N. gonorrhoeae* and *C. trachomatis* culture (NAATs are not recommended on rectal samples). Lesions suspicious for HSV should be sent for culture, and those suspicious for syphilis should be examined by direct fluorescent antibody testing (darkfield examination is not recommended for rectal lesions). Serologic testing for syphilis should be performed.

E. Treatment should be aimed at the particular infectious organism.

    1. Patients with suspected HSV should be managed in the same way as for genital herpes (see section IIIB).

    2. If an anorectal exudate is seen, empiric therapy for *N. gonorrhoeae and C. trachomatis* may be given while test results are pending. The recommended regimen in this case is ceftriaxone 125 mg intramuscularly in a single dose *plus* doxycycline 100 mg PO bid for 7 days.

F. Follow-up. Patients should be seen in 1–2 weeks to ensure resolution of disease and for further STD counseling.

G. Management of sex partners. Sex partners should be evaluated and treated for the specific disease diagnosed in the patient, as per previous sections in this chapter.

References

Centers for Disease Contol and Prevention. Sexually transmitted diseases treatment guidelines *MMWR* 2002;51:RR-6.

Golden MR, Marra CM, Holmes KK. Update on syphilis: resurgence of an old problem. *JAMA* 2003;290(11):1510–1514.

Kimberlin DW, Rouse DJ. Genital herpes. *N Engl J Med* 2004;350(19):1970–1977.

82. Human Immunodeficiency Virus (HIV)/Acquired Immunodeficiency Syndrome (AIDS)

I **INTRODUCTION.** Although HIV medicine has evolved into its own specialty at many centers, patients benefit from having a primary care provider who is knowledgeable about HIV infection, its complications, and therapy.

II **OVERVIEW OF CLINICAL HIV DISEASE**

A. **Transmission.** The most important risk factors for acquiring HIV in the United States are male-to-male sexual contact, heterosexual contact (especially among women), and injection drug use. Other less common modes of tranmission are occupational needlesticks, transfusion with contaminated blood products, and mother-to-child transmission

B. **Clinical Stages**
1. **Primary, or acute, HIV infection** is the time period from initial infection until the development of a detectable antibody response (i.e. seroconversion). Many patients have an acute viral syndrome during this time, with symptoms including fever, malaise, lymphadenopathy, maculopapular rash, and pharyngitis. Diagnosis of acute HIV infection is made by a positive viral load test (>10,000 copies/mL) in the presence of a negative or indeterminate antibody assay (or recent seroconversion). Any positive viral load test must be confirmed with documentation of subsequent antibody seroconversion.
2. **Chronic HIV Infection.** There may be little or no clinical manifestations of HIV infection during this time, although without treatment there is usually progressive loss of CD4 cells and increase in viral load. Rate of progression to AIDS varies but usually occurs over an average of 10 years.
3. **AIDS** is defined as either (1) a CD4 count <200 cells/μL, or (2) an AIDS defining illness (e.g. most opportunistic infections (OIs), certain malignancies, HIV-associated wasting or dementia).

C. Diagnosis of HIV infection

1. **Serologic testing** with an enzyme immunoassay to detect serum antibodies against HIV is the gold standard for diagnosing HIV infection. Positive tests are confirmed by Western blot assay. Antibody tests may be negative in the "window period" after initial infection, which may last a few weeks up to 6 months. Due to this risk of an early false negative, persons reporting high-risk behavior who have an initial negative test should be retested at 6, 12, and 24 weeks.

2. **Viral load tests** measure the amount of HIV RNA and are used to follow HIV disease progression, monitor treatment response, and diagnose acute HIV infection.

3. **Rapid HIV testing** is becoming more widely available. Tests can be performed on fingerstick blood or saliva samples and results can be available in less than 1 hour. Confirmatory serologic testing is required for all positive results.

4. **Disclosure of a positive test**. Newly diagnosed patients require both emotional and practical support. Enquire about the patient's support network and arrange other support services when possible. It should be emphasized to the patient that HIV can be a manageable chronic disease.

HOT KEY The key step in diagnosing acute HIV infection is to include it in the differential diagnosis. When evaluating a patient with an acute viral or mononucleosis-like syndrome, have a high index of suspicion and make sure to ask the patient about risk factors for HIV infection.

III PRIMARY CARE OF THE PATIENT WITH HIV INFECTION

A. Counseling about risk reduction (see also Table 82-1).

1. **Sexual activity.** Patients should be counselled to **use latex condoms** during sexual intercourse in order to prevent the transmission of HIV to others and to prevent exposure of the patient to STDs. Patients should **avoid oral-anal contact** in order to reduce the risk of acquiring intestinal pathogens (e.g., *Cryptosporidium*, *Campylobacter*).

2. **Injection drug use.** Patients should be encouraged to discontinue injection drug use, and referred to a substance abuse rehabilitation program or methadone clinic when approriate. Patients who continue to use injection drugs should be educated not to share or reuse needles.

TABLE 82-1. Recommended Screening Tests and Risk Reduction Strategies in Patients with HIV Infection			
Disease	Screening Test	Frequency of Screening	Risk Reduction
tuberculosis	–TST, positive at ≥5 mm of induration	–baseline –consider yearly follow-up TST in all patients but especially if have risk factors for TB	–avoid contact with known or suspected TB cases –treatment of latent TB infection (see Chapter 83)
cervical or anal squamous cell cancer*	–cervical Pap smear in women –anal Pap smear in women and MSM†	–every 6 months for the first year after diagnosis –then annually if no abnormal results are obtained	
STDs (syphilis, trichomoniasis, gonorrhea, chlamydia)	–see Chapters 48 and 81 for STD screening tests	–baseline –periodic follow-up screening based on risk factors	–use latex condoms during sexual intercourse to reduce risk of exposure to STDs
hepatitis A, B, C	–anti-hepatitis A IgG –hepatitis B surface antigen, antibody to surface antigen and core antigen –anti-hepatitis C antibody	–baseline	–consider hepatitis A and B vaccinations for all patients without prior immunity‡ –use latex condoms during sexual intercourse to reduce risk of HPV exposure –avoid oral-anal contact –injection drug users should not share needles

toxoplasmosis	–anti-*Toxoplasma* IgG	–baseline –if negative, repeat when CD4 count <100 cells/μl	–to avoid new infection: avoid eating undercooked meat and handling of cat feces, wash hands after contact with soil
CMV	–anti-CMV IgG	–baseline –if negative, repeat when CD4 count <50 cells/μL	–to avoid new infection: good handwashing; receive CMV-negative transfusions in non-emergent situations, use condoms during sexual intercourse –seropositive patients should have an ophthalmologic examination when their CD4 count is <50 cells/μL
varicella-zoster virus	–anti-varicella IgG	–baseline in patients unable to give a history of chickenpox or shingles	–seronegative patients should receive varicella-zoster immune globulin within 96 hours after exposure to a patient with chickenpox or shingles

CMV = cytomegalovirus, HPV = Human papilloma virus, MSM=men who have sex with men, RPR=rapid plasma reagin, STD = sexually transmitted disease, TB = tuberculosis, TST = tuberculin skin test, VDRL = Venereal Disease Research Laboratory

*HPV and resultant anal and cervical intraepithelial neoplasia are more common in HIV-infected patients, although it is not clear if there is an increase in anal or cervical cancer.

†There are no formal recommendations for anal HPV screening, but some experts recommend anal pap smears for HIV-infected women and MSM at the same intervals as for cervical screening.

‡Hepatitis B vaccination is recommended in all patients without evidence of immunity; hepatitis A vaccination is recommended in those with chronic liver disease, MSM, and injection drug users, but should be considered for all patients without immunity.

3. **Diet.** Patients should **avoid undercooked eggs and meat** in order to reduce the risk of infection with food-borne pathogens (e.g. *Salmonella, Toxoplasma*).

4. **Pets.** Patients should **avoid acquiring pets younger than 6 months old** because they are more likely to harbor diarrheal pathogens. To decrease the risk of exposure to *Bartonella* and *Toxoplasma*, patients should avoid cat scratches or bites and avoid contact with cat feces respectively.

B. **Baseline studies** should include a CD4 cell count, HIV viral load, complete blood count (CBC), chemistry panel, fasting blood glucose and lipid panel, liver panel, urinalysis, and chest radiograph. Check a **glucose-6-phosphate dehydrogenase** level at baseline or before initiating therapy with drugs such as dapsone or primaquine, especially in blacks and in those from the Mediterranean, India, and Southeast Asia.

C. **Ongoing laboratory monitoring**

1. **CD4 count and HIV viral load** should be repeated every 3–4 months in patients with a stable CD4 count and viral load, and more frequently in patients initiating treatment or with unstable counts.

2. Monitoring for **drug side effects** requires periodic monitoring of CBC, chemistry panel, LFTs, and fasting blood glucose and lipids.

D. **Recommended screening tests** in patients with HIV infection are shown in Table 82-1.

HOT KEY

HIV-infected patients should receive comprehensive screening for tuberculosis, CMV, toxoplasmosis, varicella zoster virus, viral hepatitis, and STDs including HPV and syphilis. Patients should be educated regarding ways to reduce their risk of exposure to these and other opportunistic infections.

E. **Vaccination**

1. Recommended vaccines include a **pneumococcal vaccine** every 5 years, **hepatitis A** and **B vaccines** in patients without immunity (see Table 82-1), and an annual inactivated **influenza vaccine**.

2. **Live vaccines** (e.g. oral polio, MMR, oral typhoid, yellow fever, varicella, intranasal influenza) are, in general, **contraindicated** in HIV-infection.

F. **Addressing end-of-life issues.** Providers should encourage patients to designate a durable power of attorney for health care, to express the degree of medical intervention desired in various circumstances, and to explore options for hospice care if appropriate.

IV OPPORTUNISTIC INFECTIONS AND OTHER COMPLICATIONS OF HIV INFECTION

A. **Complications of HIV,** in general, occur based on the degree of immunosuppression, which is reflected in the CD4 count of the patient (see Table 82-2).

B. **Presentation, diagnosis, and treatment** of the most common OIs are shown in Table 82-3.

C. **Antimicrobial prophylaxis of OIs**
   1. *Pneumocystis jiroveci* **pneumonia (PCP).** Trimethoprim-sulfamethaxazole (TMP-SMZ) (1 DS tab daily) should be given if the **CD4 count is <200 cells/μL** or for a **history of oropharyngeal candidiasis.** Alternatives include dapsone, atovaquone, and aerosolized pentamidine.
   2. *Toxoplasma gondii* **encephalitis.** TMP-SMX (1 DS tab daily) should be given if the **CD4 count is <100 cells/μL and the patient is** *Toxoplasma***-seropositive.** Alternatives include dapsone plus pyrimethamine or atovaquone with or without pyrimethamine.
   3. **Disseminated** *Mycobacterium avium* **complex (MAC).** Azithromycin (1200 mg orally [PO] weekly) or clarithromycin (500 mg PO bid) should be given if the **CD4 count is <50 cells/μL.** An alternative agent is rifabutin.

V ANTIRETROVIRAL THERAPY (ART)

A. **When to initiate treatment?**
   1. ART is **recommended** for:
      a. patients with a history of an AIDS-defining illness or severe symptoms of HIV, irrespective of CD4 count
      b. asymptomatic patients with a CD4 count <200 cells/μL
   2. ART should be **considered** for:
      a. asymptomatic patients with a CD4 count between 201–350 cells/μL
      b. asymptomatic patients with a CD4 count >350 cells/μL and HIV viral load >100,000 copies/ml, although most would defer therapy for this group
   3. ART should be **deferred** in patients with CD4 count >350 cells/μL and HIV viral load <100,000 copies/ml

B. **Types of Antiretrovirals (ARVs).** There are four main classes of ARVs: nucleoside/nucleotide reverse transcriptase inhibitors (NRTIs), non-nucleoside reverse transcriptase inhibitors (NNRTIs), protease inhibitors (PIs), and fusion inhibitors. The drugs in each class and their associated side effects are shown in Table 82-4.

C. **Which regimen to start with in a drug naïve patient?** Choice of a regimen should be made by or in conjunction with an HIV

TABLE 82-2. Correlation of CD4 Cell Count with Infectious and Noninfectious Complications of HIV Infection*

CD4 Cell Count (cells/μL)	Infectious Complications	Noninfectious Complications†
<500	bacterial pneumonia pulmonary tuberculosis herpes zoster infection	cervical intraepithelial neoplasia idiopathic thrombocytopenic purpura Hodgkin's lymphoma oral hairy leukoplakia
<200	Pneumocystis jiroveci pneumonia (PCP)‡ disseminated histoplasmosis or coccidioidomycosis miliary or extrapulmonary tuberculosis progressive multifocal encephalopathy (PML) oropharyngeal and esophageal candidiasis severe herpes simplex infections cryptosporidiosis microsporidiosis	HIV-associated dementia peripheral neuropathy Non-Hodgkin's lymphoma Kaposi's sarcoma HIV-associated wasting primary effusion lymphoma
<100	Toxoplasma encephalitis cytomegalovirus infection disseminated Mycobacterium avium complex bacillary angiomatosis cryptococcal meningitis	
<50		CNS lymphoma

*The CD4 count ranges listed here are only general guidelines for categorizing the complications by CD4 count, and should not be taken as strict definitions.

†Some neoplastic diseases listed here as "noninfectious" are associated with infectious organisms (e.g. Kaposi's sarcoma and primary effusion lymphoma are associated with human herpes virus-8) and so could also be considered as "infectious complications."

‡The taxonomy of the organism has been changed such that causative organism of Pneumocystis pneumonia in humans is referred to as Pneumocystis jiroveci, but the abbreviation is still PCP.

TABLE 82-3. Presentation, Diagnosis, and Treatment of Selected Opportunistic Infections in HIV Disease*

Disease	Presentation	Diagnosis	Treatment
Pneumocystis jiroveci pneumonia (PCP)	subacute exertional dyspnea, fever, dry cough	chest x-ray, histologic examination of induced sputum or BAL	TMP-SMX, corticosteroids if room air pO2 <70 mm Hg or Aa gradient ≥35
Toxoplasma gondii encephalitis	fever, headache, confusion, focal weakness, seizure	anti-*Toxoplasma* IgG, brain CT/MRI, biopsy	pyrimethamine plus sulfadiazine plus leucovorin
disseminated *Mycobacterium avium* complex (MAC)	fever, night sweats, weight loss, anemia, lymphadenopathy, hepatosplenomegaly	AFB blood culture, biopsy for AFB smear and culture	clarithromycin plus ethambutol +/− rifabutin
bacterial pneumonia	fever, productive cough	chest x-ray, blood and sputum cultures	same guidelines as for those without HIV infection
Salmonella, Shigella, Campylobacter	diarrhea, sepsis	stool and blood cultures	fluoroquinolones
cryptosporidiosis, microsporidiosis	diarrhea	microscopic identification of organisms in stool	ARVs with immune restoration to CD4 >100, albendazole (some microsporidia only)
bacillary angiomatosis	red, papular, vascular lesions (most commonly of skin)	biopsy for histopathology, serology	doxycycline or erythromycin
oropharyngeal and esophageal candidiasis	oral: painless thrush esophageal: retrosternal pain, odynophagia, fever	clinical appearance, KOH staining	fluconazole

(Continued)

TABLE 82-3. Presentation, Diagnosis, and Treatment of Selected Opportunistic Infections in HIV Disease* (Continued)

Disease	Presentation	Diagnosis	Treatment
cryptococcal meningitis	fever, headache, +/− neck stiffness and photophobia	CSF and serum cryptococcal antigen, CSF has high opening pressure	amphotericin B plus flucytosine for 2 wk induction then fluconazole consolidation for 8 wks then chronic maintenance therapy
cytomegalovirus (CMV)	retinitis, colitis, esophagitis	fundoscopic exam; serum antigen, PCR, or culture; CMV inclusion bodies on biopsy	IV ganciclovir or foscarnet; oral valganciclovir; ganciclovir intraocular implant
varicella zoster virus	shingles	clinical appearance, viral culture of lesion	oral or IV acyclovir; steroids not recommended
disseminated histoplasmosis, coccidioidomycosis	disseminated disease, meningitis	urine or serum *Histoplasma* antigen, *Coccidioides* serology and complement fixation, culture	amphotericin B; itraconazole, fluconazole (depending on severity and site of disease)
progressive multifocal leukoencephalopathy	rapidly progressive dementia and neurologic dysfunction	MRI, brain biopsy, CSF PCR for JC virus	some patients may benefit from starting ARVs

AFB = acid-fast bacilli, ARV = antiretroviral, BAL = bronchoalveolar lavage, CT = computed tomography, CSF = cerebrospinal fluid, IV = intravenous, MRI = magnetic resonance imaging, TMP-SMX = trimethoprim-sulfamethoxazole.
*This is a selected list of common opportunistic infections. See Chapter 83 for tuberculosis and Chapter 81 for syphilis, HSV, and other STDs.
†Only the recommended first-line treatment is shown here. Alternative regimens may be necessary when patients have an allergy to or intolerance of first line therapy

TABLE 82-4. Antiretrovirals and their Adverse Effects

Drug	Brand Name	Adverse Effects
Nucleoside/nucleotide Reverse Transcriptase Inhibitors (NRTIs)		**class effects*: hepatotoxicity, mitochondrial toxicity[†]**
abacavir (ABC)	Ziagen	nausea, vomiting, diarrhea, **hypersensitivity reaction[‡]**
didanosine (ddl)	Videx	peripheral neuropathy, pancreatitis (higher incidence than with other NRTIs), nausea, diarrhea
emtricitabine (FTC)	Emtriva	headache, nausea, insomnia, hyperpigmentation of palms/soles
lamivudine (3TC)	Epivir	headache, nausea
stavudine (d4T)	Zerit	peripheral neuropathy, lactic acidosis/hepatic steatosis (higher incidence than with other NRTIs), pancreatitis, hyperlipidemia, lipoatrophy[§]
tenofovir (TFV, TDF)	Viread	nausea, diarrhea, headache, renal insufficiency
zalcitabine (ddC)	Hivid	has recently been discontinued by its manufacturer
zidovudine (AZT, ZDV)	Retrovir	macrocytic anemia, neutropenia, myopathy, headache, nausea
AZT + 3TC + ABC	Trizivir	see individual drugs
TFV + FTC	Truvada	see individual drugs
AZT + 3TC	Combivir	see individual drugs
3TC + ABC	Epizicom	see individual drugs
Non-nucleoside Reverse Transcriptase Inhibitors (NNRTIs)		**class effects: rash, hepatotoxicity, significant drug interactions**
efavirenz (EFV)	Sustiva	CNS effects (dizziness, somnolence, insomnia, confusion, abnormal dreams), teratogenicity

(Continued)

TABLE 82-4. Antiretrovirals and their Adverse Effects *(Continued)*

Drug	Brand Name	Adverse Effects
delavirdine (DLV)	Descriptor	high pill burden and less potent so not commonly used
nevirapine (NVP)	Viramune	higher incidence of rash (including Stevens-Johnson syndrome); hepatotoxicity may be life threatening and is more common at higher CD4 counts
Protease Inhibitors (PIs)		**class effects: hepatotoxicity, metabolic complications (dyslipidemia, insulin resistance, fat misdistribution), GI intolerance (nausea, vomiting, diarrhea), significant drug interactions**
amprenavir (APV)	Agenerase	rash, oral paresthesias
atazanavir (ATV)	Reyataz	hyperbilirubinemia, PR prolongation, less lipid effects, avoid proton pump inhibitors because they need acid for drug absorption
fosamprenavir (f-APV)	Lexiva	rash, headache
indinavir (IDV)	Crixivan	nephrolithiasis, renal insufficiency, hyperbilirubinemia, rash, headache, metallic taste, alopecia
lopinavir/ritonavir (LPV/r)	Kaletra	diarrhea common, asthenia
nelfinavir (NFV)	Viracept	diarrhea very common
ritonavir (RTV)	Norvir	perioral and extremity paresthesias, taste perversion, asthenia, is a **potent inhibitor of the P450** system so drug interactions are significant (can be used to "boost" other PIs)¶

saquinavir (SQV)	Invirase	headache
tipranavir (TPV)	Aptivus	rash, has sulfa moiety so use caution in patients with sulfa allergy
Fusion Inhibitors		
enfuvirtide (T-20)	Fuzeon	T-20 is a **subcutaneous injection**, associated with injection site reactions in almost 100%; increased rate of bacterial pneumonia

*Class effects are adverse effects associated with all drugs in a certain class. Additional side effects for each individual drug are then shown.

†**Mitochondrial toxicity** includes lactic acidosis/hepatic steatosis, pancreatitis, peripheral neuropathy, and myopathy. Different NRTIs are associated with different mitochondrial toxicities. **All drugs in this class can cause a potentially life threatening lactic acidosis/hepatic steatosis** (although most common with ddI, ZDV, and in particular d4T).

‡**Abacavir hypersensitivity reaction (HSR)** occurs in about 8% of patients, usually within the first 6 weeks of therapy. Symptoms include fever, rash, nausea, vomiting, malaise, fatigue, loss of appetite, and respiratory complaints. Symptoms can worsen with continuation of the drug, and so if HSR is suspected abacavir should be discontinued. **Do not rechallenge** after suspected HSR since rechallenge reactions are usually more severe and can mimic anaphylaxis.

§Lipoatrophy is defined as a loss of subcutaneous fat in the face, arms, and buttocks.

¶Since ritonavir is a potent inhibitor of P450 cytochrome 3A4 (the enzyme that metabolizes PIs), it can be given with other PIs in order to lower their required dose, referred to as a "boost."

specialist, but in general there are 3 types of regimens, all of which include at least 3 drugs.

1. **NNRTI-based regimens (1 NNRTI + 2 NRTIs).** This is commonly used as the initial regimen due to the lower pill burden and better side effect profile of NNRTIs over PIs, and the option to "save" the PIs for future use. The main disadvantage of NNRTIs is their low barrier against resistance, and cross resistance to the entire class often develops. The preferred NNRTI is efavirenz due to its better safety profile and low pill burden.

2. **PI-based regimens (1 or 2 PIs + 2 NRTIs)** are another good option for initial ART. The preferred PI in these regimens is the co-formulated lopinavir/ritonavir due to its proven antiviral potency.

3. **Triple NRTI regimens** should not be used as first line therapy since these regimens have been shown to have lower antiviral potency, and should only be used if an NNRTI or PI-based regimen cannot be used.

D. **Regimens to avoid.** There are many potential combinations of drugs to be avoided, which underscores the importance of involving an HIV specialist in ART decisions. For example, some combinations lead to **increased toxicity** (e.g. ddI + d4T, atazanavir + indinavir) and other combinations **antagonize each other, leading to decreased efficacy** (e.g., d4T + ZDV).

E. **Limitations to Effective Therapy**
   1. **Poor adherence** can lead to virologic failure as well as resistance.
   2. **Adverse effects of ARVs** are shown in Table 82-4.
   3. **Multiple drug interactions** are possible with NNRTIs or PIs due to their interference with the hepatic P450 system. For example, some statins are contraindicated in combination with PIs because statin levels can be raised significantly, increasing the risk of toxicity. To check for drug interactions, consult with an HIV pharmacologist and/or search one of the online drug interaction databases (e.g. www.HIVinsite.com or www.aids.meds.com).

F. **Treatment Failure and Changing Therpy**
   1. Treatment failure can be defined as **virologic** (incomplete viral load suppression), **immunologic** (failure to increase the CD4 cell count), or **clinical progression** (ocurrence or recurrence of HIV-related events).
   2. **What is the cause of treatment failure?** Possibilities include poor adherence, medication intolerance, pharmacokinetic issues (e.g., drug or food interactions causing low drug levels), and drug resistance.
   3. **Changing the regimen** is a complex management decision that involves integrating the results of resistance testing and

should be performed in conjunction with an HIV specialist. Ideally, a new regimen should contain at least two fully active drugs (based on resistance testing or new mechanical class).

G. Special Situations

  1. Acute HIV infection. Beginning ARVs during acute infection is considered optional, as it is not yet known what the long-term benefits of early treatment will be.

  2. Pregnancy. Pregnancy should not preclude the use of optimal therapeutic regimens, but the safety of particular drugs in pregnancy must be considered (e.g. efavirenz is not recommended due to its known teratogenicity), and consultation with an expert is recommended. In order to prevent mother-to-child transmission, the mother's viral load should be suppressed to a goal of <1,000 copies/mL.

  3. Postexposure prophylaxis. Treatment with antiretroviral medications has been proven to reduce transmission of HIV to healthcare workers following occupational exposure. Call your local **needlestick hotline** immediately for any occupational exposure.

HOT KEY

Think about the adverse effects of ARVs by "class effect":

- All NRTIs can cause some form of **mitochondrial toxicity** (pancreatitis, peripheral neuropathy, myopathy, and lactic acidosis/hepatic steatosis). For example, peripheral neuropathy is caused by the **"d" drugs** (ddl, d4T, ddC), and pancreatitis is most common with ddl.
- All NNRTIs can cause **rash.**
- All PIs can cause **metabolic complications** (dyslipidemia, insulin resistance, fat maldistribution) and **GI intolerance** (nausea, vomiting, diarrhea).
- **All ARVs** can cause **hepatotoxicity.**

VI USEFUL WEBSITES. More detailed information regarding HIV/AIDS can be found at the free online HIV textbook from the The University of California at San Francisco (http://hivinsite.ucsf.edu/InSite), the online manual of the Johns Hopkins AIDS Service (http://www.hopkins-aids.edu), and the website for the Centers for Disease Control and Prevention (http://www.cdc.gov/hiv/).

References

Aberg JA, et al. Primary care guidelines for the management of persons infected with human immunodeficiency virus: recommendations of the HIV Medicine Association of the Infectious Diseases Society of America. *Clin Infect Dis* 2004;39:609–629.

Centers for Disease Control and Prevention. Guidelines for preventing opportunistic
    infections among HIV-infected persons—2002 recommendations of the U.S. Public
    Health Service and the Infectious Disease Society of America. *MMWR* 2002;51:
    1–51.
The Panel on Clinical Practices for Treatment of HIV Infection convened by the De-
    partment of Health and Human Services (DHHS). Guidelines for the use of an-
    tiretroviral agents in HIV-1 infected adults and adolescents. AIDSinfo Web Site
    (http://AIDSinfo.nih.gov), 2005.

83. Tuberculosis

....

I INTRODUCTION

A. **Epidemiology.** It is estimated that one third of the world's population, including 10–15 million people in the U.S., is latently infected with *Mycobacterium tuberculosis* (TB). While the number of active TB cases has declined in the United States, the global tuberculosis caseload is slowly growing, mostly due to the increase in HIV infection.

B. **Primary and latent tuberculosis.** *M. tuberculosis* is acquired via inhalation of organism-containing aerosolized particles, spread by coughing, which are ingested by alveolar macrophages in the lung. Over the course of weeks to months comprising the **primary infection** stage, granulomas form and limit the replication and spread of the organism. After this point, the bacillus can be found inside the granulomas but is considered dormant. This stage is called **latent TB infection (LTBI)**.

C. **Active TB** may occur in one of two ways:
1. If there is a defect in immunity at the initial containment stage during primary infection (e.g., in the elderly, immunocompromised, or HIV infected), then active disease can occur – this is called **primary progressive TB**.
2. Similarly, if immunosuppression occurs later in life (e.g. HIV, corticosteroid therapy, malignancy), then the latent infection can "re-activate" – this is called **reactivation TB.** The lifetime risk of reactivation is approximately 10%, and is highest in the first 1–2 years after infection.

D. **Extrapulmonary TB (EPTB)** accounts for about 15–20% of cases of active TB in HIV-negative adults and is more common in HIV-infected individuals. Common forms of EPTB include lymphadenitis, pleural effusion, spinal disease (i.e. Pott's disease), meningitis, peritonitis, genitourinary disease, and pericarditis. Disseminated TB involves multiple organs simultaneously and occurs in about 1–3% of TB cases.

II APPROACH TO THE PATIENT WITH ACTIVE TUBERCULOSIS

A. **Diagnosis**
1. **Patient history.** Patients with active tuberculosis may present with cough, hemoptysis, fever, weight loss, and night sweats.

Patients with extrapulmonary TB will have symptoms specific to the organ system involved.

HOT KEY

TB infection is sometimes called the "great mimicker" because it can cause almost any symptom, depending on where in the body infection has occurred.

---

2. **Physical examination.** Patients may appear chronically ill or have evidence of wasting. The lung examination may reveal crackles or decreased breath sounds, or may be entirely normal.
3. **Chest radiograph** may show fibrocavitary disease, pulmonary nodules, infiltrates, or pleural effusions.
   Ghon complex: evidence of prior primary TB infection may manifest as a small residual scar (often calcified) in the lung parencyhma and hilar nodes.
   a. **Primary progressive TB** usually involves the middle and lower lung fields.
   b. **Reactivation TB** usually involves the apical or posterior segments of the upper lobes.
   c. **Patients with HIV infection** may not present with the "classic" patterns of primary progressive versus reactivation disease.
4. **Tuberculin skin test (TST).** A positive TST suggests prior TB infection but does not necessarily mean active disease. Similarly, a negative TST does not completely exclude TB since false negatives may occur in up to 20–25% of patients with active TB. See section IIIA for more details about this test.
5. **Sputum testing** for acid-fast staining (i.e., smear) and culture should be done on three separate sputum samples if active TB is suspected. Smears are only positive in 50–80% of patients with pulmonary TB, while cultures are positive in 80–85% of cases. Note that cultures may take 3–8 weeks to grow.
6. **Drug-susceptibility testing** should be done on all isolates.
B. **Therapy**
   1. **General considerations.** Patients with active TB should be treated by an infectious disease or TB specialist experienced in managing the many factors that can complicate therapy for tuberculosis – in particular, drug resistance, medication side effects, and poor adherence.
      a. **Directly observed therapy (DOT)** may be used when patients have difficulty adhering to medication schedules.

Patients undergoing DOT are required to come to their provider's office or a TB clinic between two and five times times weekly to receive their medicines.

b. **Reporting.** All cases of suspected or confirmed active TB must be reported to the state or local health department.

2. **Regimen.** Accepted regimens for treating active TB generally involve an initial phase of four drugs for 2 months, followed by a continuation phase of two drugs for an additional 4 months. A multi-drug regimen is used in order to maximize killing of the bacilli while minimizing the development of resistance. An example of an appropriate regimen is shown in Table 83-1.

3. **Side effects and drug interactions.**

   a. **Isoniazid (INH).** Side effects include hepatitis, rash, and peripheral neuropathy. **Vitamin B6** (pyrazinamide 25–50 mg PO daily) should be given to patients at high risk for developing peripheral neuropathy (e.g. patients who have diabetes, uremia, alcoholism, malnutrition, HIV, or who are elderly or pregnant). INH can increase phenytoin and carbamazepine levels (but often this is offset by the effect of rifampin), and so drug levels should be monitored.

   b. **Rifampin.** Side effects include hepatitis, rash, flu-like symptoms, and thrombocytopenia. Patients should be warned that urine and other body secretions will turn orange. Rifampin can cause a significant decrease in the levels of many medications, including warfarin, oral contraceptives, anticonvulsants, and methadone. The dosages of these medications may need to be increased in order to achieve efficacy.

   c. **Ethambutol** can cause an optic neuritis resulting in decreased visual acuity or red-green color discrimination.

   d. **Pyrazinamide.** Side effects include hepatitis, arthralgias, and hyperuricemia.

4. **Baseline laboratory assessment.** All patients should have a baseline liver panel, renal panel, and complete blood count before therapy is initiated. In addition, if ethambutol will be used, patients should undergo visual acuity and red-green color perception testing.

HOT
▶
KEY
All patients with TB should be tested for HIV infection.

TABLE 83-1. Sample 4-Drug Regimen for the Initial Treatment of Active Tuberculosis in an Adult*

Drug	Dose	Schedule	Side Effects	Monitoring
Isoniazid	5–10 mg/kg, to a maximum dose of 300 mg	Once daily for 6 months†	Hepatitis, peripheral neuropathy‡	Liver function tests monthly for patients older than 35 years (optional for younger patients) Neurologic examination Monitoring of blood levels of other medications
Rifampin	10 mg/kg, to a maximum dose of 600 mg	Once daily for 6 months†	Hepatitis, rash, gastrointestinal upset, purpura	Monitoring of blood levels of other medications Liver function tests
Pyrazinamide§	15–30 mg/kg, to a maximum dose of 2 g	Once daily for 2 months	Hepatitis, arthralgias, hyperuricemia	Liver function tests Serum uric acid level (if gout occurs)
Ethambutol	5–25 mg/kg, to a maximum dose of 1 g	Once daily for 2 months	Optic neuritis, rash	Visual acuity and red-green color perception testing should be performed before starting ethambutol therapy; question patient about visual changes monthly

*This regimen assumes no drug resistance. Consult with local tuberculosis expert or the health department to ensure that this regimen is in accordance with your local resistance patterns.
†After 2 months of daily therapy, it is acceptable to change to directly observed therapy with isoniazid and rifampin administered two or three times per week.
‡Consider pyridoxine (25 mg orally) to prevent neuropathy in patients at high risk (i.e., those older than 65 years; those with diabetes, alcoholism, or chronic renal failure)
§Pyrazinamide must not be used in pregnant women.

5. **Monitoring.** Once therapy has been initiated, patients should have a monthly clinical evaluation to monitor for possible side effects. Routine follow-up labs (e.g. liver panel) are only necessary if baseline labs are abnormal, the patient has signs/symptoms of hepatitis, or if the patient has risk factors for hepatotoxicity (e.g. known liver disease, risk factors for liver disease, or alcohol abuse).

6. **Drug induced hepatitis** may result from INH, rifampin, or pyrazinamide and is defined as an elevation in transaminases ≥3 times normal with symptoms of hepatitis (e.g. fever, jaundice, anorexia, right upper quadrant pain), or ≥5 times normal without symptoms. If hepatitis is diagnosed, the potential offending agents should be stopped immediately and you should consult with a TB specialist to help assist with further management.

7. **Response to therapy.** All patients should have serial sputum examinations and culture (usually monthly until 2 consecutive specimens are negative). If the sputum cultures remain positive after 2 months of treatment, a TB specialist should be consulted.

8. **Special Circumstances.**

   a. **Multi-Drug Resistant TB (MDR-TB)** is defined as a strain of TB with resistance to at least INH and rifampin. Treatment of MDR-TB requires use of second-line medications for TB and should be undertaken by a specialist in this area.

   b. **HIV coinfection** can complicate the management of TB. For example, many antiretrovirals interact with anti-TB medications, especially rifampin. These patients should be managed by a TB or infectious diseases specialist.

III TB Screening and Prevention

A. **Screening for latent TB infection.** The goal of TB screening is to identify patients with LTBI, so they can receive drug therapy to kill the dormant organisms and prevent reactivation of disease.

1. **Who should be tested?** TB screening is indicated only for patients at *high risk* for developing active TB. With the exception of persons being tested at the start of employment in high risk settings, screening of low risk patients is discouraged. High risk patients can be divided into two groups: (1) those at risk for recent infection with TB, and (2) those with an increased risk of progression to active TB once infection has occurred (see Table 83-2).

TABLE 83-2. Interpretation of Purified Protein Derivative (PPD) Test Results

Size of Induration	Patients in Whom This Result is Considered Positive
≥5 mm	Household members and close contacts of patients with active tuberculosis
	HIV-infected patients and patients with risk factors for HIV infection and an unknown HIV status
	Patients with fibrotic lesions on a chest radiograph
≥10 mm	Foreign-born patients from countries where the incidence of tuberculosis is high
	Patients living in medically underserved, low-income areas
	Injection drug users and patients with alcoholism
	Homeless patients
	Residents of long-term care facilities
	Patients with medical conditions associated with a high risk for reactivation of tuberculosis*
	People who work in facilities where infection would put a large number of people at risk (e.g., hospitals, correctional facilities, daycare centers)
≥15 mm	All other patients

*Conditions that place a patient at high risk for reactivation tuberculosis include diabetes, chronic renal failure, malignancy, silicosis, prior gastrectomy, body weight more than 10% below the ideal, and therapy with corticosteroids or other immunosuppressive drugs.

Remember:
- Prior to performing a TST, always question the patient to ensure that he has not been previously treated for active or latent tuberculosis. These patients have known prior infection, and therefore do not require skin testing.
- TST should only be performed in those at *high risk* for developing active TB – i.e. "a decision to test is a decision to treat."

2. **The TST.** Screening is performed with the **purified protein derivative (PPD)** TST, which measures a patient's hypersensitivity reaction to an antigenic component of *M. tuberculosis* and is detectable at 2–12 weeks after infection. To perform the test, 0.1 mL of PPD solution is injected intradermally into

the volar surface of the forearm. The patient returns in 48–72 hours, and the amount of induration (not erythema) at the injection site is measured.

3. **Interpretation of TST results.** The "cut-off" for determining a positive test depends on the level of risk for developing active disease in a given patient. High-risk patients are considered to have a positive test with lower levels of induration than low-risk patients (see Table 83-2). Those who have received the bacille calmette-Guérin (BCG) vaccine (derived from an attenuated strain of *M. bovis*) may cross-react to the PPD antigen even if they have not been infected with TB. While reactions >10 mm are unusual several years after vaccination, there is no good way to differentiate between a true positive and a BCG-induced positive. Therefore, the recommendation is that prior BCG vaccination should not be taken into account when interpeting a PPD result.

4. **Follow-up**
   a. **Positive test.** All patients with a positive TST should have a chest radiograph, and if signs of pulmonary TB are seen, a full medical evaluation for active TB should be performed (see section IIA).
   b. **Negative test.** There are two potential causes for a false-negative test result:
      (1) **Loss of sensitivity to PPD** can occur over time and is regained only after re-exposure to PPD. In this case, a second test performed 1–3 weeks after an initial negative test should be positive (this is called the **"booster phenomenon"**).
      (2) **Anergy** (e.g. in HIV-infected individuals) results from a suppressed host immune response to the PPD antigen in a patient with *M. tuberculosis* infection. Although it is possible to test for anergy using control antigens (e.g., *Candida*), this is not routinely recommended.

5. **Interferon gamma release assays.** A new screening blood test has been developed that measures the amount of interferon gamma (IFN-γ) made by a patient's blood cells in response to *M. tuberculosis* antigens. This test will likely become an important part of TB screening in the future, as it has a number of advantages over the TST: it can be done on a single visit, there is less interobserver variability, and the test can better distinguish between a true positive result and prior vaccination with BCG.

B. **Treatment of LTBI**
   1. **Indications.** Treatment for LTBI is indicated for those who have a positive TST, a negative chest X-ray (or an abnormal X-ray with sufficient evaluation to exclude active TB), and

who are at high risk for development of active TB (see section IIIA-1 and Table 83-2).

 HOT KEY Active TB must be excluded before starting therapy for LTBI, because initiating single drug therapy in a patient who actually has active TB is not effective treatment and promotes drug resistance.

---

2. Regimen.

a. Drugs. INH (5 mg/kg, up to 300 mg/day maximum) daily for 9 months is the preferred regimen for all patients. Some TB specialists will use a 6 month regimen, but this should not be used if the patient has HIV or fibrotic changes on X-ray. INH can also be given 2 times per week by DOT. Alternative regimens include rifampin alone or INH/rifampin for 4 months – you should consult with a TB specialist before using these regimens.

b. Side effects of INH and the use of adjunctive vitamin B6 are discussed in section IIB-3.

c. Contraindications.

(1) **Liver disease.** Active hepatitis and end-stage liver disease are relative contraindications to INH.

(2) **Pregnancy.** Some experts prefer to defer treatment of LTBI until after delivery, since pregnancy itself does not increase the risk of progression to active TB but may increase the risk of hepatotoxicity to INH. There is no evidence to suggest that INH is harmful to the fetus.

d. Monitoring.

(1) **Baseline transaminases** are not required for all patients, but should be performed in patients with HIV, known liver disease or risk factors for liver disease, alcoholism, or women who are pregnant or in the early post-partum period.

(2) **Monthly follow-up.** Clinical evaluation for side effects should be performed monthly in all patients. A monthly liver panel should be performed in patients with abnormal baseline labs or any signs/symptoms of hepatitis, women who are pregnant or in the early post-partum period, and those at high risk for hepatotoxicity. See section IIB-6 for a discussion of drug-induced hepatitis.

References

Frieden TR, Sterling TR, Munsiff SS, Watt CJ, Dye D. Tuberculosis. *Lancet* 2003; 362:887–899.

Myers JP. New recommendations for the treatment of tuberculosis. *Curr Opin Infect Dis* 2005;18:133–140.

84. Approach to Fever

··

I INTRODUCTION

A. **Normal body temperature and fever.**
   1. **What is a fever?** The normal oral temperature is 36°C–37.4°C (average = 36.7°C), with diurnal variation such that the maximum normal temperature is 37.2°C at 6 AM and 37.7°C at 4 PM. Therefore, a temperature of >37.2°C in the morning or >37.7°C in the evening constitutes a fever.
   2. **Measuring the temperature.** The average rectal temperature is 0.5°C higher and the average axillary temperature is 0.5°C lower than the oral temperature. Tympanic membrane temperatures may be more variable than those measured by other methods.

B. **Causes of fever.** Fever is usually due to an underlying infection, but can also be caused by non-infectious processes. A systematic approach to the causes of fever is presented in Table 84-1.

C. **Fever of Unknown Origin (FUO).** FUO is defined as a temperature >38.3°C for >3 weeks, with the diagnosis uncertain after evaluation in at least 3 outpatient visits or 3 days in the hospital. The most common causes of FUO are divided into 4 categories: infection (e.g., tuberculosis, abdominal abscess), malignancy (e.g., lymphoma), inflammatory disease (e.g., Adult Still's disease, temporal arteritis), and miscellaneous (e.g., DVT, drug fever).

Remember:

HOT

KEY

- Patients who are elderly, immunocompromised, or taking steroids or nonsteroidal anti-inflammatory drugs (NSAIDs) may not mount a fever, even in the presence of a severe infection.
- Hypothermia often signals the presence of an over-whelming infection, and should therefore be evaluated as thoroughly as fever.

II APPROACH TO THE PATIENT.
A comprehensive history and physical examination is the first step, and often the key, to determining the cause of a fever.

TABLE 84-1. A Systematic Approach to Fever*

Category	Examples	Signs/Symptoms
Infection		
CNS	meningitis, brain or epidural abscess	headache, neck stiffness, photophobia, back pain, focal neurologic signs
ENT	viral URI, sinusitis, otitis, pharyngitis, dental or retropharyngeal abscess	URI symptoms, sinus or ear pain, sore throat, tooth pain, lymphadenopathy
Lungs	bronchitis, pneumonia, lung abscess, empyema, TB	cough, pleuritic chest pain, dyspnea
Cardiovascular/ Endovascular	endocarditis, pericarditis line and graft infections	recent dental work, skin lesions, chest pain
GI	gastroenteritis, liver abscess, hepatitis, cholecystitis, cholangitis, pancreatitis, abdominal abscess, appendicitis, diverticulitis, colitis, perirectal abscess	abdominal pain, diarrhea, nausea/vomiting
GU	upper and lower UTI, prostatitis, PID, STDs	dysuria, flank pain, vaginal/penile discharge, prostate tenderness, costovertebral angle tenderness
Musculoskeletal	osteomyelitis, septic arthritis, myositis	joint pain/swelling/erythema, bone or muscle pain
Soft tissue	cellulitis, soft tissue abscess	erythema, pain, swelling of soft tissues
Systemic	viral infections (acute HIV, EBV, CMV) mycobacterial infections fungal infections (histoplasmosis, coccidioidomycoses)	pharyngitis, lymphadenopathy, rash rash, weight loss, night sweats
Rheumatic	lupus, rheumatoid arthritis, vasculitides	rash, joint pain, oral ulcers
Malignancy	lymphoma, renal cell carcinoma, hepatocellular carcinoma	weight loss, night sweats, lymphadenopathy
Vascular	deep vein thrombosis, pulmonary embolism	leg swelling, pleuritic chest pain, dyspnea
Medications	antibiotics, anticonvulsants, neuroleptics, antihistamines, allopurinol, hydralazine, nifedipine	check the patient's medicine list

*This is not a comprehensive differential diagnosis for fever, but includes some of the most common causes of fever seen in the outpatient setting. CMV = cytomegalovirus, CNS = central nervous system, EBV = Epstein-Barr virus; ENT = ear, nose and throat; GI = gastrointestinal, GU = genitourinary, HIV = human immunodeficiency virus, PID = pelvic inflammatory disease, STD = sexually transmitted disease, TB = tuberculosis, UTI = urinary tract infection, URI = upper respiratory infection

A. Patient history

1. **Details of the fever.** How long has the patient had a fever? Is there any specific pattern to the fever (e.g., relapsing, sustained)? Has the patient had any sick contacts? What are the associated symptoms?

2. **Immune status.** Is the patient immunocompromised (e.g., as a result of malignancy, chemotherapy, immunosuppresive therapy including steroids, HIV)?

3. **Medical history.** Patients with a known illness may have a fever caused by their underlying disease process (e.g., tumor fever or lupus flare). However, these patients are also at risk for superimposed infection, and this must be ruled out before attributing the fever to the underlying disease.

4. **Medication history.** What prescription drugs is the patient taking? Look for medications that cause immunosuppression (e.g., steroids) and those that may result in drug fever (see Table 84-1).

5. **Social history.** What is the patient's sexual history? Is there a history of illicit drug use or other HIV risk factors? Positive answers may trigger a search for sexually transmitted diseases (STDs), abscesses, endocarditis, or HIV-related diseases.

6. **Travel history.** Has the patient traveled recently? What specific exposures did the patient have while travelling (e.g., activities, food, insect bites, sexual activity)? Ask about pre-travel immunizations and chemoprophylaxis taken during travel. These questions can help to guide the differential diagnosis in a returning traveler (see Table 84-2).

HOT KEY Fever should be presumed to be secondary to an infection until proven otherwise, because infections cause the majority of fevers and can be life-threatening.

B. Top to bottom approach. One way of determining the infectious cause of a fever is to start at the patient's head and work your way down. In Table 84-1, the various causes of infection are organized in this way – by body system from head to toe. Evaluating the patient in a systematic fashion for the corresponding signs and symptoms may help narrow your differential.

C. Physical examination. A complete physical examination should be performed. Pelvic and rectal examinations may be useful to evaluate for pelvic inflammatory disease (PID), STDs, prostatitis, or perirectal abscess.

D. Laboratory studies. The history and physical examination may provide you with enough information to make a diagnosis, but quite commonly, further testing is required.

TABLE 84-2. Fever in the Returning Traveler*

Disease	Distribution	Exposure	Signs/symptoms
Incubation <3 weeks			
malaria	tropics and subtropics†	Anopheles mosquito bite (night-biting)	fever/chills at 48–72 h intervals, splenomegaly, dark urine ("black water fever")
dengue fever	tropics and subtropics	Aedes mosquito bite (day-biting)	headache, rash, severe muscle and joint pain ("break bone fever")
typhoid fever	developing countries	fecal contaminated food or water	headache, abdominal discomfort, pulse-temperature dissociation‡
yellow fever	Africa, South America	Aedes mosquito bite (day-biting)	headache, vomiting, jaundice, bleeding
acute HIV	widespread	sexual contact, blood exposure	lymphadenopathy, pharyngitis, rash
leptosporosis	widespread	fresh water exposure	headache, myalgia, conjunctivitis
rickettsial disease (e.g., tick-borne spotted fever)	widespread	mite or tick bite	headache, myalgia, rash, painless eschar at site of bite

Incubation >3 weeks

malaria, acute HIV	as above	as above	as above
hepatitis A, E	widespread	fecal contaminated food or water	fatigue, nausea, jaundice, right upper quadrant pain
hepatitis B	widespread	sexual contact, blood exposure	fatigue, nausea, jaundice, right upper quadrant pain
schistosomiasis	Africa, Asia, Latin America	fresh water exposure	splenomegaly, ascites, gastroesophageal varices, may have bladder involvement
rabies	widespread	animal bite	headache, itching/paresthesias at site of bite; progresses to encephalitis, hydrophobia
amebic liver abscess	developing countries	fecal contaminated food or water	right upper quadrant pain

*This is not a comprehensive list, but includes some of the most common diagnoses seen in returning travelers with fever.
†subtropics: the regions adjacent to the tropics, between tropical and temperate regions
‡pulse-temperature dissociation: high fever with bradycardia

1. **Complete blood count (CBC) with differential.**
   a. **Neutropenia** with fever is a medical emergency, and requires hospitalization and broad-spectrum antibiotics.
   b. **A leftward shifted white blood cell (WBC) count refers to the presence of immature WBCs. It** often implies significant bacterial infection.
   c. **A low WBC count** may be just as worrisome as a high one. Furthermore, patients who are elderly or immunocompromised may not have an elevated WBC count, even in the presence of a serious infection.
   d. **A blood smear** should be done in cases where a hematologic malignancy is suspected.
2. **Electrolytes with blood urea nitrogen (BUN) and creatinine.** The presence of an anion gap may indicate a severe infection.
3. **A liver panel** [e.g., bilirubin, alkaline phosphatase (AP), and transaminase levels] can help evaluate the possibility of hepatobiliary disease.
4. **Amylase and/or lipase levels** may be helpful if pancreatitis is suspected.
5. **Urinalysis** should be done to evaluate the possibility of UTI.
6. **Autoimmune serologies:** Consider a rheumatoid factor or ANA if the patient has symptoms suggestive of rheumatologic disease or for unexplained fever.
7. **HIV test.** An HIV antibody test should be considered if the patient has HIV risk factors or unexplained fever. An HIV viral load test may be necessary if acute HIV is suspected.
8. A **Monospot test** is useful to diagnose infectious mononucleosis due to Epstein-Barr virus, although it may be negative early in the course of infection.
9. **Cultures**
   a. **Blood cultures** are always required in intravenous drug users presenting with fever or when endocarditis is suspected. Patients who get blood cultures require close follow-up and/or admission.
   b. **Urine cultures** should be obtained whenever the fever is unexplained.
   c. **Sputum evaluation** for acid-fast bacilli should be performed if tuberculosis is suspected (see Chapter 83).
   d. **Throat swab** for rapid streptococcal antigen testing and for strep culture may be useful when streptococcal pharyngitis ("strep throat") is suspected. Consider sending a swab for gonoccocal culture if risk factors are present for gonococcal pharyngitis (e.g., recent orogenital contact).
   e. **Cerebrospinal fluid (CSF) analysis** and **culture** is necessary in patients with suspected meningitis, fever and altered mental status, or HIV infection with headache or unexplained fever. These patients should almost always

be sent to the emergency department for further evaluation.

f. **Body fluid analysis** and **culture.** Patients with a fever accompanied by ascites, pleural effusion, or joint effusion usually need a diagnostic tap to rule out infection. Consider referring these patients to the emergency department for further work-up.

g. **Stool studies.** In patients presenting with diarrhea, consider sending stool for culture or ova and parasite testing depending on exposure history. Also, consider testing the stool for *C. difficile* if the patient has recently been on antibiotics.

HOT

▶

KEY

Patients who present with fever and rash should have a skin biopsy unless the diagnosis is straightforward.

E. **Imaging.** Imaging studies should be performed in a targeted fashion based on results of the history, physical examination, and preliminary laboratory studies.

1. **Chest X-ray** should be considered in all patients with respiratory symptoms or with unexplained fever.

2. **Computed tomography (CT) of the abdomen/pelvis** should be considered in all patients with fever and abdominal symptoms. It is also one of the first steps in the work-up of FUO since it may identify an occult abdominal abscess or malignancy.

3. **Abdominal Ultrasound** may be useful to evaluate the gallbladder and bile ducts

F. **Unexplained fever.** In the case of FUO, further evaluation (e.g., echocardiography, bone marrow biopsy, white blood cell scan) should be guided by any abnormalities discovered during the initial work-up, if possible. You should likely consult with an infectious diseases specialist at this point to help target the diagnostic evaluation.

III TREATMENT

A. **General measures**

1. **Fluids.** Patients should be encouraged to increase their fluid intake to compensate for increased insensible losses.

2. **Discontinuation of medications.** Discontinuing medications that may be responsible for a fever can be both diagnostic and therapeutic.

3. **Antipyretic therapy.** Acetaminophen (325–650 mg every 4–6 hours) is the usual first-line therapy for fever. NSAIDs can also be used to treat fever (e.g., ibuprofen 200–400 mg every 4–6 hr) but are associated with more side effects.

4. **Antibiotic therapy** is usually initiated when an infection is diagnosed. Empiric antibiotic therapy and close follow-up may also be indicated for patients with suspected infection.

HOT KEY

If blood cultures are required, they should be obtained before antibiotic therapy is initiated.

B. **Hospital admission** may be warranted when:
   1. A potentially dangerous infection is suspected
   2. The patient is elderly, immunocompromised, or has a complicating medical condition
   3. The patient is significantly dehydrated
C. **Follow-up.** Extremely close follow-up is required for outpatients with a fever.

References

Roth AR, Basello GM. Approach to the adult patient with fever of unknown origin. *Am Fam Physician* 2003;68:2223–2228.

Ryan ET, Wilson ME, Kain KC. Illness after international travel. *N Engl J Med* 2002;347(7):505–516.

PART XIII

DERMATOLOGY

85. Approach to Skin Diseases

I **DESCRIBING DERMATOLOGIC LESIONS.** Using a systematic, 3-step approach to describe a dermatologic lesion enables classification of the lesion (thereby limiting the differential diagnosis) and facilitates communication with consultants and colleagues.

A. First, classify the primary lesion, using Table 85-1. Primary lesions are early skin changes that have not yet undergone natural evolution or change caused by manipulation and often provide the most clues about the underlying etiology of the skin disorder. See Table 85-1 for major types of primary lesions.

B. Next, note any secondary changes (i.e., changes that occur after the primary lesion has appeared). Examples of secondary changes include:

1. **Scale**
2. **Crust**
3. **Excoriation**
4. **Erosion** (loss of the epidermis)
5. **Ulceration** (loss of the epidermis and dermis)
6. **Fissure** (epidermal tear, sharply defined)

TABLE 85-1. Classification of Primary Dermatologic Lesions

Appearance of Lesion	If the Lesion Is < 0.5 cm in Diameter, Then It Is a:	If the Lesion Is > 0.5 cm in Diameter, Then It Is a:
Flat and nonpalpable	Macule	Patch
Elevated and palpable	Papule	Plaque
Collection of clear fluid	Vesicle	Bulla
Collection of white or yellow fluid	Pustule	Cyst or abscess
Elevated and deep (subcutaneous)	Nodule	Tumor

TABLE 85-2. Causes, Clinical Findings, and Treatments for the Major Causes of Macules and Patches

Lesion	Cause	Clinical Findings	Treatment
Drug eruption	Side effect of various medications	Lesions are often maculo-papular, distributed on the trunk, bright red, and confluent; lesions on the palms, sores, or mucosal surfaces are worrisome for severe reactions	Withdrawal of causative agent; oral antihistamines, topical steroids, or Sarna lotion for pruritus; hospitalization may be necessary for patient with severe reactions
Viral exanthema	Skin reaction to circulating virus	Erythematous macules and papules (usually less red and less confluent than those seen in drug reactions); systemic signs and symptoms of illness are also present	Sarna lotion or topical steroids or oral antihistamines for pruritus
Lentigo ("liver spots")	Sun exposure	Hyperpigmented or brown macules	Sunscreen; bleaching agents of limited benefit
Urticaria ("hives")	Drugs, infection, autoimmune disease, foods, physical agents (cold, sun, pressure)	Recurrent wheals that last less than 24 hours	Avoidance of causative agent; oral antihistamines

Erythema multiforme	HSV, drugs (sulfonamides, phenytoin, barbiturates, penicillin), Mycoplasma infection	"Target" lesion (dark center with a clear halo); dark ring often on palms	Acyclovir suppression for HSV; withdrawal of offending drug
Toxin-mediated erythema	Group A streptococci, Staphylococcus aureus, other (unknown) agents	Confluent, erythematous macules and fine ("sand-paper") papules, accentuated in skin folds, often involving the mucous membranes and usually not pruritic; patient appears ill	Antibiotic therapy for underlying bacterial infection

HSV = herpes simplex virus.

TABLE 85-3. Causes, Clinical Findings, and Treatments for the Major Causes of Papules*

Lesion	Cause	Clinical Findings	Treatment
Basal cell cancer	Sun exposure, radiation	Pearly, translucent papules, often with a rolled border[†] Often accompanied by telangiectasias Face is a common location	Biopsy or referral for excision
Squamous cell cancer	Sun exposure, toxic exposure	Indurated papules with scale or crust; nonhealing ulcers are also suspicious[‡] Sun-exposed surfaces are common locations	Biopsy or referral for excision
Scabies	*Sarcoptes scabiei* mite infection	Burrows in finger webs and on genitals; penile itching (in men) or breast itching (in women) is very suspicious; face is usually spared, except in immunocompromised patients Eggs or mites on microscopic examination of a deep scraping of the papule confirms the diagnosis	Permethrin 5% cream applid to entire body from the neck down overnight and repeated in 1 week (treat close contacts as well) Oral anthisitamines and topical steroids (itching often persists even after adequate treatment) Laundering of clothes and bedding in hot water or isolation in a plastic bag

*Drug eruption, viral exanthema, erythema multiforme, and toxin-mediated erythema can also be popular but are discussed in Table 85-2.
[†]Basal cell cancer may also be associated with nodules.
[‡]Squamous cell cancer may also be associated with plaques or nodules.

TABLE 85-4. Causes, Clinical Findings, and Treatments for the Major Causes of Plaques

Lesion	Cause	Clinical Findings	Treatment
Actinic (solar) keratosis*	Sun exposure	Rough, dry, "sandpaper-like" lesions; sometimes easier to palpate the lesion than to see it	Liquid nitrogen, fluorouracil cream (Efudex, Carac), imiquimod cream, Diclofenac cream, chemical peel, photodynamic laser therapy
Atopic dermatitis	Unclear; associated with a history of hay fever, asthma, or allergic rhinitis	Pruritic inflammation of the skin (excoriation can place patients at risk for developing staphylococcal or viral skin infections) Erythema and scale usually occur on the flexor surfaces of the skin Skin lines become accentuated or lichenified	Topical steroids, oral antihistamines, mollients, and avoidance of soap and hot water
Contact dermatitis	External allergen	Travel and work history may be significant; inquire about toiletries and exposure to common cleaning solutions	Avoidance of causative agent Topical steroids; if the lesions are extensive, consider a short course of oral steroids (7–10 days)

(Continued)

TABLE 85-4. Causes, Clinical Findings, and Treatments for the Major Causes of Plaques *(Continued)*			
Lesion	Cause	Clinical Findings	Treatment
Psoriasis	Unknown; believed to be hereditary	Silver scale, commonly located on the extensor surfaces, in the gluteal fold, and at sites of minor trauma Nail pitting Arthritis may be present	Topical steroids, calcipoetriene cream, tazarotene gel Refer to a dermatologist for oral agents (acitretin, methotrexate, cyclosporine) or light therapy, or biologics if psoriasis is extensive
Seborrheic dermatitis	Unknown	Chronic scaling and erythema; most active in the distribution of the sebaceous glands of the face	Combined therapy with a low-potency steroid cream and an antifungal cream can be tried Anti-dandruff shampoo for scalp
Seborrheic keratosis	Unknown	Benign skin growth with a "stuck on" appearance; incidence increases with age	Curettage, laser therapy, or liquid nitrogen

Tinea	Fungal infection (dermatophytes)	Annular lesions with raised borders and central clearing	Topical antifungal agents; a systemic antifungal agent (e.g., griseofulvin, 500 mg orally daily for 4–6 weeks) may be used for severe extensive infections and infections of the scalp or face
		Fine scale at edge (or border) of lesion	
		Scrapings of scale from the border of the lesion show hyphae or budding cells on KOH preparation	
Xerosis (severe dry skin)	Aging skin, various oral medications (especially anticholesterol drugs)	Common in the elderly and during the winter; skin is often scaly, itchy, and erythematous; often seen on the legs	Emollients, low-potency steroids, and avoidance of hot water and soap

KOH = potassium hydroxide

*Actinic keratosis may also be associated with papules; it may be a precursor to squamous cell cancer.

TABLE 85-5. Causes, Clinical Findings, and Treatments for the Major Causes of Vesicles and Bullae

Lesion	Cause	Clinical Findings	Treatment
Impetigo	*Streptococcus, Staphylococcus*	Honey-colored crust	Appropriate systemic antibiotic (e.g., dicloxacillin, first-generation cephalosporin), or topical mupirocin
Herpes simplex	Herpes simplex virus (HSV), types 1 and 2	Clustered vesicles, pustules, or punched-out ulcer. Multinucleated giant cells on a Tzanck smear confirms the diagnosis	Oral acyclovir (400 mg three times daily, or 200 mg five times daily, for 10 days) for first episodes and the early treatment of recurrent disease; consider intravenous acyclovir for patients with disseminated disease and immunocompromised patients
Herpes zoster	Varicella zoster virus	Dermatomal distribution is classic	Acyclovir (800 mg orally five times daily for 7–10 days, if given within 3 days of the appearance of the lesion); consider intravenous acyclovir for immunocompromised patients with severe disease

TABLE 85-6. Causes, Clinical Findings, and Treatment for the Major Causes of Pustules and Cysts

Lesion	Cause	Clinical Findings	Treatment
Acne (disorder of the pilosebaceous units leading to increased sebum production, follicular obstruction, bacterial proliferation, and inflammation)	Multifactorial (abnormal keratinization, overgrowth of *Propionibacterium acnes*, hormones, abnormal inflammatory response to *P. acnes*)	Noninflammatory lesions (i.e., comedones, also known as "whiteheads," and "blackheads") Inflammatory lesions (i.e., pustules, papules, nodules, and cysts); may lead to scarring Hirsuitism and irregular menses in women may indicate an endocrine abnormality Medication history may reveal corticosteroid use	Noninflammatory/comedomal acne: Benzoyl peroxide 5% and/or topical retinoid cream to start; topical antibiotic may be added if the patient has mild inflammatory lesions Inflammatory acne: Oral antibiotics (e.g., tetracycline 500 mg twice daily or minocycline 50–100 mg twice daily) Nodulocystic acne: Referral to a dermatologist for isotretinoin (Accutane) therapy Acne associated with menses: Oral contraceptives with low androgenic activity (e.g., Jasmine), spironolactone *(Continued)*

TABLE 85-6. Causes, Clinical Findings, and Treatment for the Major Causes of Pustules and Cysts (Continued)

Lesion	Cause	Clinical Findings	Treatment
Folliculitis (inflammation of the hair follicle)	*Staphylococcus* infection most common cause *Pseudomonas* infection ("hot tub" folliculitis)	Follicularly based pustules, commonly in areas of friction	Systemic antibiotics (e.g., dicloxacillin, or cefazolin500 mg four times daily)
Rosacea (inflammation of the sebaceous glands of the face)*	Unknown	Flushing, sensitive skin Telangiectasias, inflammatory papules and pustules Seen in middle-aged and elderly patients Symptoms are worsened by triggers (alcohol, spicy foods, caffeine, and sunlight)	Topical metronidazole, clindamycin, or azelaic acid Systemic tetracycline or minocycline

*Can lead to rhinophyma.

TABLE 85-7. Causes, Clinical Findings, and Treatments for the Major Causes of Nodules

Lesion	Cause	Clinical Findings	Treatment
Cyst	Unknown	Solitary, round, encapsulated, subcutaneous mars with puncta	Intralesional steroids, excision
Keloid (excessive tissue growth or repair)	Trauma	Young African-Americans affected most often	Intralesional corticosteroid injections (e.g., triamcinolone, 10 mg/ml) may help lesions regress
Warts	Human papillomavirus infection	Skin lines not seen across the lesion Red-brown or black dots visible when the lesion is pared	Liquid nitrogen, salicylic acid, podophyllin, laser therapy

TABLE 85-8. Causes, Clinical Findings, and Treatments for the Major Causes of Pigmented Lesions

Lesion	Cause	Clinical Findings	Treatment
Malignant melanoma	Malignant transformation and growth of melanocytes	**A**symetry **B**order irregular **C**olor irregular **D**iameter greater than 0.6 cm (but any enlarging lesion is suspicious) **E**volution	Referral to a dermatologist for biopsy. Treatment is based on depth of invasion.
Nevi (moles)	Unknown	<5 mm well-circumscribed defined border, uniform color (beige to brown), symmetric	Clinical follow-up

    7. Lichenification (thickened epidermis, accentuated skin lines)

    8. Induration (thicked dermis)

C. Once you have identified the type of lesion and noted any secondary changes, enhance the description by detailing the lesion's:

    1. Size

    2. Color

    3. Shape

    4. Grouping: how the lesions are situated with respect to each other (e.g. solitary, clustered, serpiginous, annular, dermatomal, or linear)

    5. Distribution: where the lesions are located on the body (e.g. acral, photodistributed or generalized)

    6. Special descriptors: if present in association with the lesion in question, the following terms should be included to help narrow the differential diagnosis—telangiectasias, petechiae, burrows, purpura and comedones.

II **DIAGNOSIS AND TREATMENT OF COMMON DERMATO-LOGIC LESIONS.** The causes, clinical findings, and treatments of common dermatologic lesions are summarized according to primary lesion type in Tables 85-2 through 85-8.

Reference

Fitzpathrick TB, Johnson RA, Wolff K, Suurmond D. Color Atlas and Synopsis of Clinical Dermatology Common and Serious Diseases, 4th ed. New York; McGraw-Hill, 2001.

86. Pruritus

....

I **INTRODUCTION.** Itch is the sensation that produces the desire to scratch. A variety of dermatologic and non-dermatologic disorders can cause itch.

A. Primary dermatologic disorders. Itch is the most common symptom of skin disease. When a dermatologic disorder is the cause of itch, a primary skin lesion is usually present (See Chapter 85).

B. Systemic disorders. In the absence skin findings, severe and extensive pruritus is often associated with an underlying systemic disease.

II **COMMON CAUSES OF PRURITUS**

A. Primary Dermatologic disorders: Skin inflammation activates cutaneous itch receptors that transmit signals to the brain through afferent non-myelinated C fibers. Because dermatologic itch is a result of inflammation, a primary skin lesion (see Chapter 85) can usually be identified.

  1. Xerosis (dry skin) is a very common cause.
  2. Insect bites
  3. Infestations (e.g., scabies, pediculosis)
  4. Dermatitis (e.g., atopic dermatitis, nummular eczema, contact dermatitis, irritant dermatitis, seborrheic dermatitis)
  5. Lichen planus
  6. Urticaria, dermatographism
  7. Dermatitis herpetiformis
  8. Bullous pemphigoid
  9. Folliculitis (eosinophilic, bacterial)
  10. Prurigo (subacute, nodularis), lichen simplex chronicus
  11. Drug eruptions
  12. Superficial fungal infections

HOT
▶
KEY
The dermatologic lesions are often missed on examination of patients with insect bites, dermatitis herpetiformis, or chronic urticaria.

B. Systemic disorders

Systemic disorders that cause itch can be divided into three broad categories: Metabolic, Neuropathic and Psychogenic. Although patients with one of these disorders may manifest secondary skin changes, most commonly excoriation, crust or scaling, they do not have primary skin lesions (See Chapter 85). The presence of itch with no primary lesion is a clue that an underlying systemic disease may be present.

1. **Metabolic:** Induces itch by stimulating peripheral and/or central itch centers through chemical/metabolic mediators.
   a. **Hepatic:** Chronic obstructive liver disease, hepatitis C (with or without evidence of jaundice or liver failure) and primary biliary cirrhosis
   b. **Renal:** Chronic renal failure (incidence 15–50%) and dialysis (uremic pruritus, incidence 50–90%)
   c. **Hematologic disease:** Iron deficiency anemia, polycythemia vera (PV), lymphoma (especially Hodgkin's disease), leukemia, myeloma, mycosis fungoides and mastocytosis. The itching associated with Hodgkin's disease is often described as a "burning" sensation, especially on the lower extremities. 30–50% of PV patients develop aquagenic itch, a prickly, uncomfortable itch occurring immediately after contact with water and lasting up to 120 minutes.
   d. **Endocrine:** Hyper- or hypo-thyroidism, diabetes mellitus
   e. **Rheumatologic:** Scleroderma
   f. **Solid tumors:** Carcinoid, brain tumors and visceral adenocarcinoma
   g. **Intestinal parasites**
   h. **Drug:** Opiates, anti-malarials
2. **Neuropathic:** Induces itch by activating the afferent non-myelinated C-fibers that conduct itch signals. Characterized by episodic, intense spasms of itch or non-pruritic complaints such as stinging, burning pain, dyesthesia (diminished skin sensation) or formication (sensation of bugs crawling on skin).
   a. **Multiple sclerosis:** May present with dysethesia.
   b. **Brachioradial pruritus:** Chronic episodic pruritus of the lateral upper arm(s) from irritated radial nerves usually caused by cervical stenosis.
   c. **Notalgia paresthetica T2-6:** Sensory neuropathy involving the dorsal spinal nerves characterized by intrascapular itch and development of a well circumscribed hyperpigmented patch in the affected area.
   d. **Pruritus scroti/vulvi/ani:** Intractable, episodic itching of the scrotum, vulva or anus respectively, may be associated with a lumbar-sacral radiculopathy. Diagnosis of exclusion after primary dermatologic (e.g., psoriasis or contact

dermatitis) and infectious (e.g., dermatophyte) etiologies have been excluded. May significantly overlap with the psychogenic category of itch.

e. Post-herpetic neuralgia: Pain that persists in shingles-affected skin after the acute rash resolves.

f. Purigo nodularis, lichen simplex chronicus: Characterized by constant rubbing and itching to the point of causing skin damage. Some patients develop nodules (prurigo nodularis) others develop well-circumscribed, flat-topped skin lesions with exaggerated skin lines (lichen simplex chronicus). The etiology of these disorders is perplexing but may represent end-stage disease of a primary dermatologic, metabolic, neuropathic or psychogenic cause of itch.

3. Psychogenic: The skin is a frequent site of release for emotional tension. Primarily psychiatric disorders may manifest through self-injury or compulsive acts that produce various mutilations. The diagnosis of itch due to a psychogenic cause is one of exclusion and organic disease must be excluded. Although referral to a dermatologist is appropriate to rule out a primary dermatologic disorder, the mainstay of therapy is through psychiatric counseling.

a. Delusions of parasitosis: A firm fixation of a parasitic infection of the skin, may be a sign of an underlying psychosis

b. Neurotic excoriations: Compulsive picking that results in self-mutilation, may be associated with depression, obsessive-compulsive disorder or anxiety.

c. Factitial disorders: Patient self-injures skin for secondary gain.

d. Trichotillomania: Compulsive pulling of hair associated with depression, obsessive-compulsive disorder or anxiety. In adults, may be a sign of significant psychiatric impairment.

III APPROACH TO THE PATIENT

A. History

A thorough history should include specific details about the onset, location, distribution, duration, quality (e.g., constant, burning), severity and exacerbating or ameliorating factors of the itch. Patients should be asked about underlying medical conditions, prescription or recreational drug use, travel or occupational exposures, personal or family history of atopy or skin diseases, bathing practices and the presence of pets. A complete review of systems may provide clues of an underlying systemic disease.

Factors that suggest a non-systemic cause for itch include:

1. acute onset

   2. localized itch
   3. limitation to exposed skin
   4. presence of pruritus in other household members or close contacts

B. Physical exam

Physical examination should be centered upon identifying a primary skin disorder. The entire skin surface should be inspected. Finger and toe webs, axilla and genitals should be evaluated for burrows, a sign of scabies. Firmly scratching the skin of the inner arm or back using a tongue depressor may be used to test for induced wheals, a sign of dermatographism. Lymph nodes, liver and spleen should be palpated for lymphadenopathy or organomegally. If no specific dermatologic disorder or primary skin lesion can be identified, diagnostic screening for an underlying systemic disease may be warranted.

C. Suggested Laboratory Testing

   1. Complete blood count with differential, serum RBC-folate and B12 levels, Iron studies
   2. Thryoid studies
   3. A Liver panel, including hepatitis serologies
   4. Renal panel
   5. Fasting serum glucose
   6. If risk factors present: Consider serum protein electrophoresis, stool sample for ova and parasites, HIV testing

D. Procedures

   1. Skin scraping: If scale is present, analyze a skin scraping by KOH to rule out dermatophyte infection.
   2. Skin biopsy: Recommended to confirm or establish a definitive diagnosis especially after initial treatment has failed.

E. Imaging

   1. Chest X-ray: Rule out occult malignancy. Poor sensitivity.
   2. Spinal/Cervical X-ray: May be helpful in diagnosing itch caused by radiculopathy (See *Neuropathic Itch*).
   3. Chest and/or abdominal CT: Rule out occult malignancy. Higher sensitivity than chest X-ray. Recommended if elevated clinical suspicion or worrisome symptoms/signs present.

IV TREATMENT

Itch is best treated by providing symptomatic relief while identifying and eliminating the underlying etiology. Although the cause of itch may remain unidentified or untreatable, there are general guidelines for providing symptomatic relief.

A. Gentle skin care

Patients should be educated on proper skin care. Xerosis (dry skin) can be a primary cause of itch or exacerbate itch caused by other disorders. To treat xerosis aggressively, patients should moisterize at least twice per day. Emollients, such as Vaseline petroleum jelly or Aquaphor, moisterize more effectively than most creams or lotions and are only rarely associated with irritant or contact dermatitis reactions. If using emollients in conjuction with topical medications (e.g., steroid ointments), apply the emollient second. Emollients use should continue until the itch resolves although daily use even in absence of itch may be a helpful preventative regimen.

1. **Avoid habits that cause dry skin:** Take lukewarm showers lasting less than 15 minutes, avoid drying soaps (use gentle soaps such as Dove, Purpose, Cetaphil, or Aquanil), minimize soap use to armpits and groin, and avoid soap in areas of skin inflammation or dryness. Once out of the shower, blot dry, and immediately apply moisterizers on top of damp skin to retain moisture.

2. **Avoidance therapy:** Eliminate all non-essential skin products, medications and dietary supplements. Use frangrance-free clothing detergents and soaps and avoid fabric softners.

3. **Temperature:** Itch is generally exacerbated by heat. Stay cool, avoid hot baths or showers. Intermittent treatments with ice packs can be helpful to calm the worst areas of itch. Mentholated topical remedies (see *Menthol* below) produce a cooling sensation that is very helpful at decreasing itch for short durations.

B. **Topical antipuritic agents**

1. **Emollients:** Essential for repairing the skin barrier and part of almost all first-line therapies. Apply at least twice per day. Emollients (Aquaphor, Vaseline petroleum jelly, Eucerin) are generally more effective moisterizers than creams or lotions.

2. **Menthol:** The cooling sensation of menthol provides short-term itch relief. Mentholated skin creams are available in several inexpensive over-the-counter formulations (e.g., Sarna, Aveeno Skin Relief Moisturizing Lotion with Cooling Menthol and Eucerin Itch-Relief Moisterizing Spray.

3. **Anesthetics:** Topical formulations that numb the skin can be used for breakthrough itch or as adjunctive agents for itch that occurs in localized areas. Only in rare occasions (e.g., pruritus ani) are they used as primary, solitary treatment for itch. Pramoxine is useful for pruritus ani/scroti/vulvi. EMLA cream or lidocaine gel/patches are useful for neuropathic itch and some forms of metabolic itch (particularly uremic puritis) and itch from burn injury.

4. **Antihistamines:** Topical antihistamines have limited utility but may provide short-term relief of mild itch from eczematous disorders as well as from urticaria and dermatographism.

Diphenhydramine (Benadryl) is available over-the-counter and doxepin (Zonalon), which blocks H1-receptors with considerably higher affinity, is available by prescription. Topical doxepin can cause drowsiness and contact dermatitis.

5. **Capsaicin:** Depletes substance P and eliminates the conduction of pain signals along sensory nerves. Must be used at regular intervals over prolonged periods. The burning sensation when first applied frequently causes patients to discontinue its use. This agent is particularly effective at treating itch caused by neuropathic sources and has been also used to treat uremic pruritus.

6. **Steroids:** Topical corticosteroids are the most frequently prescribed medication for itch. They range in potency from Class I (strongest, e.g., clobetasol) to Class VI (weakest, e.g., hydrocortisone). They are most effective at treating inflammatory skin disorders and probably have only limited utility in treating itch caused by metabolic, neuropathic or psychogenic etiologies unless there is an inflammatory skin component. When improperly dosed or overused, topical steroids may cause permanent skin atrophy and abnormal blood vessel development.

7. **Immunomodulators:** Tacrolimus (Protopic) and pimecrolimus (Elidel) are topical immunosuppresents that treat many of the same inflammatory skin disorders as topical steroids, but do not cause many of the side effects. They are frequently used on the face, anogenital and axillary regions in place of steroid creams to limit side effects. Because oral tacrolimus is associated with increased risk for malignancy, topical immunodulators carry a "black-box" warning because the risk for cancer from the topical formulation is unknown. Current guidelines suggest these agents only be used for short periods, in children greater than 2 years old and in non-immunosuppressed individuals.

8. **Permethrin:** 5% permetrin cream is the first line treatment for scabies infestation except in pregnant women. When properly used, two applications spaced one-week apart is ~95% effective.

C. **Occlusion and Physical Barriers**
   Agents that form a physical barrier against external manipulation while promoting skin healing are useful for treating itch associated with neuropathic or psychogenic disorders. Examples of these include hydrocolloid dressings such as duoderm or more extensive wraps such as an UNNA boot. Codran is an adhesive tape impregnated with a potent steroid and is useful for lesions of prurigo nodularis or lichen simplex chronicus.

D. UV Light Phototherapy

Phototherapy with ultraviolet (UV) light is useful for managing conditions that cause generalized itching. This includes itch from primary skin conditions such as eczema as well as itch caused by underlying systemic diseases like renal or liver dysfunction. Although phototherapy uses UV light, it minimizes exposure to harmful radiation that can cause skin cancer. In contrast, tanning beds do not exclude such radiation and should not be considered equivalent to phototherapy.

E. Systemic treatments

1. **Antihistamines.** Antihistamines are commonly used as all-purpose anti-itch medications. However, with the exception of Doxepin, most antihistamines have limited use because they have little activity against metabolic, central or psychogenic itch. They are all very effective for treating urticaria and dermatographism, both of which are histamine-mediated, and first generation antihistamines (diphenhydramine or hydroxyzine) are useful adjunctive agents for treating nightime itch, mainly because of their sedating qualities. Oral doxepin, is probably the most useful of the antihistamines because it can reduce depression and anxiety in addition to its antihistamine affects. It can treat a wide range of itching disorders, although it can cause significant somnolence, limiting patient tolerance, and in high doses (>100 mg) can cause cardiac dysrhythmia.

2. **Other systemic medications** useful for treating itch are listed below. When itch becomes severe or incapacitating enough to require additional systemic treatment aside from antihistamines, it should most often be done in consultation with a dermatologist. Please note that many systemic medications used to treat itch are off-label uses and should be prescribed with full awareness of their risks and benefits.

   a. Naloxone: Itch associated with chronic obstructive liver disease

   b. Ondansetron: Itch associated with opioids

   c. Mirtazapine, Paroxetine: Itch related to neuropathic and psychogenic disorders. Also helpful for paraneoplastic itch and idiopathic itching disorders such as lichen simplex chronicus or prurigo nodularis.

   d. Gabapentin: For neuropathic itch, especially post herpetic neuralgia. Also helpful for uremic pruritus.

V FOLLOW-UP AND REFERRAL

A. Patients who have pruritus of unknown cause and who do not respond to treatment for xerosis or symptomatic treatment should be referred to a dermatologist.

B. Patients who continue to itch despite extensive evaluation should be frequently reassessed to ensure early detection of a potential underlying systemic disease (e.g., 2–4 times per year). Particular attention to the dermatologic examination (look for evidence of primary lesions),examination of the lymph nodes, liver, and spleen (look for enlargement, which could indicate malignancy) and a thorough review of systems should be completed at each visit.

References

Beltrani VS. Pruritus and Pruritic Dermatoses. *Contemporary Dermatology* 2003;1(10);1–8.

Etter L, Myers SA. Pruritus in systemic disease: mechanisms and management. *Dermatol Clin* 2002;20(3):459–472.

Pruritus and Neurocutaneous Disorders. In James WD, Berger TB, Elston DE, eds: *Andrews' Diseases of the Skin*, 10th ed. Philadelphia, PA: Elsevier: 2006:51.

87. Palpable Purpura

I INTRODUCTION

A. Palpable purpura is the cutaneous manifestation of small and mixed medium and small vessel vasculitis. The clinical term describes small (1 to 2 mm) red-purple, non-blanching papules that are raised and have substance. They usually occur as clustered lesions or "crops" and most commonly involved area are the lower legs, however, both distal and proximal extremity involvement may occur.

    1. Lesions may progress to become confluent, hemorrhagic plaques that can ulcerate

    2. Purpuric lesions may frequently be accompanied by urticaria

    3. Variants occur with pustules, vesicles and necrosis

B. Vasculitis is the general term to describe inflammation and necrosis of blood vessels. Vasculitis can be a primary process (no known cause or association) or can be secondary to an infection, drug, or systemic illness (e.g. lupus). The clinical morphology correlates with the vessel size affected, therefore vasculitides are classified by the vessel size affected.

    1. Small vessels (urticaria and palpable purpura)

    2. Medium sized vessels (subcutaneous nodules)

    3. Mixed medium and small sized vessels (end-organ damage, livedo reticularis, palpable purpura and mononeuritis)

    4. Large vessels (ischemic claudication and necrosis)

HOT KEY

Palpable purpura refers to the clinical presentation of a particular type of vasculitis, most commonly small vessel vasculitis, less freqently, the mixed medium and small vessel vasculitides.

    Small and mixed medium and small vasculitides are the focus of this chapter.

II DIFFERENTIAL DIAGNOSIS

A. Vasculitis

B. Petechiae (see Chapter 71)

C. Pigmented purpuric eruptions (benign capillaritis)

D. Septic emboli

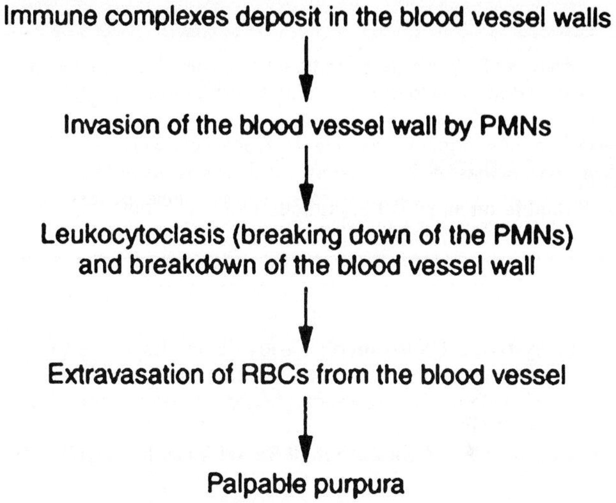

Immune complexes deposit in the blood vessel walls

↓

Invasion of the blood vessel wall by PMNs

↓

**Leukocytoclasis (breaking down of the PMNs)
and breakdown of the blood vessel wall**

↓

Extravasation of RBCs from the blood vessel

↓

Palpable purpura

FIGURE 87-1. Pathogenesis of vasculitis. PMNs = polymorphonuclear neutrophils; RBCs = red blood cells.

III APPROACH TO THE PATIENT

A. **Small vessel vasculitis** predominantly affects the post capillary venules.
  1. **Pathogenesis:** circulating antigen/antibody immune complexes are deposited on the endothelium of small vessels found most frequently in the skin, intestine and kidneys. These immune complexes activate complement, resulting in vessel damage, thrombosis, hemorrhage and occlusion (see Figure 87-1)
  2. **Histology:** although the underlying cause may differ, small vessel vasculitides all share the histological finding of leukocytoclastic vasculitis (LCV); the transmural infiltration and disruption of post capillary venules by neutrophils accompanied by leukocytoclasia (neutrophilic dust), extravasated erythrocytes and fibrinoid necrosis of vessel walls.
  3. **Patient history:** patients may complain of itch, sting, or burn. They may also have malaise, fever and arthralgias.
  4. **Physical examination**
    a. **Skin:** lesions favor dependent areas and may occur in areas of trauma (pathergy). There may be evidence of palpable purpura and urticaria. Variants may have vesicles, bullae, pustules or ulceration.

TABLE 87-1. Systemic Manifestations of Vasculitides

Constitutional symptoms (e.g., fever, fatigue, weight loss, anorexia)
Musculoskeletal symptoms (e.g., arthritis, arthralgias, proximal muscle pain)
Symptoms from organ ischemia (e.g., abdominal pain)
Symptoms suggestive of pulmonary, renal, or nervous system involvement (e.g., hemoptysis, dyspnea, dark urine, peripheral edema, peripheral neuropathy)

   b. Systemic involvement: varies depending on underyling etiology but pulmonary, renal, gastrointestinal, and neurologic involvement should be ruled out (see Table 87-1).
5. **Common Etiologies of Small Vessel Vasculitis (DrIINR)**

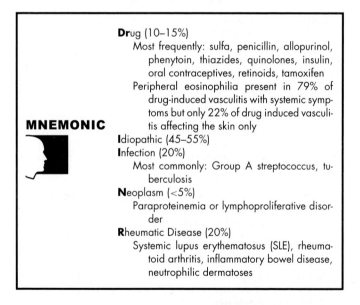

MNEMONIC

Drug (10–15%)
   Most frequently: sulfa, penicillin, allopurinol, phenytoin, thiazides, quinolones, insulin, oral contraceptives, retinoids, tamoxifen
   Peripheral eosinophilia present in 79% of drug-induced vasculitis with systemic symptoms but only 22% of drug induced vasculitis affecting the skin only
Idiopathic (45–55%)
Infection (20%)
   Most commonly: Group A streptococcus, tuberculosis
Neoplasm (<5%)
   Paraproteinemia or lymphoproliferative disorder
Rheumatic Disease (20%)
   Systemic lupus erythematosus (SLE), rheumatoid arthritis, inflammatory bowel disease, neutrophilic dermatoses

6. **Subtypes of Small Vessel Vasculitis**
   a. Cutaneous small vessel vasculitis is confined only to the skin without systemic involvement. It is a diagnosis of exclusion, but may be caused by any of the etiologies listed above.

HOT KEY

Density of purpuric lesions increase from head to toe.

  b. Cryroglobulinemic vasculitis (CV): Cryoglobulin immune complexes become deposited in the walls of small vessels inciting acute inflammation.
   (1) Cryoglobulins are immunoglobulins that precipitate at low temperature
   (2) Associated medical conditions: Hepatitis C virus (most common), HIV, autoimmune or lymphoproliferative disorders.
   (3) Findings might include palpable purpura, most commonly precipitated by cold, prolonged standing, trauma or a reaction to a drug or infection.

HOT KEY

Cryoglobulinemia is a cause of cold-induced acrocyanosis of the helices of the ear

  c. Henoch-Schönlein purpura (HSP): Vasculitis with IgA dominant immune deposits affecting vessels in skin, gut and glomeruli.
   (1) It is the most common systemic vasculitis in children; rare in adults.
   (2) Often occurs 1–2 weeks following an upper respiratory tract infection.
   (3) The diagnostic tetrad is
      – Palpable purpura (buttocks and lower extremities)
      – Arthritis (especially knees and ankles)
      – Colicky abdominal pain
      – Nephritis (5% have progressive renal disease)

HOT KEY

Patients with spread of purpura above waist, fever and elevated ESR are at higher risk for renal involvement

  d. Urticarial vasculitis presents as recurrent raised edematous wheals that burn rather than itch. The distribution favors trunk and proximal extremities. It can become confluent and form very large lesions. Individual lesions take >24 hours to resolve. Associated conditions: chronic urticaria, Sjögren's syndrome and SLE

HOT KEY

Patients with low complement levels have higher incidence of systemic disease (arthritis, pulmonary or gastrointestinal symptoms).

---

    e. Paraneoplastic vasculitis is most often due to lymphoproliferative disorders or paraproteinemias

B. Mixed medium and small vessel vasculitis

  1. ANCA-associated (Anti-Neutrophilic Cytoplasmic Antibody:

    a. Microscopic polyangiitis (MPA): Necrotizing vasculitis with few or no immune deposits affecting small vessels. Necrotizing glomerulonephritis is common and hemorrhagic pulmonary capillaritis may occur. Necrotizing arteritis involving small and medium sized arteries may also be present.

      (1) Positive P- or C-ANCA (myeloperoxidase [MPO] or anti-proteinase-3 [AP3]) serologies >90%

      (2) Skin: palpable purpura

    b. Wegener's granulomatosis (WG): Granulomatous inflammation involving the upper and lower repiratory tract and necrotizing vasculitis affecting small-to-medium sized vessels. Necrotizing glomerulonephritis is common.

      (1) Positive ANCA serologies 75–80%, more commonly AP3

      (2) Skin: Palpable purpura, oral ulcers, papulonecrotic lesions, subcutaneous nodules, ulcers

    c. Allergic granulomatosis (Churg-Strauss syndrome): Eosinophil-rich, granulomatous inflammation involving the respiratory tract and necrotizing vasculitis affecting small-to-medium sized vessels. Associated with asthma and peripheral eosinophilia.

      (1) Positive MPO serologies 60–70%

      (2) Skin: Palpable purpura, papulonecrotic lesions, subcutaneous nodules

      (3) Inflammation of the myocardium is common and is the leading cause of mortality

2. **Autoimmune disorders:** SLE, systemic sclerosis, and rheumatoid arthritis may cause a vasculitis due to deposition of circulating immune complexes.
3. **Septic vasculitis:** Vascular injury results from embolization of organisms and activation of complement. Implicated microbial pathogens include meningococcus, staphylococcus, Group A streptococcus, pneumococcus, pseudomonas, *Vibria vulnificus*, rickettsia and candida.

IV TREATMENT

A. Establish diagnosis with a biopsy: Usually, patients are referred emergently to a dermatologist for a skin biopsy.
   1. Hematoxylin and Eosin (H&E)
      Assess for leukocytoclastic vasculitis
   2. Direct immunofluorescence
      Assess for Ig complement/fibrin in venule wall
B. Determine extent of systemic involvement: Perform a thorough history and physical and review of systems. In particular, assess for skin, pulmonary, renal, gastrointestinal and joint involvment. Elicit history of recent medications, infections, neoplasms and autoimmune disorders.
C. Recommended baseline laboratory testing
   1. Complete blood count with differential
   2. Creatinine, liver chemistry test, ESR
   3. Anti-streptolysin O titers (ASO), Hepatitis B/C serologies
   4. Rheumatic work-up: ANA, ANCA, rheumatoid factor, cryoglobulins
   5. Complement levels (C3, C4)
   6. Urine analysis w/ microcsopy
   7. Stool guiac
   8. Throat culture
   9. If there is suspicion for a lymphoproliferative disorder:
      a. Serum protein electrophoresis (SPEP)
      b. Urine protein electrophoresis (UPEP)
      c. Immunofixation electrophoresis (IFE)
D. Design therapeutic intervention based on all of the above

V FOLLOW-UP AND REFERRAL

Palpable purpura usually represents a medical emergency. Often, patients are admitted to the hospital for expeditious evaluation. Follow-up depends on the underlying cause and the extent of systemic involvement. In general, patients should be seen frequently until symptoms abate and systemic involvement resolves.

References

Crowson AN, Mihm MC Jr, Magro CM. Cutaneous vasculitis: a review. *J Cutan Pathol* 2003;30(3):161–173.

Fiorentino DF. Cutaneous vasculitis. *J Am Acad Dermatol* 2003;48(3):311–340.

Jennette JC, Falk RJ. Small-vessel vasculitis. *N Engl J Med* 1997;337(21): 1512–1523.

PART XIV

PSYCHIATRY

88. Depression

I INTRODUCTION

A. Depression is **extremely common:** the lifetime incidence of major depression is 10% in men and 20% in women.

B. In the medical setting, the **diagnosis** of depression is **missed in 30%–50% of patients.**

C. Risk factors for depression include:
   1. Age 35–45 years in women, or greater than 55 years in men
   2. Female gender
   3. Personal or family history of depression
   4. Presence of a serious medical condition
   5. Presence of social stressors and a lack of social support
   6. Substance abuse (e.g., alcoholism)

II CLINICAL MANIFESTATIONS OF DEPRESSION. Patients may present in many different ways, which may account for the high incidence of missed diagnoses. The following findings may suggest depression:

A. Weight loss (especially common in elderly patients)
B. Unkempt appearance
C. Irritable or depressed affect
D. Vagueness
E. Anxiety
F. Multiple somatic complaints
G. Failure of appropriate treatment regimen for a medical illness

III DIFFERENTIAL DIAGNOSIS

HOT KEY

Depression may coexist with most of the conditions in the differential diagnosis.

A. Psychiatric disorders
   1. Other mood disorders, such as dysthymia or bipolar disorder
   2. Anxiety disorder
   3. Personality disorder, especially borderline or obsessive-compulsive disorder
B. Normal bereavement. Approximately 5% of patients with normal bereavement may develop a mood disorder.
C. Neurologic disorders
   1. Parkinson's disease
   2. Cerebrovascular disease
   3. Seizure disorder
   4. Dementia
   5. Head trauma
D. Substance abuse
E. Endocrine disorders (e.g., thyroid or adrenal disorders)
F. Medications
   1. Corticosteroids or hormone replacement therapy (HRT)
   2. Antihypertensives
   3. Analgesics, especially narcotics
   4. Any drugs acting on the central nervous system (CNS)

IV APPROACH TO THE PATIENT

A. Establish the diagnosis
   1. The diagnosis of depression is made using the *Diagnostic and Statistical Manual of Mental Disorders,* 4th edition (DSM-IV) diagnostic criteria. The mnemonic "1, 2, 3, 4, 5" can help you remember how to diagnose depression.

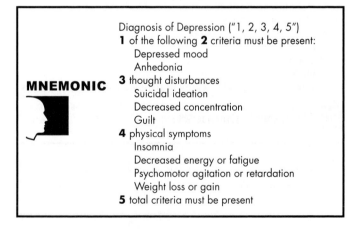

MNEMONIC

Diagnosis of Depression ("1, 2, 3, 4, 5")
1 of the following **2** criteria must be present:
  Depressed mood
  Anhedonia
3 thought disturbances
  Suicidal ideation
  Decreased concentration
  Guilt
4 physical symptoms
  Insomnia
  Decreased energy or fatigue
  Psychomotor agitation or retardation
  Weight loss or gain
5 total criteria must be present

2. Make sure to rule out other psychiatric and medical conditions and evaluate whether certain medications or substance abuse may be contributing to the illness.

B. Assess the patient's risk factors for suicide

1. Patients who have a history of attempting suicide (e.g., more than 4 or 5 previous attempts) are more likely to attempt suicide in the future, but are much less likely to succeed. This pattern may indicate an underlying personality disorder.

2. Asking patients about suicidal ideation does not lead patients to commit suicide; rather, it identifies patients at risk. The risk factors for committing suicide can be remembered by the mnemonic, "SAD PERSONS."

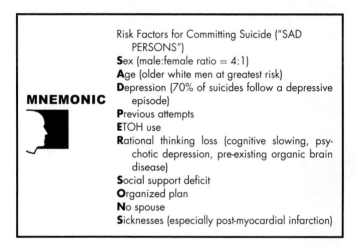

MNEMONIC

Risk Factors for Committing Suicide ("SAD PERSONS")

Sex (male:female ratio = 4:1)
Age (older white men at greatest risk)
Depression (70% of suicides follow a depressive episode)
Previous attempts
ETOH use
Rational thinking loss (cognitive slowing, psychotic depression, pre-existing organic brain disease)
Social support deficit
Organized plan
No spouse
Sicknesses (especially post-myocardial infarction)

V **TREATMENT.** Seventy percent of patients with major depression improve with initial treatment. However, a single episode may last for 2 years or longer, and relapses occur in most patients.

A. Selective serotonin reuptake inhibitors (SSRIs) are the most commonly prescribed medications for major depression, given their relatively benign side effect profiles, and few untoward effects in patients who attempt to overdose.

1. Agents (Table 88-1). Although fluoxetine has been around the longest, other agents have fewer side effects and drug interactions and are therefore preferred.

2. Side effects. The most common side effects of SSRIs include **agitation**, **gastrointestinal problems** (e.g., nausea, vomiting, diarrhea), **sexual dysfunction** (e.g., decreased libido,

TABLE 88-1. Selective Serotonin Reuptake Inhibitors

Generic Name	Brand Name	Advantages	Disadvantages	Dosing
Paroxetine	Paxil	Most sedating	Need to taper gradually if discontinuing	**Starting dose:** 10 mg daily in elderly patients, 20 mg daily otherwise **Maximum dose:** 40 mg daily
Sertraline	Zoloft	Less activating than fluoxetine; less sedating than paroxetine	Most gastrointestinal side effects	**Starting dose:** 25 mg daily in elderly patients, 50 mg daily otherwise **Maximum dose:** 150–200 mg daily
Fluoxetine	Prozac	Most activating May decrease appetite	May cause insomnia or jitteriness Long half-life Most inhibition of the cytochrome p-450 system	**Starting dose:** 10 mg daily in elderly patients, 20 mg daily otherwise **Maximum dose:** 40 mg daily
Escitalopram	Lexepro	Nonsedating Available in elixir form	Need to taper gradually if discontinuing	**Starting dose:** 10 mg daily **Maximum dose:** 20 mg; 10 mg if hepatic impairment, caution in renal failure
Citalopram	Celexa	Nonsedating Available in solution form	Need to taper gradually if discontinuing	**Starting dose:** 20 mg daily **Maximum dose:** 60 mg daily; 40 mg in elderly and those with hepatic impairment, caution in renal failure
Fluvoxamine	Luvox (brand discontinued in the United States)	Approved for pediatric population	Need to taper gradually if discontinuing	**Starting dose:** 50 mg at night, decrease if hepatic impairment **Maximum dose:** 300 mg daily, divide dose if over 100 mg

erectile dysfunction), and possibly an increased risk of suicide, although this is controversial. SSRIs also inhibit the
cytochrome P-450 system and therefore **may affect warfarin,
phenytoin,** and **tricyclic antidepressant levels.**

HOT **KEY** Achieving the maximal antidepressive effect may take 4–6
weeks with SSRIs. Patients should be made aware of this delayed effect so that they do not stop taking the medication
prematurely.

B. **Tricyclic antidepressants,** which are inexpensive and very effective, have been available for many years. Patients who have severe agitation, insomnia, migraines, or concomitant neuropathic
pain, or who have failed SSRIs may benefit the most from tricyclic antidepressants.
   1. **Agents** (Table 88-2)
      a. **Amitriptyline** is the most well-recognized of the tricyclic
         antidepressants, but its anticholinergic side effects are
         poorly tolerated.
      b. **Nortriptyline** and **desipramine** are equally as efficacious as
         amitriptyline, both for use as antidepressant as well as for
         the treatment of neuropathic pain. These agents should be
         used in favor of amitriptyline.
   2. **Side effects.** Because the side effect profile is daunting (espe-
      cially in elderly patients) and there is a narrow therapeutic
      index, tricyclic antidepressants are favored less than SSRIs
      for the treatment of depression.
C. **Atypical antidepressants** are summarized in Table 88-3.

HOT **KEY** Bupropion has also been approved by the Food and Drug
Administration (FDA) as an aid for smoking cessation.

D. **Monoamine oxidase (MAO) inhibitors** are almost never used in
the primary care setting because of the absolute need for adherence to the regimen and the possibility of causing a hypertensive
crisis in the presence of sympathomimetics. MAO inhibitors include isocarboxazid (Marplan), tranylcypromine (Parnate), and
phenelzine (Nardil).
E. **Psychostimulants** are typically prescribed by psychiatrists for
terminally ill patients or as adjunctive agents in people who
have only partially responded to antidepressants. These agents

TABLE 88-2. Tricyclic Antidepressants				
Generic Name	Brand Name	Advantages	Disadvantages	Dosing
Nortriptyline	Pamelor	Associated with least orthostasis Twice as potent as other tricyclic antidepressants	Anticholinergic effects	**Starting dose:** 25 mg daily **Maximum dose:** 150–200 mg daily
Desipramine	Norpramin	Least sedating Least anticholinergic	Can be activating; can cause insomnia	**Starting dose:** 50 mg daily **Maximum dose:** 200–300 mg daily
Amitriptyline	Elavil	—	Highly anticholinergic	**Starting dose:** 50 mg daily **Maximum dose:** 200–300 mg daily

TABLE 88-3. Atypical Antidepressants

Generic Name	Brand Name	Mechanism	Advantages	Disadvantages	Dosing
Bupropion	Wellbutrin	Weak dopamine and norepinephrine inhibitor	Good for patients older than 65 years Few side effects	Contraindicated in patients with organic brain disease or seizure disorder	**Starting dose:** 75 mg twice daily (150 mg once daily if using slow-release formula) **Maximum dose:** 150 mg three times daily (150 mg twice daily if using slow-release formula)
Nefazodone	Serzone	Serotonin receptor antagonist and reuptake inhibitor	Low incidence of sexual side effects Less sedation Difficult to overdose	Inhibition of the cytochrome P-450 system	**Starting dose:** 100 mg twice daily **Maximum dose:** 150–250 mg twice daily
Venlafaxine	Effexor	Serotonin and norepinephrine reuptake inhibitor	Can be activating Mild side effect profile Low incidence of sexual side effects	Can cause dose-dependent increases in blood pressure	**Starting dose:** 37.5 mg twice daily **Maximum dose:** 375 mg daily in divided doses
Duloxetine	Cymbalta	Exact mechanism not known; norepinephrine and serotonin reuptake inhibitor	Some patients may respond better to this dual medication	May cause high blood pressure	**Starting dose:** 40–60 mg daily or divided daily **Maximum dose:** 60 mg daily
Mitrazapine	Remeron	Exact mechanism not known; adrenergic and serotonin inhibitor	Sedative effects make it useful for sleep aid and for patients with anxiety Lacks GI and sexual side effects	Antihistamine effects can cause sedation, dry mouth, increased appetite, and weight gain	**Starting dose:** 15 mg daily **Maximum dose:** 45 mg daily

include dextroamphetamine (Dexedrine) and methylphenidate (Ritalin).

VI FOLLOW-UP AND REFERRAL

A. Follow-up

1. Patients receiving pharmacologic therapy should be seen every 1–4 weeks. Medication should be maintained for 9–12 months; at this point, tapering of the dose may be tried. Patients with chronic or frequently recurrent depression and those with severe delusions or suicidal ideation may be kept on medications for a longer period of time or indefinitely.

2. Most patients eventually relapse; if this occurs, a second 1-year trial can be undertaken. A second relapse usually indicates the need for lifelong medical therapy.

B. Referral to a psychiatrist is indicated for patients with an unclear diagnosis or psychotic features, and for patients who fail treatment or may require atypical therapy. Patients who may be at risk for suicide should undergo immediate psychiatric evaluation.

References

Fancher T, Kravitz R. In the clinic: depression. *Ann Intern Med* 2007;146:ITC5-1–ITC5-16.

Gelenberg AJ, Hopkins HS. Assessing and treating depression in primary care medicine. *Am J Med* 2007;120:105–108.

89. Alcohol Abuse and Dependence

 INTRODUCTION

A. Alcohol abuse and dependence are extremely common, with a lifetime prevalence approaching 10%.

1. One hundred thousand Americans die each year from complications of alcohol use.
2. Almost 25% of Americans say that drinking has been a source of trouble in their families.

B. Alcohol abuse and dependence are often underdiagnosed and undertreated, despite the fact that effective treatment is available.

CLINICAL MANIFESTATIONS. The patient, or one of his family members or friends, may express concern about health or behavioral problems related to drinking. Often, however, the discussion is not patient-initiated; therefore, the physician should be aware of social issues and medical complications that may become apparent during the office visit and could suggest alcohol abuse.

A. Social issues

1. Arrests for driving while intoxicated, fighting, or other behaviors associated with alcohol use
2. Absence from work or loss of jobs due to drinking
3. Relationship problems
4. Repeated bouts of intoxication and "blackouts"

B. Medical complications. Many medical complications can result from excessive alcohol use. Some of the most common are:

1. **Gastrointestinal disorders** (e.g., gastritis, hepatitis, cirrhosis, esophageal varices, hepatoma, pancreatitis, malabsorption)
2. **Neurologic disorders** (e.g., ataxia, peripheral neuropathy, Wernicke's encephalopathy, dementia)
3. **Cardiovascular disorders** (e.g., hypertension, tachycardia, cardiomyopathy)
4. **Hematologic disorders** (e.g., anemia, thrombocytopenia)

    5. Endocrine disorders (e.g., hypoglycemia, ketoacidosis, hypokalemia, hyponatremia)

    6. Trauma (e.g., automobile accidents, falls, domestic violence)

III PATTERNS OF USE. A drink is defined as 1 ounce (30 ml) of distilled alcohol (e.g., brandy, gin, rum, vodka, whiskey), 4 ounces of wine, or 12 ounces of beer.

A. Low-risk. These patients have fewer than 1–2 drinks per day (less than 1 drink per day in women and people older than 65 years) and no more than 3–4 drinks per occasion. They practice abstinence in high-risk situations (e.g., when pregnant, before driving, or when taking medications that should not be taken with alcohol).

B. High-risk. For men, "high risk" is defined as more than 14 drinks per week, or more than 4 drinks per occasion. For women, the definition is more than 7 drinks per week, or more than 3 drinks per occasion.

C. Alcohol abuse. A patient can be said to have a "drinking problem" if any of the following criteria are met:

    1. The patient has been arrested for driving while intoxicated

    2. The patient has experienced impaired social functioning or disrupted relationships with friends and family as a result of alcohol use

    3. The patient has lost a job as a result of alcohol use

D. Alcohol dependence. These patients are dependent on alcohol and meet at least three of the following seven *Diagnostic and Statistical Manual of Mental Disorders,* 4th edition (DSM-IV) criteria for substance dependence:

    1. They drink more than they intend

    2. They have a persistent desire to drink, or have been unsuccessful in attempts to stop drinking

    3. They spend a significant amount of time procuring alcohol

    4. They have given up social and occupational activities because of alcohol

    5. They drink despite physical or psychological problems

    6. They exhibit tolerance (a sign of physical dependence)

    7. They exhibit withdrawal (a sign of physical dependence)

IV APPROACH TO THE PATIENT. All patients should be screened for alcohol use, given the high prevalence of alcohol-related problems and the proven effectiveness of intervention. All three of the following screening techniques should be implemented:

A. **Engage the patient in a discussion regarding his use of alcohol** with questions such as "Do you drink alcohol? If not, what made you decide not to drink?" or "Please tell me about your use of alcohol."

B. **Use the CAGE questionnaire,** a simple and well-validated screening tool for the detection of alcohol abuse.
   1. Have you ever felt that you should cut down on your drinking?
   2. Have people annoyed you by criticizing your drinking?
   3. Have you ever felt guilty about drinking?
   4. Have you ever needed an eye-opener in the morning to calm your nerves or to get rid of a hangover?

MNEMONIC

Screening Questions for the Detection of Alcohol Abuse ("CAGE")
Cut down on your drinking?
Annoyed by others?
Guilty about drinking?
Eye-opener to counteract a hangover?

C. **Ask questions about the patient's pattern of use.**
   1. How many drinks do you have in an average week?
   2. On a typical day, how many drinks do you have?
   3. What is the maximum number of drinks that you have had on any occasion in the past month?

HOT KEY

Because alcohol abuse and dependence are highly associated with depression and anxiety, care should be taken to diagnose and initiate treatment for depression.

V TREATMENT

HOT KEY

Much of the strategy used to help patients reduce or quit drinking applies to patients with other types of substance abuse disorders as well.

A. **Counseling.** Although not all patients with a positive screening test have an alcohol abuse disorder, all patients with a positive screening test should receive counseling about alcohol use and its associated problems. Brief counseling interventions (e.g., lasting 5–15 minutes) are associated with a two-fold decrease in alcohol consumption by heavy drinkers. Counseling "FRAMES" an effective cessation program.

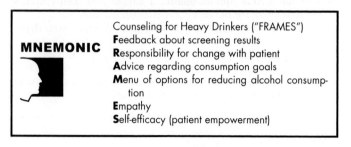

MNEMONIC

Counseling for Heavy Drinkers ("FRAMES")
Feedback about screening results
Responsibility for change with patient
Advice regarding consumption goals
Menu of options for reducing alcohol consumption
Empathy
Self-efficacy (patient empowerment)

1. **Provide feedback about screening results**
   a. Be straightforward and nonjudgmental.
   b. State your concerns about the potential or actual detrimental effects of drinking on the patient's health.
   c. Use neutral, nonstigmatizing language (e.g., avoid labels such as "alcoholic" or "addict").
2. **Educate the patient about safe consumption limits (or abstinence).** Most high-risk or heavy drinkers do not realize that they are using alcohol abnormally. Clearly state your recommendations regarding consumption goals (e.g., "I recommend that you limit your alcohol use to 1–2 drinks per day" or "I don't think it is safe for you to drink any alcohol.") Telling patients about the dangers of driving while intoxicated, including death of themselves and loved ones and criminal prosecution, is also important.
3. **Provide a "menu" of options for reducing alcohol consumption.** Ask the patient what measures she thinks will work. Possibilities include:
   a. Set a date to quit drinking or reduce the amount of alcohol consumed
   b. Keep a diary
   c. Make a written agreement
   d. Enlist help from an alcohol or substance abuse counselor
   e. Attend group counseling sessions
   f. Join a self-help program, such as Alcoholics Anonymous
   g. Enroll in an inpatient detoxification program
4. **Provide empathy and encouragement.** Support the patient's efforts by letting him know that you understand the difficulties involved. Empower the patient by helping him to realize that he can change (e.g., "I'm impressed by your motivation to stop drinking. Your resolve will help you reach this goal.")

B. Outpatient pharmacotherapy
  1. General considerations
    a. Eligibility for outpatient treatment. Patients may exhibit impaired short-term memory, poor judgment, and decreased motor skills while undergoing detoxification. In order for patients to be successful with outpatient treatment, they should have all of the following:
      (1) A network of family and friends to provide psychological support
      (2) No history of severe withdrawal symptoms, severe alcohol dependence, or other drug use
      (3) A willingness to avoid driving and operating heavy machinery
      (4) The ability to attend a day treatment program or an intensive outpatient substance abuse treatment program
    b. Contraindications to outpatient treatment include the following:
      (1) A history of hallucinations, seizures, or delirium as a result of alcohol withdrawal
      (2) A documented history of very heavy alcohol use and tolerance
      (3) Concomitant abuse of other drugs
      (4) Pregnancy
      (5) A high risk for suicide
      (6) A lack of a reliable social support system
  2. Detoxification can be achieved using benzodiazepines, carbamazepine, or phenobarbital.
    a. Benzodiazepines
      (1) Contraindications. Relative contraindications include age greater than 60 years and chronic obstructive pulmonary disease (COPD).
      (2) Side effects include decreased consciousness, ataxia, impaired short-term memory, slurred speech, and agitation.
      (3) Agents (Table 89-1)
        (a) Chlordiazepoxide is the drug of choice because of its long-acting, "self-tapering" nature; however, it is contraindicated in patients with liver disease.
        (b) Oxazepam or **lorazepam** are used for patients with liver disease.
    b. Carbamazepine is widely used in Europe, but may not prevent withdrawal seizures or delirium. In short treatment protocols, carbamazepine has not been shown to cause significant hematologic or hepatic toxicity. The dosing regimen is 200–400 mg orally twice daily for 7 days.

TABLE 89-1. Dosing Regimens for Outpatient Pharmacologic Detoxification Therapy with Benzodiazepines*

Drug	Dosing Regimen
Chlordiazepoxide	Give 25–50 mg every 6 hours until tremulousness decreases, the pulse rate is lowered to less than 100 beats/min, and withdrawal symptoms have resolved. Decrease the dose to 25 mg every 6 hours on the second and third days, and taper the dose by approximately 20% each subsequent day until withdrawal is complete.
Oxazepam	Give 30 mg every 6 hours on day 1; hold for sedation. Decrease the dose by 20% daily until withdrawal is complete.
Lorazepam	Give 2 mg every 6 hours on day 1; hold for sedation. Decrease the dose by 20% daily until withdrawal is complete.

*If symptoms of withdrawal cannot be controlled with these doses of medication, hospital admission should be considered.

    c. Phenobarbital is not recommended as an initial choice because there is less evidence of its efficacy. The potential for abuse is low, but there is a greater risk of respiratory depression than with benzodiazepines, and the margin of safety may be lower than that of benzodiazepines when high doses are required.

3. Adjunctive therapy

    a. Adrenergic agents (e.g., atenolol, 50 mg daily for 3–7 days or clonidine, 0.1 mg twice daily for 3–7 days) may be useful as adjunctive therapy in patients with high heart rate or blood pressure. These agents do not treat alcohol withdrawal.

    b. Nutritional support should be provided, as well as replenishment of vitamins:

        (1) Thiamine, 100 g orally daily

        (2) Folic acid, 1 mg orally daily

        (3) Multivitamins that include pyridoxine and ascorbic acid

4. Relapse prevention

    a. Disulfiram interferes with the metabolism of acetaldehyde, which accumulates in the blood after alcohol use.

If alcohol is used while on the medication, the patient will experience unpleasant symptoms (e.g., flushing, vasodilation, headache, tachycardia, diaphoresis, hyperventilation, nausea, vomiting) for 1–3 hours.

   (1) Dosing regimen. Initiate therapy after the patient is alcohol-free for 4–5 days with a dose of 0.5 g orally daily for 1–3 weeks. The maintenance dosage is 0.25–0.5 g daily. The effects of disulfiram may last for 3–7 days after the last dose.

   (2) Side effects include optic neuritis, peripheral neuropathy, rash, and hepatitis (rare). Psychotic reactions, which are also rare, are associated with a high dosage or combined drug toxicity (particularly metronidazole or isoniazid use).

   (3) Contraindications include acute hepatitis, significant cardiac disease, pregnancy, severe chronic lung disease, schizophrenia or bipolar affective disorder, suicidal ideation, rubber allergy, occupational exposure to solvents or alcohol, and the concurrent use of metronidazole or isoniazid.

b. Naltrexone interferes with the pleasurable effects of both alcohol and opiates. The best candidates for naltrexone therapy are patients with high levels of alcohol dependence or craving or a family history of alcoholism.

   (1) Dosing regimen. Initiate therapy as soon as withdrawal symptoms have resolved. The dose is 25 mg daily with food early in the day; this dose may be increased to 50 mg daily.

   (2) Side effects. Naltrexone is generally well tolerated, although nausea or abdominal cramping may occur about 1 hour after taking the medicine. Anxiety, malaise, and insomnia are less common.

   (3) Contraindications. The following patients are not candidates for naltrexone therapy:

      (a) Patients who are dependent on opioids, or who have stopped opioid use within the past 2 weeks

      (b) Patients who require opioid analgesics for pain

      (c) Patients with acute hepatitis

      (d) Pregnant patients

c. Campral (Acamprosate) may be used to help patients avoid a relapse after they have stopped drinking. Treatment is generally done in conjunction with counseling and support. Campral is not effective in patients who are still drinking at the start of treatment. While the mechanism of action is not completely known, it is thought that the medication helps balance excitatory and inhibitory neurotransmitters.

(1) Dosing regimens. Typically, patients have not been able to tolerate or have had an insufficient response to naltrexone. Initiate therapy after the patient is alcohol free for 4–5 days with a dose of 666 mg orally three times per day (the dose is halved in patients with renal impairment).

(2) Side effects. Currently known side effects are usually transient and mild and include diarrhea, dyspepsia, anxiety, sleep problems, nausea and vomiting, and rash and itching. Because judgment and motor skills may be impaired, patients should not drive a car or operate dangerous machinery until they know how they are affected by the medication. Patients should also be monitored for symptoms of depression or suicidal ideation.

(3) Contraindications. Campral should not be used or should be used with caution in patients with allergies to the medication, pregnant or lactating women, and patients with kidney or liver disease.

VI FOLLOW-UP AND REFERRAL

A. Follow-up. Patients who begin a trial of alcohol use reduction or abstinence should be followed closely (i.e., once a week to once a month) during the initial phases so that the physician can provide support and encouragement, and assess continued drinking.

B. Referral. Patients who fail to respond to a brief intervention session or who meet the criteria for alcohol dependence should be strongly considered for referral to a substance abuse treatment program.

References

Room R, Babor T, Rehm J. Alcohol and public health. *Lancet* 2005;365:519–530.

Williams SH. Medications for treating alcohol dependence. *Am Fam Phys* 2005;72:1775–1780.

90. Psychosis

....

I **INTRODUCTION.** The defining feature of psychosis (i.e., the inability to distinguish what is real from what is not) is **impaired reality testing** (i.e., an inability to test subjective ideas and experiences against objective facts of the external world).

II **CLINICAL MANIFESTATIONS OF PSYCHOSIS.** The most common symptoms are:

A. Disorders of thought content (delusions)
B. Disorders of perception (hallucinations)
C. Bizarre forms of speaking and behavior

III **CAUSES OF PSYCHOSIS.** All psychoses are ultimately organic and fall within the realm of both general medicine and psychiatry. However, there are two general categories of psychoses: **primary** and **secondary.**

A. Primary psychosis is not caused by another condition.
  1. Schizophrenia is a lifelong disease characterized by psychotic symptoms with intermittent exacerbations and a deterioration in social functioning.
    a. The **prevalence** is estimated at 1%.
    b. The **cause** remains unknown, although evidence suggests a strong genetic component and malfunctioning of the dopamine systems.
    c. Phases
      (1) The **prodromal phase** typically starts between adolescence and early adulthood and may persist for years before the first acute psychotic episode occurs. Patients withdraw from social relationships, become indifferent to grooming, develop suspicious attitudes, and have a gradual deterioration in scholastic and vocational abilities.
      (2) **Acute psychotic episodes** are marked by delusions, hallucinations, a flattened or inappropriate affect, disorganized speech, bizarre posturing or behavior, and an inability to carry out goal-directed behavior. Between episodes, the psychosis may resolve completely,

601

although impaired social and occupational function often persists.

2. **Mood disorder with psychotic features.** Psychosis occurs only during episodes of the mood disorder (i.e., depression or mania).

3. **Schizoaffective disorder.** Psychosis occurs at times where there are no prominent mood symptoms, as well as during episodes of the mood disorder.

4. **Schizophreniform disorder** is identical to schizophrenia, except that the disorder only lasts for 1–6 months, and there may not be a decline in social functioning.

5. **Brief psychotic disorder.** The duration of illness is less than 1 month and there is no prodromal phase.

6. **Delusional disorder** is characterized by one or more non-bizarre (i.e., conceivable) delusions (e.g., "someone is stealing my clothes").

7. **Schizotypal personality disorder.** Prominent symptoms include magical thinking, paranoia, and odd behavior.

8. **Psychosis not otherwise specified.** The psychosis cannot be categorized.

HOT **KEY**   Familiarity with the primary psychoses is important to the generalist for two principal reasons: these patients often present to a generalist first, and the generalist can provide much of the care for patients with chronic psychiatric disorders.

B. **Secondary psychosis** is caused by the presence of another condition. Key features include disturbances in consciousness (i.e., delirium); disorientation of person, place, or time; and impaired intellectual function (e.g., impaired calculation or memory).

1. **Psychosis resulting from a medical condition** (e.g., hypercalcemia, hypoxia, tumor). In this situation, the psychosis is a direct physiologic effect of the medical condition.

2. **Psychosis in association with dementia.** Severe dementia frequently causes an individual to lose touch with reality, but even mild forms of dementia can induce psychosis. Features of psychosis in dementia often include suspiciousness, paranoia, or persecutory delusions.

3. **Substance-induced psychosis** can occur in association with intoxication or withdrawal from a drug.

IV APPROACH TO THE PATIENT

A. **Perform a mental status examination.** The mental status examination is crucial for two reasons: it helps to establish the cause of the psychosis, and it can be used as a tool for monitoring the patient's condition over hours, days, or months. Pay careful attention to the following areas:

1. **Speech.** For example, is the patient's speech unusually rapid or slow?
2. **Affect** is the observed emotional state of the patient during the interview. Words used to describe affect include "depressed," "euphoric," "agitated," and "anxious."
3. **Mood** is the patient's emotional state over the past few days, weeks, or months.
4. **Thought process.** Words used to describe the patient's thought process include "incoherent," "tangential," and "loose."
5. **Thought content.** Is the patient experiencing delusions or hallucinations?
6. **Cognitive function** is assessed using the Mini Mental State Examination (see Chapter 65, Table 65-1).

B. **Attempt to determine whether the psychosis is secondary or primary.**
1. **Patient history.** With the exception of psychosis in association with dementia, secondary psychosis often presents with delirium (see Chapter 65 III A). The hallmark features of secondary psychosis include clouding of consciousness, inattentiveness, cognitive impairment, and rapid fluctuations in mental state. If hallucinations or delusions are present, they are fleeting and poorly systemized, unlike those of primary psychosis.

HOT

▶ Psychosis is frequently a sign of a medical illness, especially if it first presents late in life.

KEY

---

2. **Physical examination and laboratory studies.** Perform a complete physical examination and obtain appropriate laboratory and imaging studies to evaluate for delirium or dementia (see Chapter 65 IV A 2, B 2–3).

C. **Assess the urgency of the situation.** Clearly, more than one 15-minute session may be required to determine the cause and nature of the patient's psychosis. Is it safe to send the patient home? If any of the following features are present, the patient needs immediate psychiatric consultation or hospitalization, regardless of the cause of the psychosis:
1. The patient is agitated and/or has significant suicidal or homicidal ideation.

2. The patient inadvertently is a danger to himself or others.

3. The patient cannot provide food, shelter, or clothing for himself.

D. Consult with a psychiatrist if the psychosis is primary. In nearly all cases of new-onset primary psychosis, consultation with a psychiatrist is indicated.

 TREATMENT. Patients should be managed in consultation with a psychiatrist.

A. Primary psychosis

1. Acute therapy. Consultation with a psychiatrist should be obtained for patients with acute psychotic episodes.

2. Chronic therapy may be handled by a generalist. The goal is to minimize the patient's psychosis using the lowest dose of neuroleptic possible. "Atypical" neuroleptics should be tried first (to minimize side effects). The equivalent of 1–6 mg/day of risperidone often suffices.

a. Specific situations

(1) Mood disorder with psychotic symptoms. Add an antidepressant (to treat depression) and a mood stabilizer (to treat mania), as indicated. Taper the dose of the neuroleptic when the psychotic symptoms have resolved.

(2) Dementia. Use a low dose of neuroleptics (e.g., risperidone, 0.5–1.0 mg once or twice daily) only if a specific symptom (e.g., agitation, delusions, aggression, hallucinations) is causing distress or presents a danger to the patient or others.

b. Ensuring patient compliance. Noncompliance with psychiatric medications may be the greatest factor leading to repeat hospitalizations. The following strategies may improve patient compliance:

(1) Schedule frequent follow-up visits (at least one per month).

(2) Educate the patient and her family members about the disease.

(a) Schedule a meeting with the family.

(b) Recommend resources, such as Torrey: *Surviving Schizophrenia: A Manual for Families, Consumers, and Providers,* 3rd edition.

(3) Recruit family members and friends to aid the patient.

(4) Adjust therapy to minimize side effects.

(5) Try a long-acting intramuscular neuroleptic (e.g., fluphenazine, 25–50 mg every 2–4 weeks) instead of oral medications.

B. Secondary psychosis. The general approach is to diagnose and treat the underlying condition. Often, these patients require hospitalization. The treatment of psychosis in association with dementia is similar to that of primary psychosis (see V A).

C. Treatment of side effects from neuroleptic agents

1. **Early side effects** include sedation, anticholinergic symptoms (e.g., dry mouth, stuffy nose), orthostatic hypotension, drug-induced Parkinson's syndrome, acute dystonias (contractures), akathisia (motor restlessness), and neuroleptic malignant syndrome (characterized by muscle rigidity and a high fever). Early side effects often decrease or resolve after 1–2 months.

HOT KEY Low-potency neuroleptics (e.g., chlorpromazine) are more likely to cause sedation and less likely to cause extrapyramidal symptoms; the reverse is true for high-potency agents (e.g., haloperidol).

---

2. **Late side effects** include tardive dyskinesia (involuntary movements of a choreiform nature), Parkinsonian syndrome, and akathisia.

3. **Motor disorders** can be treated with the following measures:
   a. **Anticholinergic agents** (e.g., benztropine, 1 mg twice daily or diphenhydramine, 25–50 mg four times daily)
   b. **Anti-Parkinson agents**
   c. **Reduction of the neuroleptic dose**
   d. **Switching from a conventional to an "atypical" neuroleptic,** such as olanzapine or risperidone

VI FOLLOW-UP AND REFERRAL. A variety of programs and professionals are available to assist the psychotic patient, including:

A. Vocational rehabilitation programs, sheltered workshops, or day treatment programs

B. Psychotherapists (may help the patient to focus on behavior modification and compliance)

C. Occupational therapists

D. Social workers (may help locate sources of financial support)

References

Bryne P. Managing the acute psychotic episode. *BMJ* 2007;334:686–692.

Gardner DM, Baldessarini RJ, Waraich P. Modern antipsychotic drugs: a critical overview. *CMAJ* 2005;172:1703–1711.

Index

618